Head and Neck Surgery for General Surgeons

Bruce Ashford
Editor

Head and Neck Surgery for General Surgeons

Springer

Editor
Bruce Ashford
Department of Medicine
University of Wollongong
Wollongong, Australia

ISBN 978-981-19-7899-9 ISBN 978-981-19-7900-2 (eBook)
https://doi.org/10.1007/978-981-19-7900-2

This Springer imprint is published by the registered company Springer Nature Singapore Pte Ltd.
The registered company address is: 152 Beach Road, #21-01/04 Gateway East, Singapore 189721, Singapore

Foreword

Head and neck surgery has evolved as a specialty with contributions from reconstructive surgeons, otolaryngologists, general surgeons, maxillofacial surgeons, and other allied surgical specialties, such as neurosurgery, thoracic surgery, and vascular surgery. Thus, it is not possible for a trainee in any one of the above specialties to have a grasp on the diseases and disorders occurring in this part of the body. In addition, the complex anatomy and the expression of higher senses such as smell, vision, hearing, taste, speech, and swallowing and expression of emotions are all clustered in this compact region of human anatomy that any trauma, disease, disorder, or deformity and its treatment can have serious esthetic, emotional, and functional consequences. Clearly, there are numerous textbooks and monographs on each of the above topics and on all of the abovementioned specialties available in the literature.

Head and neck surgery forms only a small but important and essential component of the curriculum of training in general surgery. It is, however, impossible for a trainee in general surgery to peruse the vast sea of literature on a variety of topics and issues in the head and neck and have enough practical knowledge on the etiology, pathology, diagnosis, workup, and management of these conditions. In addition, surgical nuances, and the role of multidisciplinary teams, continue to evolve. While survival from cancer remains the ultimate goal, advances in surgical techniques and management of esthetic and functional sequela of surgery are an important component of the treatment algorithm.

Dr. Bruce Ashford and his colleagues have taken a bold step to distill the essential information from a vast body of literature, in a single textbook geared for the general surgical trainee, to acquaint him/her with the commonly encountered clinical problems and give the fundamental information on anatomy, clinical diagnosis, workup, and management, including special tips for surgery in an up-to-date, easy-to-understand, and succinct overview. This book should be of tremendous value to trainees and practitioners of general surgery, to arm them with a quick understanding of the diagnostic and management issues in patients who may need head and neck surgery. The authors of each chapter are established experts in their areas of contribution who have emphasized and highlighted important points to remember in each clinical scenario. Further, this book would be a very valuable resource for candidates preparing for their board or fellowship examinations. Clearly, this book fills a void and fulfills an unmet demand for a quick compendium of head and neck surgery for the general surgeon.

Memorial Sloan Kettering Cancer Center
New York, NY, USA

Jatin P. Shah

Acknowledgments

To the editorial team who have ushered this project from inception to completion, I would apologize for my deficiencies and thank for their patience.

I would like to give special thanks to Prof. Julio Mayol of Madrid and the late Prof. Sherif Hanna of Toronto. Both were instrumental in the genesis of this text. Without their encouragement, this project would not have proceeded.

To all my colleagues who provided their wisdom and insights to the writing of this book, I am so grateful. This book again represents your commitment to training and the future of high-quality head and neck surgery.

And finally, as for all surgeons, for their love and support, I would wish to acknowledge and thank my family.

Introduction

The surgical management of diseases of the head and neck demands much of the surgeon. The interplay between complex anatomy and lethal disease is unforgiving, with complications and the unexpected the order of the day. But just like other fields of surgery, sound practice delivering optimal outcomes for our patients is based on knowledge and a dedication to medical and technical excellence.

General surgery is the parent of all surgical specialties. Some of the most renowned head and neck surgeons have been general surgeons, including George Crile, Hayes Martin, and more recently Jatin Shah. In many parts of the world, general surgeons provide a very high standard of care in head and neck surgery.

Within general surgery training programs, the teaching of head and neck surgery for both benign and malignant disease can be patchy. The coverage of key topics is often left to others, and unsatisfying gaps in the syllabus leave our junior colleagues to pursue other training or to abandon the field as too difficult to even begin to master. The provision of graduating surgeons with a firm handle on the topic is generally incomplete.

We have therefore compiled a collection covering key topics in head and neck surgery, written by an international multidisciplinary and multispecialty group of surgeons, each an expert in their field. Our aim has been to distill the essence of each topic, with applicable workup and both operative and nonoperative approaches to management, with key takeaways and limited but essential references for further reading. Relevant anatomy is reviewed as this is the basis for safe surgery in a minefield of critical structures. We have tried to cover technical pearls of the pertinent operations, but to not serve as a step-by-step operative surgery manual.

My hope is that this book provides a context and a template for the syllabus of head and neck surgery topics to be adequately taught, studied, and revisited by both trainees and surgeons alike. And by concisely dealing with the complex and demanding, I hope the gaps in training can be demystified, shedding light on the path and making sense of the obscure and opaque.

Contents

Imaging in Head and Neck Surgery

1

Grace Aw and Jennifer Gillespie

1.1 Imaging Modalities

	Advantages	Disadvantages
US	Inexpensive Quick, easy to access Biopsy guidance	Operator dependent Small field of view Limited assessment of deep tissues, bone
CT	Easy access Quick to perform Excellent spatial resolution IV contrast can help identify disease Assess bony structures Assess lymph nodes	Dental amalgam causes beam hardening artefact Radiation dose Limited contrast resolution Adverse reactions to intravenous contrast
MRI	No radiation dose Excellent contrast resolution Assess perineural spread and bone marrow involvement Assess lymph nodes	Difficult access Long scan time Movement artefact Claustrophobia Ferromagnetic restorations can cause significant artefact Safety limitations with prostheses, stents, clips, cardiac pacemaker, shrapnel etc.
PET/CT	Detection of distant metastases Detection of adenopathy Useful in the investigation for carcinoma of unknown primary	Limited access Radiation dose Requires expert interpretation – normal tissues and benign pathologies also take up FDG Misregistration of PET and CT

1.2 Trauma

The assessment of neck trauma can be challenging, as this anatomical region contains many vital structures. For this purpose, the neck is divided into three zones, and each zone has anatomic, diagnostic and management implications. Imaging plays a key role in the evaluation of traumatic neck injuries [1].

G. Aw (✉)
Department of Medical Imaging, Royal Brisbane and Women's Hospital, Herston, QLD, Australia
e-mail: grace.aw@health.qld.gov.au

J. Gillespie
Department of Medical Imaging, Royal Brisbane and Women's Hospital, Herston, QLD, Australia

Faculty of Medicine, University of Queensland, Herston, QLD, Australia
e-mail: jennifer.gillespie2@health.qld.gov.au

B. Ashford (ed.), *Head and Neck Surgery for General Surgeons*,
https://doi.org/10.1007/978-981-19-7900-2_1

	Boundaries	Contents at risk
Zone 1	Cricoid process to sternoclavicular notch	Innominate vessels Proximal common carotid arteries Subclavian and vertebral arteries Internal jugular veins Recurrent laryngeal and vagus nerves Brachial plexus Trachea Oesophagus Lung apices Thoracic duct
Zone 2	Angle of the mandible to the cricoid process	Vertebral arteries Distal common carotid arteries, proximal internal and external carotid arteries Jugular veins Vagus nerve Larynx and pharynx
Zone 3	Base of the skull to the angle of the mandible	Extracranial internal carotid and vertebral arteries External carotid arteries Jugular veins Cranial nerves IX–XII Pharynx

(a) Chest radiography—Anterior and lateral neck and chest radiographs to look for haemothorax, pneumothorax or pneumomediastinum.
(b) CT angiography—Initial study to evaluate for vascular injury and surrounding structures.
(c) Digital subtraction angiography—"Gold standard" for evaluating vascular injury and should include examination of the aortic arch and branches, carotid and vertebral vessels.
(d) Duplex ultrasound—May be obtained in stable patients; however, it is operator-dependent. Non-occlusive injuries may be missed if the flow is preserved, e.g. intimal flaps and pseudoaneurysms. Its role in Zone 3 injuries is limited.
(e) Contrast swallow—Should be performed if an oesophageal perforation is suspected.

1.3 Neck Spaces: Anatomy of the Suprahyoid and Infrahyoid Neck

The neck is divided by the hyoid bone into the suprahyoid (to the base of the skull) and the infrahyoid neck (to the sternoclavicular notch). The suprahyoid neck (Fig. 1.1) is further divided into compartments or "spaces", including the visceral (pharyngomucosal), parapharyngeal, parotid, masticator (suprazygomatic and infrazygomatic), buccal, submandibular and sublingual. Other spaces cross the suprahyoid and infrahyoid neck, including the carotid, visceral, retropharyngeal and prevertebral spaces [2]. A brief summary of the contents of each space is included below; however, a full anatomical description is beyond the scope of this chapter.

1.3.1 Visceral Space

The visceral space contains the nasopharynx and oropharynx in the suprahyoid neck and the hypopharynx, larynx and thyroid gland in the infrahyoid neck.

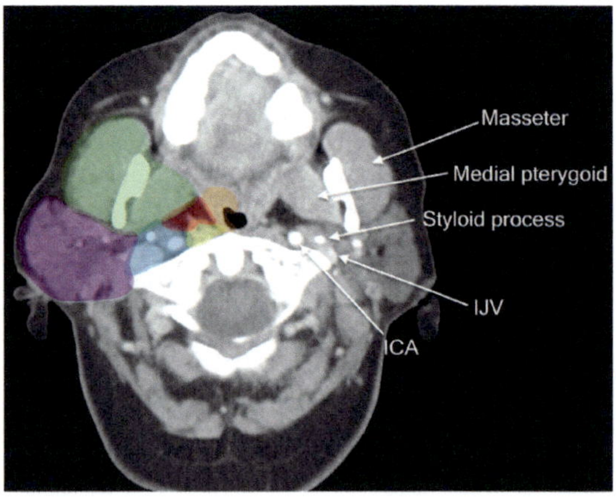

Fig. 1.1 Spaces of the suprahyoid neck. Contrast-enhanced CT of the neck at the level of the oropharynx demonstrates the spaces of the suprahyoid neck – parapharyngeal space (red), pharyngeal mucosal space (orange), retropharynx (yellow), carotid space (blue), parotid space (purple) and masticator space (green)

1.3.2 Retropharyngeal Space

The retropharyngeal space extends from the skull base to the superior mediastinum. The anterior border is formed by the visceral fascia and the posterior border by the prevertebral fascia. It contains fat and retropharyngeal lymph nodes.

1.3.3 Prevertebral Space

The prevertebral space lies posterior to the retropharyngeal space and is enclosed by the prevertebral fascia. It contains the prevertebral muscles, vertebral bodies and intervertebral discs, spinal canal, vertebral artery and phrenic nerve.

1.3.4 Parapharyngeal Space

The prestyloid parapharyngeal space (PPS) contains fat, neurovascular structures (a small branch of V3 supplying the tensor veli palatini muscle, internal maxillary artery, ascending pharyngeal artery and pterygoid venous plexus) and minor/ectopic salivary gland/rests. Primary PPS masses displace the lateral wall of the visceral space medially, the deep lobe of the parotid gland laterally and the contents of the carotid sheath posteriorly.

1.3.5 Carotid Space

The carotid space, or carotid sheath, extends from the jugular foramen superiorly to the aortic arch inferiorly. It is bordered anteriorly by the styloid process and parapharyngeal space, laterally by the anterior belly of the digastric muscle and the parotid space and medially by the lateral margin of the retropharyngeal space. The carotid sheath contains the carotid artery, the internal jugular vein and cranial nerves IX to XII.

1.3.6 Masticator Space

The masticator space extends superiorly to the skull base and inferiorly to the attachment of the medial pterygoid and masseter muscles to the mandible. It is bordered anteriorly by the buccal space, posterolaterally by the parotid space and medially by the parapharyngeal space. It contains the muscles of mastication (medial and lateral pterygoid, masseter and temporalis), mandibular ramus and the mandibular division of the trigeminal nerve.

1.3.7 Parotid Space

The parotid space is a pyramidal space with a broad base facing laterally and formed by the superficial layer of the deep cervical fascia overlying the superficial lobe of the parotid gland. The pyramid apex points medially. The parotid space is bordered medially by the parapharyngeal space, laterally by the superficial space and subcutaneous tissue, posteriorly by the carotid space and anteriorly by the masticator space. It contains the parotid gland and is divided into superficial and deep lobes by the facial nerve. The PS also contains the retromandibular vein, external carotid artery and intra-parotid lymph nodes.

1.3.8 Buccal Space

The buccal space is bordered medially by the buccinator muscle, posteriorly by the masticator space and anterolaterally by the parotid space. It contains fat, minor salivary gland tissue, parotid duct, lymph nodes, facial and buccal artery, facial vein, buccal branch of the facial nerve and buccal division of CNV3.

1.3.9 Submandibular Space

The submandibular space is located below the mandible, inferior to the mylohyoid muscle. Posteriorly, the submandibular space communicates with the posterior aspect of the sublingual space. It contains fat, the anterior belly of the digastric muscle, the superficial portion of the submandibular gland, submandibular and submental lymph nodes, the facial artery and vein, and the inferior loop of the hypoglossal nerve.

1.3.10 Sublingual Space

The sublingual space is also referred to as the "floor of mouth". The mylohyoid muscle separates the sublingual and submandibular spaces. The sublingual space is bordered superiorly by the intrinsic tongue muscles, inferolaterally by mylohyoid, anteriorly by the mandible and medially by the geniohyoid and genioglossus muscles. It freely communicates with the submandibular and parapharyngeal spaces along the posterior border of the mylohyoid muscle. The sublingual space contains the sublingual gland and ducts, the deep portion of the submandibular gland and duct, the lingual artery and vein, the lingual nerve, branches of the glossopharyngeal and hypoglossal nerves, a portion of the hyoglossus muscle and lymph nodes.

1.4 Evaluation of a Neck Lump

The roles of imaging in the investigation of neck masses include:

- Localisation
- Characterisation
  - Cystic or solid
  - Presence of calcification, fat
  - Contrast enhancement
- Anatomical relationships: vessels, salivary glands, thyroid gland, bone and cartilage
- Evidence of malignancy
  - Invasion of surrounding structures
  - Perineural spread
  - Lymphadenopathy

1.4.1 Salivary Gland

Focal or diffuse salivary gland swelling may be due to inflammation, systemic disease or tumour.

Ultrasound is the initial imaging investigation of choice for salivary gland pathologies.

- Differentiate intraglandular from extraglandular masses
- Visualise dilated salivary gland ducts
- May be able to visualise calculi
- Guide fine needle/core biopsy

CT and MRI may be required for assessment of deep or large masses, such as those that involve the deep lobe of the parotid gland, floor of the mouth, etc. CT is also useful for localisation of intraductal calculi and for assessment of lymphadenopathy in presumed malignancy, whilst MRI is used for assessment of perineural spread.

Sialography may be performed for salivary duct assessment; however, it is contraindicated in the presence of acute salivary gland inflammation. Given the ease of access to and resolution of modern cross-sectional imaging, sialography no longer plays a significant role in clinical practice.

1.4.1.1 Tumour

Primary salivary gland tumours may be classified as benign or malignant. Benign tumours include benign mixed tumour (pleomorphic adenoma), lymphomatous papillary cystadenomas (Warthin tumour), lipoma and neuroma. Malignant tumours include adenoid cystic carcinoma and mucoepidermoid carcinoma. SCC and melanoma metastases may also be found in the salivary glands. Figure 1.2 demonstrates two common lesions arising in the parotid glands.

Pleomorphic Adenoma

Pleomorphic adenoma, also previously known as benign mixed tumour, are benign epithelial neoplasms that commonly occur in salivary glands but can arise in any tissue that has glandular myoepithelial tissue (e.g. lacrimal glands, skin, breast and vulva).

About 84% of pleomorphic adenomas in the salivary glands arise in the parotid gland, followed by 8% in the submandibular gland and 6.5% in minor salivary glands (nasal cavity, pharynx, larynx and trachea) [3].

Tumours typically appear as well-defined rounded masses with bosselated margins, typically in the superficial lobe of the parotid gland. When they arise from the deep lobe of the parotid, they may appear entirely extra-parotid in the prestyloid parapharyngeal space without a fat plane

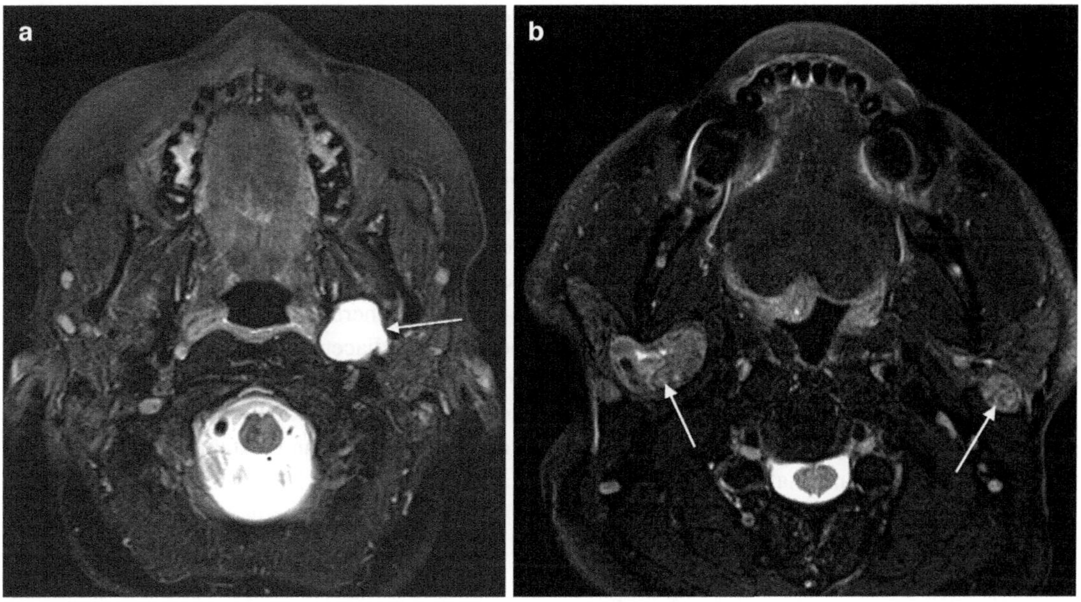

Fig. 1.2 Parotid lesions. (**a**) Pleomorphic adenoma of the deep lobe of the left parotid gland (arrow), which demonstrates marked T2 hyperintensity on T2 fat-saturated (T2 FS) MRI. (**b**) Bilateral Warthin tumours (arrows), which are well-defined and mildly hyperintense on the T2 FS sequence

between it and the parotid gland. On ultrasound, lesions are typically hypoechoic and may show posterior acoustic enhancement. Small lesions on CT demonstrate homogeneous attenuation and prominent enhancement, although larger lesions may appear more heterogeneous, with foci of necrosis and small regions of calcification. On MRI, lesions are usually T1 hypointense with intense T2 hyperintensity (CSF bright) with homogeneous enhancement post gadolinium administration.

Warthin Tumour

Lymphomatous papillary cystadenomas, more commonly known as Warthin tumours, are the second most common benign parotid tumour and represent up to 10% of all parotid tumours. They are bilateral or multifocal in up to 20% of cases and the most common neoplasm in multiple solid parotid masses.

Most tumours are well-defined, with multiple small irregular spongiform anechoic areas on ultrasound. They are often hypervascular. The classic appearance on CT is a well-defined heterogeneous solid and cystic, moderately enhancing lesion within the superficial lobe or in the parotid tail. The presence of a mural nodule is strongly suggestive of a Warthin tumour. On MRI, it is low to intermediate T1 signal with cholesterol components containing focal high signal; heterogeneous T2 signal and enhancing solid components. Warthin tumours may incidentally show uptake with Tc-99m-pertechnetate and FDG-PET/CT [4].

Mucoepidermoid Carcinoma

Mucoepidermoid carcinoma accounts for up to 15% of all salivary gland tumours, up to 10% of all major salivary gland tumours, and up to 41% of minor salivary gland tumours. They are the most common malignant primary neoplasm of the parotid gland (with or without facial nerve involvement) [5]. Ultrasound demonstrates a well-circumscribed hypoechoic lesion with a partially or completely cystic appearance. On CT, low-grade tumours appear as well-circumscribed masses with cystic components and occasional calcification, whereas high-grade tumours appear more solid with poorly defined margins

, and features of local infiltration. MRI appearances are dependent on grade, but typically low to intermediate T1 signal and variable T2 signal (low-grade have intermediate to high T2 signal, whereas high-grade have lower T2 signal and poorly defined margins). MR neurogram is essential to assess for perineural spread along the trigeminal and facial nerves [6]. FDG-PET/CT may be used for staging.

Adenoid Cystic Carcinoma

Adenoid cystic carcinoma is the second most common malignancy involving the parotid gland and the minor salivary glands. They arise more commonly in the minor salivary glands (55%) and tend to be locally aggressive with a penchant for perineural spread. On ultrasound, low-grade tumours tend to be more well-defined, with high-grade tumours appearing more infiltrative. On CT, both subtypes enhance homogeneously post contrast administration. On MRI, tumours are T1 hypo- to isointense, and mildly T2 hyperintense to hypointense depending on grade [7]. Again, there is relatively homogeneous enhancement on MRI, and MR neurogram is extremely important to assess for perineural spread. FDG-PET/CT may be used for staging.

1.4.1.2 Infection/Inflammation

Bacterial aetiologies usually cause unilateral salivary gland inflammation, whereas viral aetiologies commonly cause bilateral gland involvement. A calculus may cause non-infectious inflammatory sialadenitis due to obstruction of the salivary duct.

Bilateral parotid gland swelling may be caused by systemic diseases, such as Sjogren syndrome, sarcoidosis and HIV.

1.4.2 Cervical Lymphadenitis

Patients with cervical lymphadenitis typically present with a painful cervical mass and symptoms and pathology consistent with infection. Ultrasound is typically the first line of investigation, and in uncomplicated cases, this would demonstrate a nodal conglomerate with homogeneously low echogenicity of nodal parenchyma and preservation of the normal fatty hilum. Further cross-sectional imaging is not usually required.

Features of complication or abscess formation include thickened and irregular walls, central heterogeneous echogenicity suggesting necrosis, central complexity with debris, septae or hyperechoic foci of air, obliteration of the normal fatty hilum, peripheral increased vascularity and oedema of adjacent soft tissues. Cross-sectional imaging may be indicated to assess for adjacent complications, e.g. extent of infection, arterial or venous thrombosis and distant complications.

1.4.3 Thyroid

Differentials for a thyroid mass are reasonably extensive and include inflammatory, benign and malignant aetiologies. Again, ultrasound is the initial imaging investigation of choice to evaluate for the presence and characteristics of thyroid nodules, as well as to assess the background thyroid parenchyma and guide fine needle aspirate biopsy.

Thyroid nodules on ultrasound are assessed and reported using the American College of Radiology Thyroid Imaging Reporting and Data System (TI-RADS) in order to ensure standardisation of reporting, classification and follow-up recommendations [8]. Scoring is determined from five categories of ultrasound findings. The higher the cumulative score, the higher the TI-RADS level and the likelihood of malignancy. If multiple nodules are present, only the four highest-scoring nodules are scored, reported and followed up.

Scoring

- Composition
  - Cystic or spongiform: 0 points
  - Mixed cystic and solid: 1 point
  - Solid or almost completely solid: 2 points
- Echogenicity
  - Anechoic: 0 points
  - Hyper- or isoechoic: 1 point
  - Hypoechoic: 2 points

  - Very hypoechoic: 3 points
- Shape (assessed on transverse plane)
  - Wider than tall: 0 points
  - Taller than wide: 3 points
- Margin
  - Smooth: 0 points
  - Ill-defined: 0 points
  - Lobulated/irregular: 2 points
  - Extra-thyroidal extension: 3 points
- Echogenic foci
  - None: 0 points
  - Large comet-tail artefact: 0 points
  - Macrocalcifications: 1 point
  - Peripheral/rim calcifications: 2 points
  - Punctate echogenic foci: 3 points

Classification and recommendations

- TR1: 0 points. Benign. No FNA required
- TR2: 2 points. Not suspicious. No FNA required
- TR3: 3 points. Mildly suspicious
  - ≥1.5 cm: follow up 1, 3, 5 years
  - ≥2.5 cm: FNA
- TR4: 4–6 points. Moderately suspicious
  - ≥1.0 cm: follow up 1, 2, 3, 5 years
  - ≥1.5 cm: FNA
- TR5: ≥7 points. Highly suspicious
  - ≥0.5 cm: follow up, annually for 5 years
  - ≥1.0 cm: FNA

1.4.3.1 Thyroid Carcinoma

Papillary carcinoma accounts for 70% of all thyroid neoplasms and 85% of all thyroid cancers. It usually appears as a solitary subcapsular thyroid mass with an irregular outline, vascularity and small punctate echogenic regions representing microcalcifications (psammoma bodies). It tends to metastasise early to regional lymph nodes (levels 3, 4 and 6), and a reasonable proportion of lymph node metastases have central cavitation, relatively thick walls, septations and mural nodules. Lymphatic spread is more common than haematogenous spread. Figure 1.3 demonstrates the typical ultrasound and CT appearances of papillary thyroid carcinoma.

Follicular thyroid cancer is the second most frequent thyroid gland malignancy after papillary

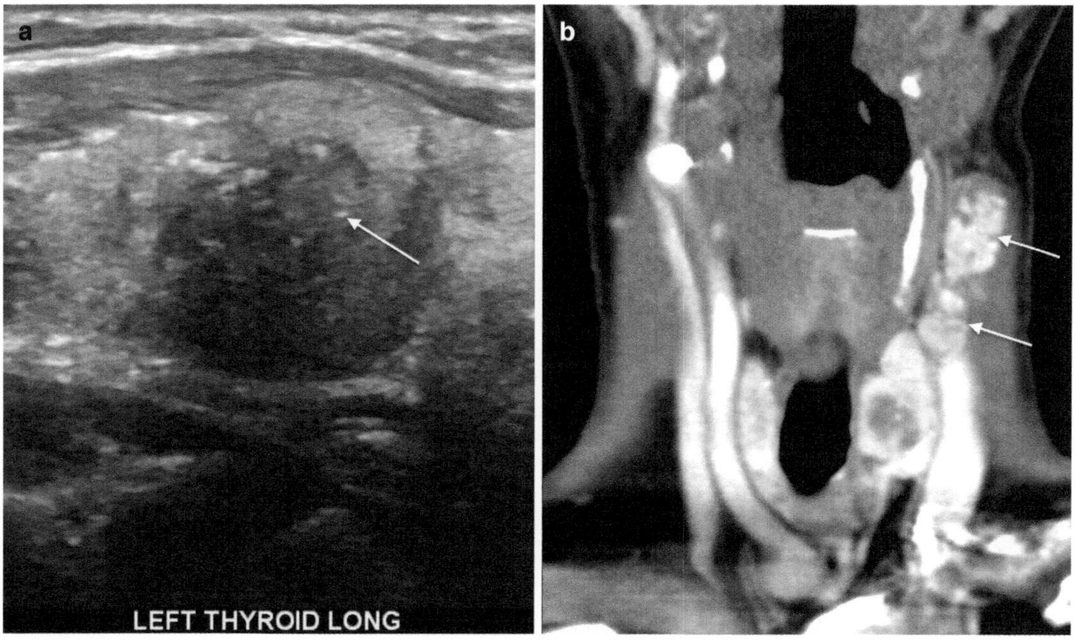

Fig. 1.3 Papillary thyroid carcinoma. (**a**) Ultrasound of the left lobe of the thyroid demonstrates a solid, lobulated, very hypoechoic mass with punctate echogenic foci (arrow) consistent with a TI-RADS 5 nodule. Coronal contrast-enhanced CT neck (**b**) shows multiple enhancing left-sided metastatic neck nodes

cancer and accounts for 10–20% of all thyroid neoplasms. Lesions are typically hypoechoic and usually lack cystic change [9]. It tends to metastasise late to lymph nodes, with haematogenous spread being much more common.

Anaplastic thyroid carcinoma is a highly aggressive form of thyroid cancer and accounts for 1–2% of primary thyroid malignancies. Ultrasound typically shows an infiltrative lesion, with some lesions containing microcalcification. CT is useful for the assessment of extrathyroidal tumour invasion of surrounding critical structures, such as the carotid artery, jugular vein, bone and muscle, as well as lymph node involvement and distant metastatic disease [10].

Ultrasound is the imaging modality of choice for the initial assessment of the thyroid gland and to guide fine needle aspirate biopsy [11]. CT of the neck and chest is subsequently used for staging lymph node involvement and to assess for pulmonary or bone metastases. 99mTc-sestamibi imaging was previously frequently performed in patients with differentiated thyroid cancer but has been replaced by other imaging modalities, such as FDG-PET/CT. The role of FDG-PET/CT lies mainly in the assessment of recurrent or aggressive disease rather than at initial diagnosis. Radioactive iodine scintigraphy is useful for the completion of post-operative staging and accurate risk stratification of patients with thyroid cancer and has demonstrated a role in guiding I-131 therapy [12]. However, anaplastic carcinoma usually shows no uptake with radioiodine.

1.4.4 Parathyroid

Parathyroid adenomas are benign tumours of the parathyroid glands and the most common cause of primary hyperparathyroidism. The majority of parathyroid adenomas are juxtathyroid and located immediately posterior and inferior to the thyroid gland (Fig. 1.4). Superior gland parathyroid adenomas may lie posteriorly in the tracheo-oesophageal groove or in a paraoesophageal location. Up to 5% of adenomas may lie in an ectopic location, such as the mediastinum, retropharyngeal, carotid sheath or thyroid gland.

Ultrasound is the most commonly used initial imaging modality. However, most nodules need to be $\geq$1 cm to be confidently visualised on ultrasound. Parathyroid adenomas tend to be homogeneously hypoechoic compared to the thyroid gland, and Doppler ultrasound may demonstrate a characteristic extrathyroidal arterial feeding vessel arising from the inferior thyroid artery.

Tc-99m-sestamibi scintigraphy has a 65–95% sensitivity in locating a single-gland adenoma, with the protein and radioactive tracer taken up by the overactive enlarged parathyroid gland whilst normal parathyroid glands are inactive in the presence of hypercalcemia. However, there are a small number of false-negative results, with some patients who have a negative sestamibi study at surgical exploration are found to have a single adenoma causing hyperparathyroidism [13].

Hybrid imaging with single photon-emission computed tomography, which combines functional data with three-dimensional anatomical data, improves lesion localisation, particularly in the presence of ectopic glandular or multiglandular disease, concomitant nodular thyroid disease, and recurrence or persistence of disease after surgery.

False-positive findings of a hyperfunctioning parathyroid gland can occur, the most frequent cause of which is a solitary solid nodule thyroid adenoma or a multinodular goitre. Benign or malignant tumours that also take up the radiotracer include breast, lung, and head and neck carcinomas, and associated nodal and osseous metastases, as well as bronchial carcinoids. Delayed washout of Tc-99m-sestamibi is also seen in some well-differentiated thyroid carcinomas, primary thyroid lymphoma, a remnant thymus and a PTH-secreting paraganglioma. However, in the clinical setting of hyperparathyroidism, false-positive findings are uncommon.

Multiphase (or 4D) parathyroid CT has been shown to be more sensitive than ultrasound or

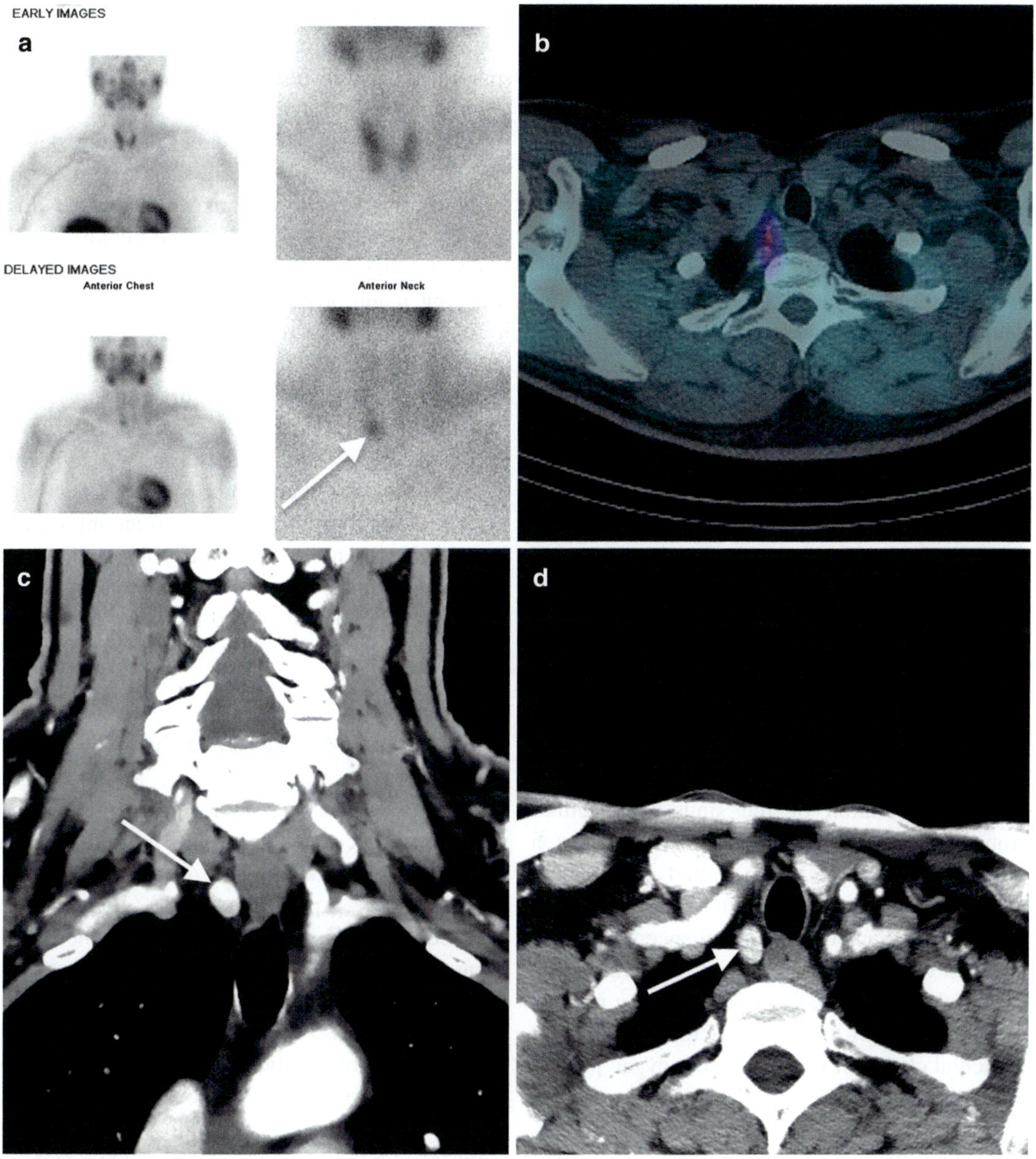

Fig. 1.4 Parathyroid adenoma. (**a**) Tc-99m sestamibi planar images and SPECT (**b**) show a right para-oesophageal nodule that shows radiotracer uptake on the delayed scans. Coronal (**c**) and axial (**d**) 4D CT neck confirms an arterially enhancing lesion corresponding to the parathyroid adenoma

scintigraphy to precisely localise adenomas prior to minimally invasive parathyroidectomy. "4D" refers to imaging performed in multiple phases of contrast, with time being the fourth dimension in addition to the multiplanar format of CT. The classic pattern of parathyroid adenomas, with low attenuation on non-contrast imaging, intense arterial enhancement and contrast washout on delayed phase, is present in only a minority of cases [14, 15].

MRI is infrequently used in initial workup due to lower spatial resolution and artefacts, with the reported sensitivity of MR imaging for the detection of parathyroid adenomas ranging from 65% to 80%. MRI is more commonly used in patients with persistent or recurrent hyperparathyroidism, in whom it has been shown to be effective in locating remaining abnormal parathyroid tissue [16].

Parathyroid carcinomas are extremely rare and often present with profound hyperparathyroidism. Early metastasis is not uncommon. Imaging typically uses a combination of ultrasound and CT. FDG-PET/CT has described avidity in case reports and may have a role in staging of proven parathyroid carcinoma [17].

1.4.5 Branchial Cleft Anomalies

Branchial cleft anomalies comprise a spectrum of congenital defects in the head and neck. Anomalies include a cyst, a fistula or a sinus.

First branchial cleft anomalies are seen above the level of the mandible near the external auditory canal within or close to the parotid gland. Cysts usually manifest as recurrent abscesses or other inflammation of the sinus tract, either around the ear or at the angle of the mandible. On CT, they appear as a thin-walled cystic mass within, superficial to or deep to the parotid gland. Cyst wall thickness and enhancement may increase with recurrent infection. It is important to note that neither CT nor MR imaging is characteristic enough to allow differentiating a first branchial cleft cyst from any other cystic parotid mass.

Second branchial cleft anomalies are mostly located in the submandibular space; however, they can occur anywhere along a line from the oropharyngeal tonsillar fossa to the supraclavicular neck. The cyst usually appears as a painless fluctuant mass in the lateral neck adjacent to the anteromedial border of the sternocleidomastoid muscle at the mandibular angle, lateral to the carotid space and at the posterior margin of the submandibular gland. It may become painful and tender with repeated infection. If a fistula is present, the ostium is usually noted at birth just above the clavicle in the anterior neck.

On ultrasound, a second branchial cleft cyst is well-defined, round to ovoid, centrally anechoic mass with a thin peripheral wall. The mass is compressible and shows distinct posterior acoustic enhancement. Internal echoes represent debris within the cyst. Cysts on CT appear well-circumscribed, homogeneously hypodense with a uniformly thin wall, although wall thickness may increase after infection. Figure 1.5 demonstrates the typical appearance of a second branchial cleft cyst, as opposed to a necrotic nodal metastasis. MRI is useful for assessing the deep tissue extent of the cyst to allow for accurate preoperative planning. The cyst contents vary from T1 hypointense to slightly hyperintense and T2 hyperintense, with wall enhancement [18].

Third and fourth branchial cleft anomalies are rare and present in the infrahyoid neck, with fourth branchial cleft cysts usually adjacent to the thyroid gland. There are no fifth branchial cleft anomalies.

1.4.6 Thyroglossal Duct Cyst

Thyroglossal duct cysts are located in the midline in 75% of cases and slightly off-midline in 25% in the anterior neck. They are always within 2 cm of the midline. Approximately 80% of cysts are located either at or below the level of the hyoid bone, with the remaining 20% located above the hyoid bone. A thyroglossal duct cyst may rarely present as a mass in the floor of mouth. The duct and cyst characteristically move upward with tongue protrusion [19].

On ultrasound, a thyroglossal duct cyst appears as a thin-walled anechoic or hypoechoic structure with posterior acoustic enhancement in the characteristic location. A few internal septations may be seen, and internal echoes reflect proteinaceous fluid within the cyst. Comparison with the normal thyroid gland should suffice to exclude ectopic thyroid tissue. On CT, thyroglossal duct cysts appear as a thin-walled hypodense cystic structure with peripheral rim enhancement. On MRI, an uncomplicated thyroglossal duct cyst demonstrates a low T1 signal and high T2 signal, which reflects its fluid content.

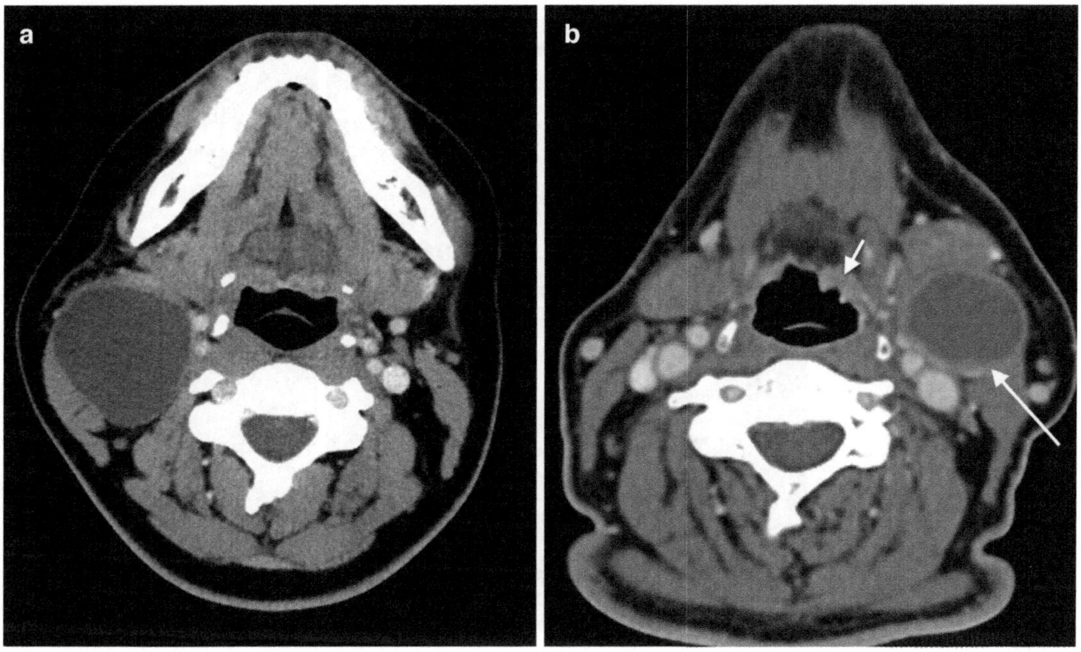

Fig. 1.5 Cystic neck lesions. (**a**) Second branchial cleft cyst with a smooth, non-enhancing rim and internal low density positioned deep to the SCM, lateral to the carotid sheath and posterior to the submandibular gland. (**b**) SCC nodal metastasis (arrow), which is predominantly cystic but has a thickened enhancing margin. The primary lesion was a small tumour in the right base of the tongue (short arrow)

1.4.7 Carotid Body Tumour

A carotid body tumour, also known as chemodectoma, is a highly vascular glomus tumour that arises from paraganglion cells of the carotid body. They are the most common type of paraganglioma in the head and neck (60–70%) and are bilateral in 10% of cases. A small number are familial (up to 10%) with an autosomal dominant inheritance and associated with multiple endocrine neoplasia (MEN IIa and IIb), phakomatoses (neurofibromatosis type 1, tuberous sclerosis complex and von Hippel–Lindau disease) and Carney triad [20].

Carotid body tumours are located at the carotid bifurcation, with characteristic splaying of the ICA and ECA (the "lyre" sign), see Fig. 1.6. On CT, they demonstrate vivid contrast enhancement. On MRI, carotid body tumours appear T1 iso- to hypointense, and T2 hyperintense, with a "salt and pepper" appearance on both T1 and T2 whereby punctate regions of haemorrhage (salt) are intermingled with small flow voids (pepper). Lesions enhance intensely following gadolinium administration.

The splaying of the carotid vessels or the "lyre" sign is nicely demonstrated on digital subtraction angiography, with an intense tumour blush and early venous drainage due to arteriovenous shunting. The ascending pharyngeal artery generally constitutes the main arterial supply to the tumour. As with other paragangliomas, carotid body tumours will show uptake with 68Ga-DOTATATE PET/CT as well as metaiodobenzylguanidine (MIBG), which is useful in assessing multicentric tumours. MIBG is comparatively more costly and has decreased spatial resolution compared to 68Ga-DOTATATE PET/CT but may be useful in some tumours that are negative on PET/CT.

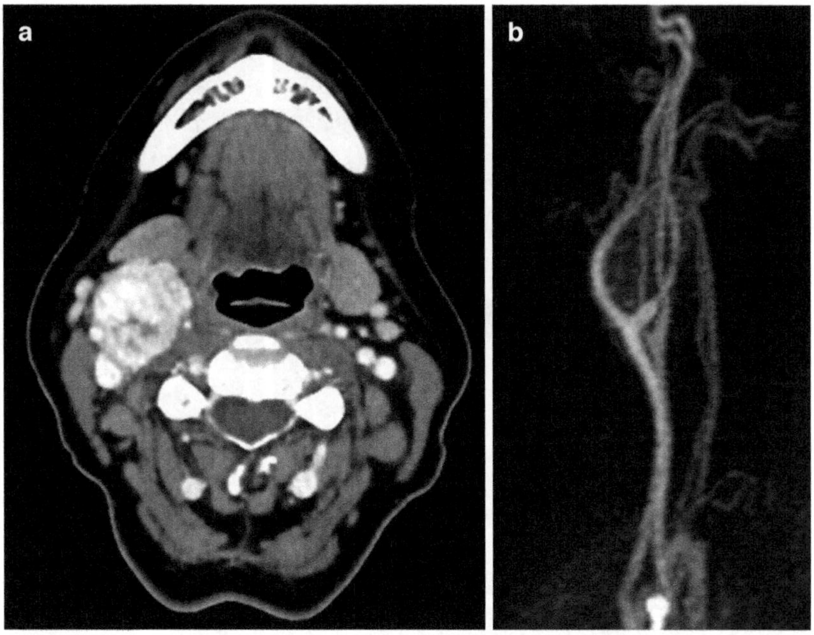

Fig. 1.6 Carotid body tumour. (**a**) Axial contrast-enhanced CT (CECT) demonstrates an avidly enhancing lesion within the right carotid space, splaying the internal and external carotid arteries. (**b**) The sagittal image from time-resolved MRA shows the "lyre sign"

1.5 Skin Cancer

Most non-melanoma skin cancers can be managed without any imaging prior to treatment. However, tumours that are large or in difficult anatomical sites, such as the eyelid, lip or ear, may require imaging to assess for deeper invasion. The histology of the primary tumour may also alter the need for staging.

In patients with squamous cell carcinoma (SCC), high-risk features, such as recurrent tumours, >2 cm in diameter, poorly differentiated histology, perineural invasion and lymphovascular invasion, may prompt further staging with CT given the increased risk of nodal and distant metastases. Merkel cell carcinoma (MCC) is a neuroendocrine tumour of the skin. Although these tumours are rare, they are highly aggressive with a high incidence of nodal and distant metastases. It is now generally accepted to include FDG-PET in the staging of patients with MCC [21, 22].

CT should be the initial imaging modality for large tumours that are fixed to underlying structures. Bony invasion is well demonstrated on thin slice, high-resolution bone windows. If there is a concern for invasion through the calvarium, then MRI may be required. MRI is also useful in lesions where there is suspicion of orbital invasion, especially tumours around the medial canthus.

The other feature that should prompt imaging with MRI is if there are clinical features suggestive of perineural tumour spread (PNS). This occurs when tumour spreads along the perineurium of peripheral sensory and motor nerves and is associated with dysaesthesia or motor dysfunction depending on the nerve involved, most commonly the trigeminal and facial nerves. It can occur years after prior treatment of a skin cancer. Therefore, any new symptoms of cranial neuropathy should prompt a dedicated, high-resolution skull base MRI (MR neurogram) to assess for PNS. Imaging features (Fig. 1.7) include thickening and abnormal enhancement of the nerve, with loss of the normal fat pads around the skull base foramina and expansion or erosion of the foramina [23]. There may also be secondary signs of nerve involvement with denervation changes in the muscles of facial expression or mastication.

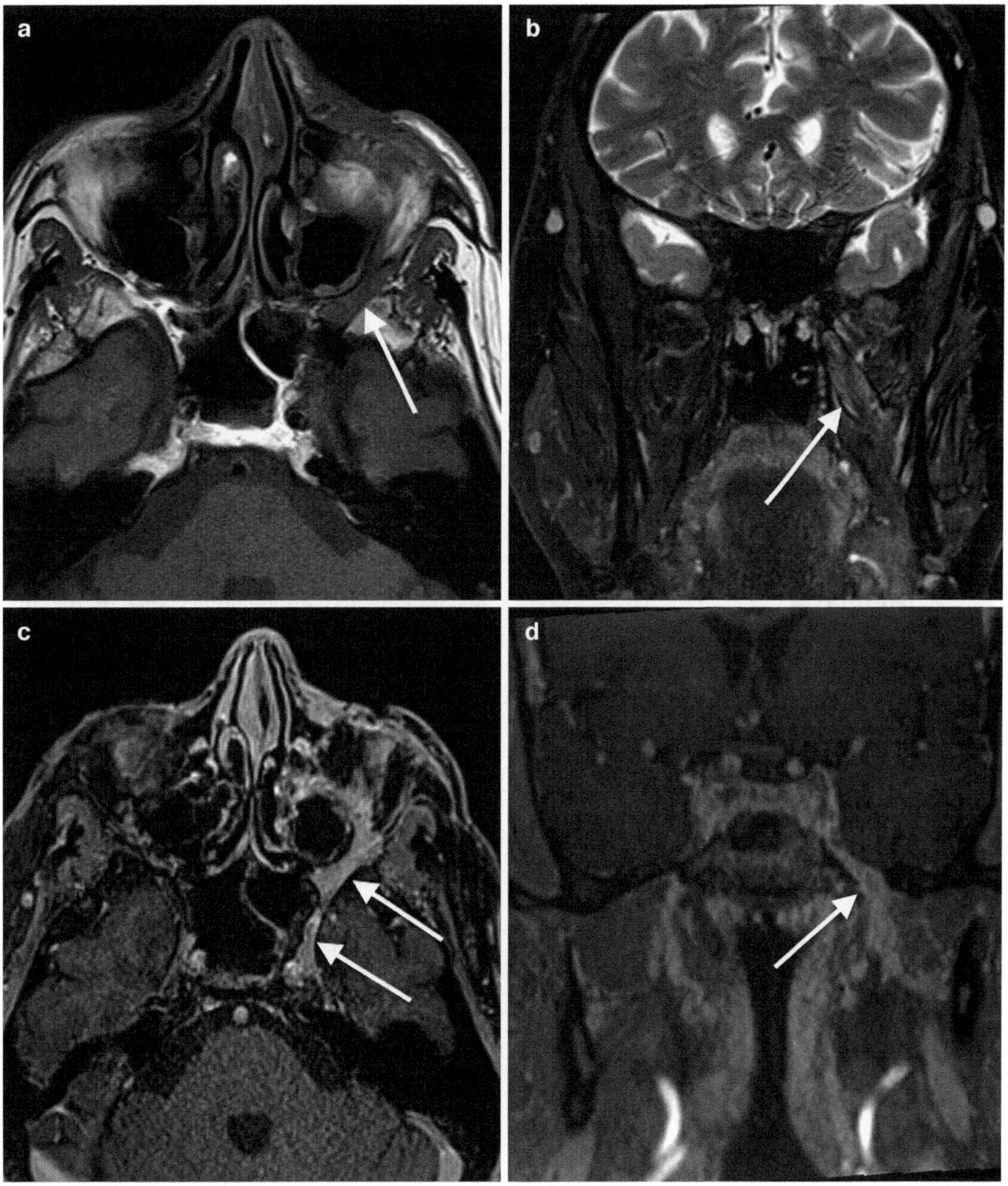

Fig. 1.7 Perineural tumour spread. (**a**) Axial T1-weighted MRI demonstrates loss of the normal fat within the left pterygopalatine fossa (arrow). (**b**) Coronal T2 FS sequences show high signal intensity and volume loss within the muscles of mastication (arrow) consistent with subacute denervation change. T1 post contrast FS sequences in axial (**c**) and coronal (**d**) planes show abnormal enhancement and thickening of the maxillary and mandibular divisions of the left trigeminal nerve (arrows)

In patients with Stage III or IV melanoma, PET-CT is the imaging method of choice to assess for nodal or visceral metastases. High-resolution CT performed alongside the PET can detect small pulmonary nodules (<8 mm) that may not demonstrate FDG uptake due to their small size. Contrast-enhanced MRI of the brain is the most sensitive modality for the detection of intracranial metastases and should be considered in patients with Stage IV disease if there are no contraindications to MRI [24]. Due to the presence of melanin, which causes T1 shortening, cerebral metastases may demonstrate high signal intensity on T1-weighted sequences. They may also be low signal intensity on T2-weighted sequences due to the presence of haemorrhage.

1.6 Upper Aerodigestive Tract Neoplasia

Neoplasms of the upper aerodigestive tract may come to the attention of the general surgeon due to the detection of an enlarged lymph node in the neck. The vast majority of these will be SCC, although other malignancies, such as adenoid cystic carcinoma or adenocarcinoma, can rarely arise from the mucosa of the upper aerodigestive tract.

Size is one of the key features that may arouse suspicion for a pathological node. The standard measurement to determine if a node is enlarged or not is the short-axis diameter, measured in the axial plane, with 10 mm generally accepted as the cut off for most neck nodes, or up to 12 mm in the jugulodigastric (level 2) nodes. However, it is important to remember that there are multiple imaging features to consider when evaluating pathological lymph nodes. These include the morphology of the node (with loss of the normal fatty hilum), presence of necrosis or cystic change, increased enhancement and calcification [25]. These features are demonstrated in Fig. 1.8.

Extranodal extension (ENE) is a finding on clinical examination in which the nodes are fixed to adjacent muscles, there is invasion of the skin or features of invasion into other structures (brachial plexus or sympathetic trunk) [24]. This may be supported by radiological evidence of ENE with nodes demonstrating poorly defined or spiculated margins with encasement of vessels and direct invasion into the adjacent musculature.

In a patient with a pathological node (palpable or detected on imaging), one of the first imaging steps is to perform an ultrasound-guided fine needle aspirate or core biopsy, including testing for p16 staining (to assess for HPV status). CT is used to detect a primary lesion and also stage the nodal disease in the neck [26]. At the same time, the patient should undergo a comprehensive clinical assessment including nasendoscopy to assess for a primary lesion. MRI is typically reserved for specific tumours such as a small oropharyngeal primary tumour being considered for trans-oral robotic surgery (TORS) as seen in Fig. 1.9. FDG/PET is particularly helpful in HPV positive tumours and can help to localise the primary site and is also important in assessing for treatment response following radiotherapy (± chemotherapy).

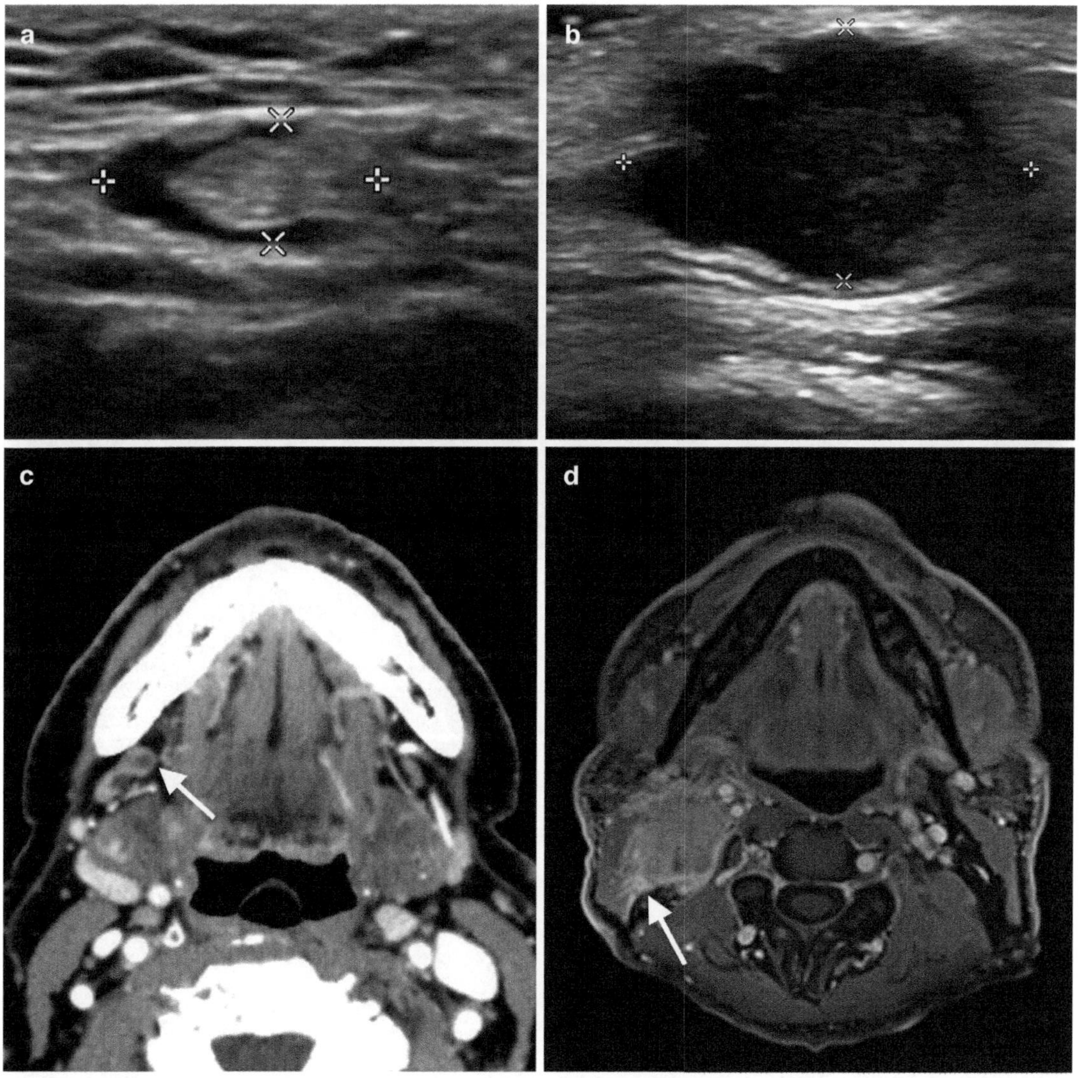

Fig. 1.8 Neck nodes. (**a**) Normal node on ultrasound with a fat-containing echogenic hilum and thin cortex with reniform shape. (**b**) SCC nodal metastasis on ultrasound demonstrating loss of the normal fatty hilum, lobulated margins and loss of the normal reniform shape. (**c**) A small focus of necrosis (arrow) in a right level Ib node on CT was confirmed to be a metastasis from an SCC of the ventral tongue. (**d**) T1 post contrast FS MRI of a large nodal mass demonstrating evidence of ENE with spiculated margins (arrow) and infiltration into the adjacent sternocleidomastoid muscle

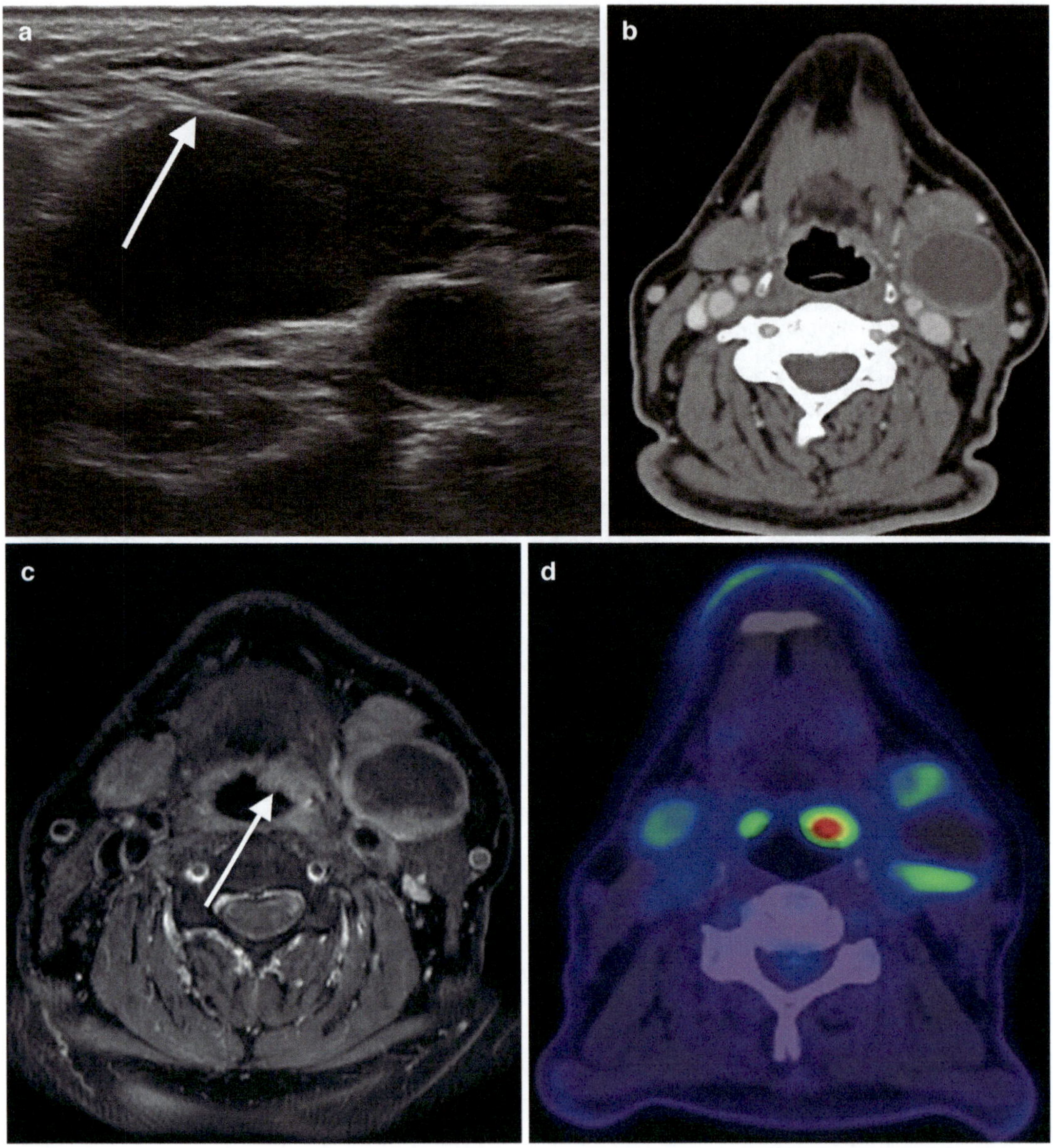

Fig. 1.9 Oropharyngeal SCC. (**a**) Ultrasound-guided FNA of a left level II lymph node. The arrow demonstrates the needle within the node. (**b**) CECT of the left level II node with internal necrosis. Subtle thickening and enhancement of the left base of the tongue represents the primary oropharyngeal tumour (arrow), better demonstrated on the contrast-enhanced T1 FS axial MRI (**c**) and PET (**d**). Note the central photopaenia within the node on FDG-PET due to necrosis of the node

1.7 Conclusion

Imaging plays an essential role in the evaluation of both benign and malignant head and neck conditions, with a combination of CT, MRI, ultrasound, nuclear medicine and angiography playing complementary roles to assist the physician and surgeon in making diagnostic and therapeutic decisions.

Acknowledgements The authors thank Dr. Patrina Campbell for her review of this chapter.

References

1. Alao T, Waseem M. Neck trauma. Treasure Island, FL: StatPearls; 2021.
2. Mukherji SK, Castillo M. A simplified approach to the spaces of the suprahyoid neck. Radiol Clin N Am. 1998;36(5):761–80. v
3. Zhan KY, Khaja SF, Flack AB, Day TA. Benign parotid tumors. Otolaryngol Clin N Am. 2016;49(2):327–42.
4. Koch BL, Hamilton BE, Hudgins PA, Harnsberger HR. Diagnostic imaging: head and neck E-book. Philadelphia, PA: Elsevier Health Sciences; 2016.
5. Som PM, Curtin HD. Head and neck imaging E-book. Elsevier Health Sciences; 2011.
6. Yousem DM, Kraut MA, Chalian AA. Major salivary gland imaging. Radiology. 2000;216(1):19–29.
7. Yih WY, Kratochvil FJ, Stewart JC. Intraoral minor salivary gland neoplasms: review of 213 cases. J Oral Maxillofac Surg. 2005;63(6):805–10.
8. Tessler FN, Middleton WD, Grant EG. Thyroid imaging reporting and data system (TI-RADS): a user's guide. Radiology. 2018;287(3):1082.
9. Sillery JC, Reading CC, Charboneau JW, Henrichsen TL, Hay ID, Mandrekar JN. Thyroid follicular carcinoma: sonographic features of 50 cases. AJR Am J Roentgenol. 2010;194(1):44–54.
10. Takashima S, Morimoto S, Ikezoe J, Takai S, Kobayashi T, Koyama H, et al. CT evaluation of anaplastic thyroid carcinoma. AJR Am J Roentgenol. 1990;154(5):1079–85.
11. Wunderbaldinger P, Harisinghani MG, Hahn PF, Daniels GH, Turetschek K, Simeone J, et al. Cystic lymph node metastases in papillary thyroid carcinoma. AJR Am J Roentgenol. 2002;178(3):693–7.
12. Donohoe KJ, Aloff J, Avram AM, Bennet KG, Giovanella L, Greenspan B, et al. Appropriate use criteria for nuclear medicine in the evaluation and treatment of differentiated thyroid cancer. J Nucl Med. 2020;61(3):375–96.
13. Eslamy HK, Ziessman HA. Parathyroid scintigraphy in patients with primary hyperparathyroidism: 99mTc sestamibi SPECT and SPECT/CT. Radiographics. 2008;28(5):1461–76.
14. Hoang JK, Sung WK, Bahl M, Phillips CD. How to perform parathyroid 4D CT: tips and traps for technique and interpretation. Radiology. 2014;270(1):15–24.
15. Bahl M, Sepahdari AR, Sosa JA, Hoang JK. Parathyroid adenomas and hyperplasia on four-dimensional CT scans: three patterns of enhancement relative to the thyroid gland justify a three-phase protocol. Radiology. 2015;277(2):454–62.
16. Johnson NA, Tublin ME, Ogilvie JB. Parathyroid imaging: technique and role in the preoperative evaluation of primary hyperparathyroidism. AJR Am J Roentgenol. 2007;188(6):1706–15.
17. Evangelista L, Sorgato N, Torresan F, Boschin IM, Pennelli G, Saladini G, et al. FDG-PET/CT and parathyroid carcinoma: review of literature and illustrative case series. World J Clin Oncol. 2011;2(10):348–54.
18. Koeller KK, Alamo L, Adair CF, Smirniotopoulos JG. Congenital cystic masses of the neck: radiologic-pathologic correlation. Radiographics. 1999;19(1):121–46; quiz 52–3
19. Zander DA, Smoker WR. Imaging of ectopic thyroid tissue and thyroglossal duct cysts. Radiographics. 2014;34(1):37–50.
20. Lee KY, Oh YW, Noh HJ, Lee YJ, Yong HS, Kang EY, et al. Extraadrenal paragangliomas of the body: imaging features. AJR Am J Roentgenol. 2006;187(2):492–504.
21. Enzenhofer E, Ubl P, Czerny C, Erovic BM. Imaging in patients with merkel cell carcinoma. J Skin Cancer. 2013;2013:973123.
22. Humphreys TR, Shah K, Wysong A, Lexa F, MacFarlane D. The role of imaging in the management of patients with nonmelanoma skin cancer: when is imaging necessary? J Am Acad Dermatol. 2017;76(4):591–607.
23. Gandhi M, Sommerville J. The imaging of large nerve perineural spread. J Neurol Surg B Skull Base. 2016;77(2):113–23.
24. Amin MB, Greene FL, Edge SB, Compton CC, Gershenwald JE, Brookland RK, et al. The eighth edition AJCC cancer staging manual: continuing to build a bridge from a population-based to a more "personalized" approach to cancer staging. CA Cancer J Clin. 2017;67(2):93–9.
25. Hoang JK, Vanka J, Ludwig BJ, Glastonbury CM. Evaluation of cervical lymph nodes in head and neck cancer with CT and MRI: tips, traps, and a systematic approach. AJR Am J Roentgenol. 2013;200(1):W17–25.
26. Civantos FJ, Vermorken JB, Shah JP, Rinaldo A, Suarez C, Kowalski LP, et al. Metastatic squamous cell carcinoma to the cervical lymph nodes from an unknown primary cancer: management in the HPV era. Front Oncol. 2020;10:593164.

2 Thyroid

Steven Craig

2.1 Introduction

Thyroid surgery is commonly encountered in modern general surgery training and practice, but it was not always so. In the early 1900s, thyroid surgery was banned in France and parts of the United States because of high mortality rates associated with bleeding, unrecognised bilateral nerve injuries and unrecognised severe hypocalcaemia. At that time, thyroid surgery could not be conducted safely because of a lack of detailed understanding of the anatomy and physiology of the thyroid gland.

Although modern thyroid surgery is now safe and low risk, with a near zero mortality rate, it should not be entered into lightly. Easy access to medical imaging in Australia has increased the detection of thyroid pathology, particularly asymptomatic thyroid nodules and low-risk papillary thyroid cancer. To prevent unwarranted surgical risk to patients, it is imperative to understand the nuanced indications for thyroid surgery, and the extent of surgery required.

S. Craig (✉)
Illawarra Shoalhaven Local Health District, Wollongong, NSW, Australia

Graduate School of Medicine, University of Wollongong, Wollongong, Australia
e-mail: steven@drstevencraig.com.au

2.2 The Basics: Essential Anatomy, Embryology and Physiology

2.2.1 Embryology and Anatomy

2.2.1.1 Origin

The follicular cells of the thyroid develop from the foramen caecum, an embryological midline diverticulum in the floor of the mouth that originates between the first and second pharyngeal pouches.

The parafollicular C-cells develop from neural crest cells that derive from the ultimobranchial body and migrate into the superolateral margins of the gland. The embryological remnant of this migration is the Tubercle of Zuckerkandl.

Failure of descent of all or part of the thyroid from the foramen caecum results in ectopic thyroid tissue. In adults, the fibrous remnant of the foramen caecum is located between the anterior 2/3 and posterior 1/3 of the tongue. This is the most common location for the ectopic thyroid tissue (lingual thyroid), and when present, it represents the sole thyroid tissue in 75% of cases.

2.2.1.2 Thyroglossal Duct

Differential growth of the embryo causes elongation of the embryological thyroid diverticulum and its subsequent descent into the lower neck, forming the thyroglossal duct. The duct descends in the midline, closely associated with the hyoid

B. Ashford (ed.), *Head and Neck Surgery for General Surgeons*,
https://doi.org/10.1007/978-981-19-7900-2_2

bone. The thyroid gland comes to rest in the lower neck and begins to mature by week 7.

The thyroglossal duct is usually obliterated between weeks 7 and 10. Failure of obliteration can result in a persisting thyroglossal duct or cyst. Thyroglossal cysts can enlarge, become infected and carry a 1% lifetime risk of malignancy. Cysts are generally located between the hyoid bone and thyroid isthmus but can lie anywhere between the base of the tongue and the thyroid.

When present, the pyramidal lobe is located at the apex of the thyroid isthmus. It is a remnant of the thyroglossal duct.

2.2.1.3 Thyroid Anatomy

The thyroid is a butterfly-shaped organ located immediately anterior to the trachea. In adults, a normal gland extends from the cricoid cartilage down to the level of the sixth tracheal ring. The gland comprises two lobes (each lobe measures roughly 4 cm × 2 cm × 1 cm), a mid-section (the isthmus), a lateral projection of varying size (Tubercle of Zukerkandl) and a pyramidal lobe. The normal thyroid weighs between 20 g and 25 g. It is enveloped by the pre-tracheal fascia and is attached to the trachea by strong fibrous tissue, the ligament of Berry.

Blood Supply

Superior Thyroid Artery (STA) and External Branch of Superior Laryngeal Nerve

The superior thyroid artery (STA) is the first branch of the external carotid artery (ECA). It branches from the ECA beneath the anterior border of the sternocleidomastoid muscle (SCM) at the level of the hyoid cartilage. At the superior pole of the thyroid, the STA has a close relationship to the external branch of the superior laryngeal nerve (EBSLN).

The superior laryngeal nerve (SLN) of the vagus divides into an internal branch (purely sensory to the supra-glottic larynx) and an external branch. The EBSLN is the sole motor supply to the cricothyroid muscles. These muscles tense the vocal cords to produce pitch.

Inferior Thyroid Artery (ITA)

The ITA originates from the thyrocervical trunk (majority) or directly from the subclavian artery. It passes superomedially, anterior to the vertebral artery and deep to the carotid sheath before entering the thyroid. The ITA is a close relation to the recurrent laryngeal nerve (RLN) at the mid-pole of the thyroid. The ITA provides the sole blood supply to the superior and inferior parathyroid glands, via secondary and tertiary branches.

Thyroidea IMA

The thyroidea IMA is an infrequent vascular variant that arises commonly from the brachiocephalic trunk and extends to the lower border of the thyroid in the midline. It can also arise from the common carotid artery or the right subclavian artery.

Venous Drainage

The thyroid is drained by a venous network that ultimately forms the paired superior, middle and inferior thyroid veins. The superior and middle veins drain directly into the internal jugular vein. The inferior vein drains into the brachiocephalic vein.

The middle thyroid vein is an important operative landmark. The middle thyroid vein is the only important structure that crosses the anterior surface of the common carotid, and it must be ligated safely during the lateral exposure of the thyroid gland. An important point to note is that while the superior and inferior thyroid are paired veins and arteries, there is no middle thyroid artery.

2.2.1.4 Recurrent Laryngeal Nerve (RLN)

Anatomy and Function

The RLN branches off the vagus nerve in the superior mediastinum. The left RLN passes posteromedially beneath the aortic arch, whereas the right RLN passes posteromedially around the subclavian artery. Both nerves then ascend in the tracheo-oesophageal groove.

The RLN on each side divides into a lateral (sensory) and a medial (motor) branch within the larynx, although branching is sometimes seen proximal to the larynx where the branches appear more as posterior (sensory) and anterior (motor). The RLN is related closely to the posterior surface of the thyroid gland, branches of the ITA and Berry's ligament.

The RLN provides the sole motor supply to the intrinsic muscles of the larynx, with the exception of the cricothyroid muscles. As such, the RLN is the sole nerve for voice control, and identification and protection of these nerves are of utmost importance during thyroid surgery.

Embryology

The RLN is a derivative of the sixth pharyngeal arch, and in contrast, the SLN is a derivative of the more cranial fourth pharyngeal arch. The vascular derivatives of the fourth pharyngeal arch include the aorta (left) and subclavian artery (right). Linear growth of the embryo displaces these vessels into the mediastinum, dragging both RLN inferiorly.

Arteria Lusoria and the Non-recurrent Laryngeal Nerve

In 1/200 patients, the right subclavian artery fails to develop in its normal position. Instead, the right subclavian artery branches off the aorta (usually the fourth branch) to pass to the right behind the oesphagus to supply the upper limb. As a result, the right RLN is then non-recurrent and branches immediately from the right vagus nerve around the level of the cricoid cartilage to supply the larynx. It is particularly at risk of injury during thyroidectomy. The finding of a retro-oesophageal right subclavian artery on cross-sectional imaging is a clue to a non-recurrent right-sided RLN.

2.2.2 Physiology

2.2.2.1 Thyroid Hormone Synthesis

Ingested iodine is taken up into the follicular cell by the basolateral sodium/ iodine (Na^+/ I^-) symporter. Iodine diffuses into the follicular colloid via pendrin.

Thyroglobulin (Tg) is produced in the endoplasmic reticulum and exocytosed into the follicular colloid. Thyroid peroxidase (TPO) catalyses the oxidation of iodine and its binding to thyroglobulin tyrosine residues (a process called organification).

Organified thyroglobulin is cleaved into thyroxine (T4) and small amounts of triiodothyronine (T3). The majority of circulating T3 is derived from the peripheral conversion of T4 to T3.

2.3 Thyroid Nodules and Basic Thyroid Work-up

Thyroid nodules are discrete lesions within the thyroid gland that appear radiologically different from the surrounding thyroid parenchyma. They are very common in the general population and become more prevalent with age. The common term 'goitre' describes an enlarged thyroid gland of any cause. Hence, a multi-nodular goitre is an enlarged thyroid caused by the presence of more than one nodule. Thyroid nodule assessment and work-up are perhaps the most common initial thyroid presentation encountered by general surgeons.

There are numerous differential diagnoses for thyroid nodules. Three key questions that should always be kept in mind during the assessment of thyroid nodules to guide work-up, diagnosis and management decisions are as follows:

- Is the nodule hyperfunctional? This is the first question asked, as fine needle aspiration biopsy (FNAB) should not be performed on hyperfunctioning nodules, as less than 1–2% of hyperfunctional nodules are malignant.
- Is the nodule malignant? This is the second question asked, as the treatment of malignancy would occur regardless of symptoms.
- Is the nodule causing symptoms? This is the third question asked. This is often the hardest to determine, as many of the common thyroid nodule symptoms can also be caused by other pathologies.

The answers to these questions should be determined from a thorough history and examination, biochemistry, relevant imaging and cytopathology, where appropriate.

2.3.1 History and Examination

In addition to a standard medical history, the following points will help to address the three key questions.

2.3.1.1 History

Is the Nodule Hyper Functional?

New onset palpitations, headaches and tremors, recent weight loss, hair and skin changes, etc. suggestive of excess thyroid hormone from a functional nodule.

Is the Nodule Malignant?

A history of head and neck radiation or occupational exposure to ionising radiation.

A family history of thyroid malignancy.

A known genetic predisposition to thyroid cancer, such as MEN II (described later).

A personal history of other cancers known to metastasize to the thyroid.

The rapid evolution of a thyroid nodule.

A painful mass can be suggestive of an advanced, invasive malignancy.

Is the Nodule Causing Symptoms?

Dysphagia can result from localised oesophageal compression by an enlarging thyroid mass. The duration and progression of dysphagia should be characterised.

Positional dyspnoea and orthopnoea may be experienced.

Change in the character of the voice, the development of a hoarse voice, or a dry cough can be due to irritation of the recurrent laryngeal nerve by compression or invasion. This is often noted by a family member rather than the patient themselves.

Tender thyroid nodules, which are not suspicious for malignancy, can be associated with thyroiditis or cyst haemorrhage.

2.3.1.2 Examination

A thyroid is best examined with the patient seated on a chair and palpation performed standing behind the patient. The clinical findings below can help to answer the three key questions.

Is the Nodule Hyperfunctional?

Hypertension and tachycardia may suggest hyperthyroidism.

The patient's hands are outstretched to assess for a tremor, palmar erythema and diaphoresis.

Clubbing of the fingers (thyroid acropachy) may be suggestive of chronic hyperthyroidism.

Eye signs are seen Graves' ophthalmopathy. They include exophthalmos, lid lag and lid retraction. These are best appreciated from a side and/or top view of the face.

Is the Nodule Malignant?

Assess the size and characteristics of the nodule and the thyroid gland.

In sequence, palpate all six cervical lymph node levels for lymphadenopathy.

Is the Nodule Causing Symptoms?

Look for facial plethora at rest. Then assess for Pemberton's sign by asking the patient to raise both hands above head height for 1 min. Note the development of central cyanosis, facial plethora and dyspnoea. These can occur due to venous compression at the thoracic inlet secondary to retro-sternal goitre.

Ask the patient to speak. Neuropraxia of the RLN gives a distinct voice quality, which is weaker, deeper and hoarser than normal. There may be a reduced phonation time (see also Chap. 14).

Palpate the trachea and comment on its position relative to the midline.

Feel for the inferior extent of the thyroid gland relative to the thoracic inlet. If unable to palpate the lower border (even on swallowing), this indicates a significant retrosternal component.

2.3.2 Thyroid Biochemistry and Imaging for Nodules

A serum thyroid stimulating hormone (TSH) is the first investigation performed (assuming imaging has not already been done). The initial TSH is used to direct further imaging and assessment.

- A normal or elevated TSH indicates no thyroid hormone excess. The appropriate first scan should be an ultrasound (US) ± FNA to assess the malignant potential of the nodule.
- A low TSH indicates hyperthyroidism with TSH suppression via the feedback loop. The appropriate first scan should be a functional radionuclide scan.

2.3.2.1 Ultrasound for Thyroid Nodules (in Normal or Elevated TSH)

The American College of Radiology Thyroid Imaging Reporting and Data System committee classification (ACR TI-RADS) is the most commonly used thyroid nodule ultrasound system in Australia (Fig. 2.1). This system allows for standardised reporting and interpretation, risk stratification and subsequent management decisions. A helpful mnemonic to remember the features on ultrasound is COMSEC (**CO**mposition/ **M**argin/ **S**hape/ **E**chogenicity/ **C**alcifications). According to the TI-RADS classification and the nodule size, a nodule can be recommended for one of three options: no further investigation, surveillance with imaging or FNA.

Ultrasound assessment of the central and lateral cervical lymph node chains should also be performed whenever a thyroid nodule is being imaged. The lymph node features of concern in

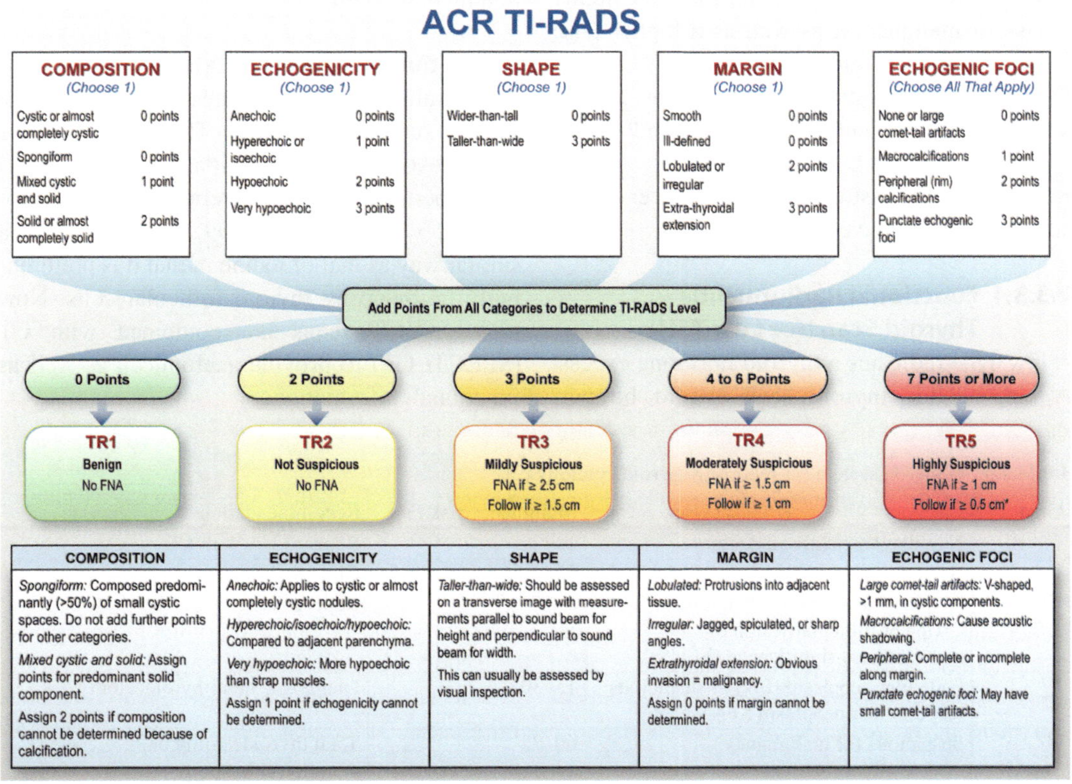

Fig. 2.1 American College of Radiology Thyroid Imaging Reporting and Data System (ACR TI-RADS) [1]

US include size >1 cm, round (not oval), loss of fatty hilum, microcalcification and peripheral vascularity.

2.3.3 Cytopathology

Thyroid cytology is classified into one of six standardised categories according to the Bethesda System (Table 2.1). This classification system has an associated 'risk of malignancy' for each category. The estimated risk of malignancy can then be used to guide management decisions.

Although ultrasound, FNAB and standardised reporting is the most sensitive initial diagnostic process for assessing malignancy, there are some caveats to the recommended management described in Table 2.1. Diagnostic thyroidectomy may also be required for nodules in the following scenarios:

- Larger thyroid nodules (typically considered to be >4 cm). They have an inherent higher risk of malignancy, as well as a higher false negative biopsy rate.
- Suspicious retrosternal nodules that are not amenable to percutaneous biopsy and/ or US surveillance.
- Strong family history of thyroid cancer or predisposing genetic condition.

2.3.3.1 Functional Radionuclide Thyroid Scan (for Low TSH)

A low TSH indicates a thyroid hormone excess. A radionuclide thyroid scan should be performed to investigate for functional thyroid lesion/s. Conducting a biopsy of a functional nodule is futile. The resultant level of inflammatory cell infiltrate on subsequent histology is difficult to interpret, and less than 2% of differentiated thyroid malignancies are found to be functional.

MIBG 123 and 131

Iodine 123-meta-iodobenzylguanidine (MIBG) is a nuclear medicine scan that utilises radiolabelled iodine. Thyroid follicular cells will preferentially take up radiolabelled iodine to create a dispersion pattern within the gland that can be associated with various disease processes.

Radioactive iodine 123 (RAI^{123}) emits low-energy gamma waves and is not considered to be cytotoxic. This is in contrast to RAI^{131}, which emits higher energy beta-radiation that is cytotoxic to thyroid follicular cells. For this reason, $RAI^{123}$is useful for whole body imaging, whilst RAI^{131} is used more commonly as an adjuvant treatment modality.

Technetium 99 Pertechnetate

In Australia, T^{99} pertechnetate SPECT scans have largely supplanted RAI^{123}. This is due to the lower cost and lower radiation dosing associated with a pertechnetate scan. Pertechnetate is radiolabelled with technetium 99. It functions in a similar way as that of iodine in that it is preferentially taken up by thyroid follicular cells. Now most SPECT scans are combined with CT (SPECT/ CT) to provide anatomical, as well as functional, information.

Table 2.1 Bethesda system for reporting thyroid cytology [2]

Grade	Category	Malignancy risk (%)	Recommendation
I	Non-diagnostic/unsatisfactory	1–4	Repeat FNA with US
II	Benign	0–3	Clinical follow up
III	Atypia of undetermined significance (AUS) or follicular lesion of undetermined significance (FLUS)	5–15	Repeat FNA
IV	Follicular neoplasm (FN) or suspicious for follicular neoplasm SFN	15–30	Diagnostic hemithyroidectomy
V	Suspicious for malignancy	60–75	Total thyroidectomy or hemithyroidectomy
VI	Malignant	97–99	Total thyroidectomy or hemithyroidectomy

2.3.4 Multinodular Goitre

Many patients who develop multinodular goitre (MNG) have a family history of enlarged thyroids. A multinodular goitre that gives substantial symptoms or has an unwanted appearance can be considered for thyroidectomy. Additionally, a rapid change in the nature of a nodule within MNG should prompt consideration of the potential for malignancy and for cytological assessment. Pressure effects from MNG are progressive with enlargement of the gland and can be more pronounced when left-sided enlargement is prominent.

2.3.5 Thyroid Cysts

Thyroid cysts are common and can be classified as simple thyroid cysts or partially cystic nodules. Thyroid cysts are thought to arise from the degeneration of solid thyroid nodules, and as such, partially cystic nodules with a mixed cystic-solid component are more common.

Purely cystic thyroid nodules (without a solid component) are almost always benign and do not require biopsy. The workup of a partially cystic nodule follows the same investigation and management algorithms as for thyroid nodules described above. Nodules with a >50% cystic component have a higher rate of non-diagnostic or false-negative cytology on FNA [3], and therefore, FNA biopsy targeting both the solid and fluid component of the nodule should be performed.

Thyroid cysts can also present with discomfort and compressive symptoms. A rapid increase in the size of a thyroid cyst can occur secondary to infarction and haemorrhage into a nodule. Ultrasound-guided aspiration drainage of thyroid cysts is an effective and low-risk procedure to relieve symptoms, but there is a high rate of recurrence. For recurrent, symptomatic thyroid cysts a hemithyroidectomy may be required for definitive treatment (usually considered after 2–3 aspirations).

2.4 Malignant Thyroid Conditions

There are five distinct groups of thyroid cancers, roughly based on their origin, behaviour and frequency:

1. Differentiated thyroid cancers (Papillary, Follicular and Hurthle cell)
2. Medullary thyroid cancer
3. Anaplastic thyroid cancer
4. Thyroid metastases
5. Rare thyroid cancer variants (lymphoma, teratoma, paraganglioma, SCC and CASTLE)

Table 2.2 provides a summary and aide de memoire for some of the key features of the five most frequent types of thyroid cancer.

2.4.1 Differentiated Thyroid Cancers (DTC): Papillary, Follicular and Hurthle Cell

Papillary thyroid cancer (PTC) is by far the most common thyroid cancer, accounting for about 80% of thyroid malignancies (see Table 2.2). Typically, PTC typically follows an indolent course with a cure rate of about 90% and an overall survival rate of 98% at 5 years. Lymph node metastases are common at diagnosis in PTC but do not necessarily impact overall survival. Follicular thyroid cancer accounts for approximately 10–15% of all thyroid malignancies. The overall 5-year survival for follicular thyroid cancer (FTC) is slightly worse than PTC and varies between 85% and 95%. Hurthle cell thyroid cancer (HCTC) is the least common of the three differentiated thyroid malignancies, but it carries the worst prognosis.

2.4.1.1 Risk Factors for DTC

- Female
- Family history of thyroid cancer
- Obesity
- Ionising radiation to the neck (especially as a child)

Table 2.2 Thyroid malignancies. Credit for this teaching table to Dr. Janice Pasieka, Endocrine Surgeon and Clinical Professor of Surgery and Oncology at The University of Calgary

	Incidence (% of thyroid cancers)	Sex	Age	Differentiation	Common mechanism of spread	RAI sensitivity	5-year OS
Papillary	80%	W >> M	3rd–5th decades	Well-differentiated	Lymphatic	90%	98%
Follicular	10%	W >> M	5th decade	Well-differentiated	Haematogenous	80%	90%
Hurthle	5%	W > M	6th decade	Intermediate	Lymphatic + haematogenous	30%	85%
Medullary	3–4%	W = M	6th–7th decades	N/A	Lymphatic + haematogenous	0%	80%
Anaplastic	1–2%	W = M	7th–8th decades	Very poorly differentiated	Highly invasive (all mechanisms)	0%	<5%

- Genetics
  - RET proto-oncogene
  - Cowden's disease
  - Familial adenomatous polyposis syndrome (FAP)
  - Peutz–Jegher's disease

2.4.1.2 Essential Histology

PTC: A well-differentiated malignancy composed of thyroid follicular (cuboidal) cells. The term 'papillary' denotes a growth pattern of finger-like projections of neoplastic cells in between, or arising from, thyroid follicles.

- 'Orphan Annie' nuclei are seen in 80% of PTC specimens. They are described as larger, clear, oval-shaped nuclei where nuclear chromatin has been pushed to the periphery of the nuclear envelope.
- Nuclear grooves arise from irregularities in the nuclear envelope with the resultant 'buckling' of the inner layer to form invaginations.
- Nuclear overlapping occurs when multiple nuclei from adjacent neoplastic follicular cells overlap.
- Psammoma bodies (seen in 60%) develop from the lamellation (layering) of calcium in each malignant papilla due to progressive apoptosis.

FTC: The defining histological feature is a follicular growth pattern without the typical nuclear features seen in PTC. The majority of cancers present as encapsulated solitary nodules, and malignancy is defined by capsular invasion.

HCTC: Histologically, Hurtle cells are larger than those seen in PTC/ FTC with pink staining cytoplasm. Oncocytic (mitochondria rich) cell types predominate.

2.4.2 Workup, Management and Surveillance of Differentiated Thyroid Cancers

As described above in basic thyroid work-up, the gold-standard for the assessment of differentiated thyroid cancer is neck ultrasound, FNAB and standardised reporting with the Bethesda System.

Suspicious central or lateral neck nodes on imaging should be biopsied, and a thyroglobulin needle rinse performed:

- Multiple passes of a biopsy needle are made into the node.
- Cells are blown onto a slide mixed with 1 mL of normal saline and the thyroglobulin level is measured (any detectable thyroglobulin in the sample indicates metastases).

2.4.2.1 Extent of Thyroidectomy

In surgical candidates, thyroidectomy is recommended for confirmed or suspected DTC. Traditionally, total thyroidectomy was considered the standard of care for DTC >1 cm. More recently, the ATA has changed its guidelines for the management of 'low-risk' DTC to include either hemithyroidectomy or total thyroidectomy. This change was based on several retrospective studies that showed equivalent survival outcomes in patients undergoing lobectomy or total thyroidectomy for low-risk cancer.

The decision to progress to a total or hemi thyroidectomy is dictated by disease and patient factors. As a guide, the ATA recommends the following [4]:

A total thyroidectomy should be performed in any of the following:

- Thyroid cancer >4 cm
- Gross extra-thyroidal extension
- Evidence of metastatic disease

A hemithyroidectomy may be considered if:

- The thyroid cancer is <4 cm AND
- There is no evidence of gross extra-thyroidal extension AND
- There is no evidence of metastatic disease AND
- The primary lesion is a low-risk papillary or follicular carcinoma AND
- There is no history of head and neck irradiation

Other factors that may influence the extent of surgery include:

- The presence of nodules in the contralateral lobe
- Compliance with on-going imaging surveillance and hormone replacement
- Anaesthetic risk is viewed in the possibility of requiring a completion thyroidectomy

In HCTC, a total thyroidectomy is also generally preferred over a hemithyroidectomy due to the more aggressive nature of the disease and lower RAI-sensitivity.

2.4.2.2 Neck Dissection

Cervical lymph node involvement is common (estimates vary between 20% and 90% depending on the sensitivity of the detection process), but this is mostly micrometastatic disease with unclear prognostic significance.

Prophylactic central neck dissection is no longer routinely recommended because it has not been shown to significantly influence overall survival and because central neck dissection increases the risk of hypoparathyroidism and RLN injury. The ATA currently recommends a central neck dissection when the central compartment nodes are positive (clinically or on biopsy) when the lateral compartment nodes are involved, and may be considered for T3/T4 tumours.

Lateral neck dissection (typically levels 2–4/5) is only indicated where lateral compartment nodes are involved. *There is no evidence that prophylactic lateral neck dissection improves survival measures, and it should not be performed.*

2.4.2.3 Postoperative Levothyroxine

Following total thyroidectomy, patients are usually commenced on a weight-based dose of levothyroxine (1.6 μg/kg daily). As well as replacing T4 loss following total thyroidectomy, levothyroxine suppresses TSH release and its trophic action on any residual thyroid cells. The ideal TSH level should be <0.1 mIU/L following total thyroidectomy.

The TSH half-life is 65 h. The half-lives of levothyroxine and T4 in the euthyroid patient are approximately 6–7 days, with the biological effect lasting longer. Dose adjustments of levothyroxine should, therefore, occur at 4–6 weeks postoperatively.

2.4.2.4 Systemic Therapy

All patients with thyroid cancer should be presented with a multidisciplinary team for consideration of adjuvant radioactive iodine. Clinical practice may vary greatly between institutions, both in terms of indications for treatment and doses used. Some of the more commonly accepted indications for RAI^{131}include:

- Extra-thyroidal extension.
- Primary tumour >4 cm.
- Unstimulated Tg level >10 ng/mL.
- Bulky nodal disease or >5 involved nodes.
- Multicentric, multifocal or bilobar disease.
- Age >45 years where the patient has at least T3 disease.

2.4.2.5 Postoperative Surveillance

Patients should be followed up at six monthly intervals for the first year and then annually. Serum biochemistry (Tg, TSH and anti-thyroglobulin antibodies) and neck ultrasound should be performed at each visit. Abnormal serum biochemistry or ultrasound findings should be further assessed with functional imaging (RAI^{131} whole body scan/ FDG-PET). Be aware that some differentiated thyroid cancers, especially HCTC, may not be iodine avid and FDG-PET is a reliable second-line investigation for suspected metastatic disease.

2.4.3 Medullary Thyroid Cancer (MTC)

Medullary thyroid cancer is an uncommon thyroid tumour of neuroendocrine origin. MTC can occur as part of a familial syndrome, but most cases (around 75–80%) are sporadic. In aggressive familial forms of MEN2a, it can occur as early as the first year of life. MTC generally shows more aggressive clinical behaviour than DTC. In patients with localised intra-thyroidal

MTC in pre-operative staging, LN metastasis is found in 70–80% of patients who undergo central and lateral neck dissection.

2.4.3.1 Classification

MTC is classified as sporadic or familial. This is an important distinction, as the clinical behaviour can differ, and it is important to exclude associated tumours in familial cases. Familial MTC encompasses MEN IIa, MEN IIb, FMTC, von-Hippel Lindau Disease and neurofibromatosis (see *Genetic Syndromes*).

Risk Factors

A family history of MTC is the single greatest risk factor for developing MTC. The RET oncogene is seen in both sporadic and familial cases. Approximately 10% of sporadic diseases will have a de novo mutation.

Essential Histology

MTC is derived from the parafollicular c-cells of the thyroid. Microscopy demonstrates sheets of spindle cells with stroma containing amyloid. C-cell hyperplasia is considered a pre-malignant condition.

2.4.3.2 Workup

All suspicious thyroid nodules are investigated as described in the TI-RADS and Bethesda stratification systems. In confirmed cases of MTC on FNA, the following additional workup should be performed:

- Serum calcitonin level and serum carcinoembryonic antigen (CEA)
- Serum calcium because (1) elevated serum calcitonin may result in hypocalcaemia, and (2) the association of MTC with the parathyroid disease in MEN2a can cause hypercalcaemia
- Urinary metanephrines as screening for phaeochromocytoma (due to the strong association with MEN II)
- Screening for a germline RET proto-oncogene mutation
- Whole body imaging is not performed routinely and should only be performed if distant metastatic disease is clinically suspected
- MTC is not iodine avid so staging imaging should comprise contrast-enhanced CT or MRI of the head and neck for investigation of regional disease, and dedicated liver imaging with CT or MRI and DOTATATE PET/CT if disseminated disease is suspected

2.4.3.3 Treatment and Surveillance

Surgery

Surgery is the only means of a potential cure for MTC, and hence, surgical management is more aggressive than for DTC. Total thyroidectomy with central neck dissection is generally accepted as the appropriate initial surgical management for all confirmed cases of sporadic and familial MTC.

Lateral neck dissection is indicated for suspected nodal disease in the cervical compartments. There is no clear consensus on the role of prophylactic lateral neck dissection in cN0 disease or on the role of dissection of the contralateral lateral neck compartments when the ipsilateral lateral neck nodes are involved. Decisions around lateral neck dissection in cN0 disease are made based on calcitonin levels and individual prognostic factors such as age.

In sporadic cases where MTC is diagnosed incidentally during hemithyroidectomy, evidence suggests that completion thyroidectomy is unnecessary unless there is a known germline RET mutation, an elevated postoperative serum calcitonin level or radiological evidence of residual disease in the neck [5].

Surveillance

Patients are followed-up at 6 months postoperatively with a physical examination, serum calcitonin and CEA levels. If calcitonin is undetectable, follow-up can continue annually.

If calcitonin is elevated, imaging should be performed to detect structural metastases. If there is on-going evidence of biochemical recurrence (i.e. elevated calcitonin but no evidence of metastasis on imaging), calcitonin should be measured every 3 months to determine the 'calcitonin doubling time', which is an established prognostic factor for MTC.

In patients with evidence of locoregional recurrence but no disseminated disease, resection by compartmental dissection is recommended. Other modalities such as external beam radiation therapy (EBRT) may be considered for inoperable disease or non-operative candidates.

In patients with evidence of disseminated disease, systemic therapy with tyrosine kinase inhibitors targeting RET and VEGFR is the first-line therapy.

2.4.4 Anaplastic Thyroid Cancer (ATC)

Anaplastic thyroid cancer is rare, accounting for <2% of thyroid malignancies. ATC is the most lethal thyroid malignancy and can be rapidly fatal, with a 5 year survival of <10% and median survival from diagnosis of 6 months. Patients are usually symptomatic at presentation and can have a painful, rapidly expanding thyroid mass and/or signs and symptoms of local invasion of the RLN, airway, blood vessels, lymphatics and oesophagus.

2.4.4.1 Histology

Most appear to originate within a well-differentiated thyroid malignancy. It is thought that ATC may represent a de-differentiation of these malignant cells, due to the accumulation of somatic mutations. Cells appear 'undifferentiated', having lost all of the characteristic functions of follicular thyroid cells.

2.4.4.2 Workup and Management

On confirmation of ATC with FNA, patients should undergo:

- Whole body imaging with CT of neck, chest, abdomen and pelvis
- Whole body FDG PET/CT
- Molecular tumour profiling: BRAF and next-generation sequencing (the results of which may direct the use of targeted therapies)

Establishing the goals of care-expedient review and decision-making are essential due to the aggressive nature of the disease. Resectability should be determined, and the perceived benefit from surgery should be carefully balanced against the anticipated morbidity of the operation (especially for locally invasive disease) and overall poor prognosis. Targeted therapy (BRAF/MEK inhibitors) has been used in some cases to downstage tumours to become surgically resectable. Non-surgical options include targeted inhibitors (e.g. BRAF), primary or palliative chemo therapy and/or radiotherapy, or supportive care.

2.4.5 Rare Variants

The following conditions, briefly summarised for completeness, are rare in daily clinical practice. Diagnosis or suspicion of one of these conditions should always prompt expedient referral to a specialist thyroid surgeon.

2.4.5.1 Lymphoma

Primary thyroid lymphoma presents clinically as a rapidly growing mass often with compressive symptoms. Treatment depends on staging, but it is rarely surgical. Thyroid lymphoma responds very quickly to chemotherapy and/or radiotherapy.

2.4.5.2 Teratoma

A germ-cell tumour comprised all three ectodermal, mesodermal and endodermal elements in varying contributions. These tumours can present from birth through to late adulthood. They are generally benign, although malignant transformation, when it does occur, is seen almost exclusively in adults.

2.4.5.3 Thyroid Paraganglioma

These tumours derive from the laryngeal paraganglia cells adjacent to the false vocal folds. Thyroid paragangliomas represent a diagnostic challenge because they are histologically similar to FTC and MTC.

2.4.5.4 Squamous Cell Carcinoma of the Thyroid

Primary thyroid SCC is an aggressive thyroid malignancy that presents with fairly rapid, progressive growth resulting in compressive symptoms. Treatment is by a total thyroidectomy with adjuvant radiotherapy. It is essential to consider metastatic SCC as a differential.

2.4.5.5 Castle

Thyroid Carcinoma Showing Thymic-Like Differentiation (CASTLE) histologically resembles a thymic tumour or an aggressive primary thyroid malignancy. However, the prognosis is much more favourable.

2.4.6 PET Positive Nodules and Thyroid Gland Metastases

With the increasing availability of PET scans, the detection of suspected or confirmed thyroid gland metastases is increasing. FDG-PET uptake in a thyroid lesion is found in 1–2% of PET scans performed for staging of non-thyroid malignancy. Studies have shown that 30–40% of PET-positive thyroid lesions are cancerous. As such, we recommend FNA biopsy of all PET-positive lesions in patients who are fit for active treatment.

Biopsy of a PET-positive thyroid lesion in a patient with a non-thyroid malignancy may result in one of three scenarios;

1. Confirmed or suspected metastasis. Lung and kidney are the most frequent tumours to metastasise to the thyroid. Others known to metastasise to the thyroid include breast, GI and cutaneous sources. Any thyroid gland metastasis should be managed in an appropriate oncology MDT setting. For aggressive primary malignancies (such as lung cancer), the main treatment is supportive care. For less aggressive malignancies with isolated metastatic deposits to the thyroid (such as renal cell carcinoma and malignant melanoma), thyroidectomy may improve overall survival.
2. Confirmed or suspected incidental primary thyroid cancer: PET-positive thyroid cancers detected incidentally on scans performed for another primary malignancy have little impact on short-term (1–5 year) survival for patients with more advanced non-thyroid malignancies. As such, the treatment of the thyroid cancer should not interfere with, or delay, the treatment of the initial non-thyroid malignancy. Active surveillance of thyroid cancer is recommended until patients have recovered from their primary cancer treatment.
3. Benign appearance on US and biopsy: Simple surveillance as per ACR-TIRADS guidelines.

2.4.7 Thyroid Cancer in Pregnancy

The initial workup for suspected thyroid cancer in pregnancy is the same as for the non-pregnant state, with the exception that the use of radioactive thyroid scintigraphy is restricted. The surgical management of suspected or confirmed DTC can be deferred until after pregnancy, due to the indolent nature of the disease, particularly in younger age groups. Surgery may be required to be performed earlier in the case of rapidly growing malignant nodules (>20% increase in size in 3 months), the development of lymphadenopathy or confirmation of aggressive cancer types (medullary, anaplastic). The ideal timing of surgery is the second trimester when the anaesthetic and endocrine complication risks to the mother and foetus are lower. The ATA recommends that patients who are not managed surgically be commenced on suppressive therapy (levothyroxine) during pregnancy to maintain TSH in the range of 0.3–2.0 mU/L.

2.4.8 Genetic Syndromes Relevant to Thyroid Cancer

Only 5% of all thyroid malignancies occur in the context of a familial condition. The majority of these are non-medullary familial thyroid cancers

Table 2.3 Genetic conditions associated with increased risk of thyroid malignancy

	Genetics	Age of increased risk	Incidence	Clinical manifestation
NMFTC				
FAP	AD; APC gene mutation Chr 5	>25yo	1/50	GIT polyposis syndrome Thyroid cancer = PTC (cribriform/hobnail variants)
Cowden's disease	AD; PTEN tumour suppressor gene mutation	4th–5th decades of life	1/200,000	GIT hamartomatous syndrome Thyroid cancer = PTC
Peutz-Jegher's syndrome	AD; STK-11 tumour suppressor gene mutation	Late teens	Up to 1/50,000	GIT hamartomatous syndrome Thyroid cancer = PTC and FTC
fMTC				
MEN IIa	Germline mutation RET proto-oncogene Chr 10	Early teens	1/30,000	C-cell hyperplasia + MTC (nearly all patients) Phaeochromocytoma (50%). Hyperparathyroidism (20–30%)
MEN IIb	Germline mutation RET proto-oncogene Chr 10	Early childhood (<10yo)	1/30,000-50,000	MTC (100% of patients) Phaechromocytoma (40–50%) Marfanoid stature, mucosal neuromas, GIT ganglioneuromatoses
Non-MEN familial MTC	Germline mutation RET proto-oncogene Chr 10 (50% of patients)	4th–5th decades of life		MTC (relatively indolent clinical course)

(NMFTC). Although medullary thyroid cancer is uncommon, it is estimated that 20–25% of MTCs are familial (fMTC). Table 2.3 demonstrates the incidence and clinical characteristics of each disease.

2.5 Hyperthyroid Conditions

Hyperthyroidism affects 2–3% of the population. The most common cause in Australia and other iodine-replete countries is Graves' disease. Other causes include neoplasia (multinodular goitre and solitary toxic nodules), autoimmune (Hashimoto's, Riedel's, and De Quervain's disease), pregnancy and medications (amiodarone and contrast). Most cases of hyperthyroidism are managed medically, but there are some specific scenarios detailed below, which may require surgical involvement.

2.5.1 Graves' Disease

Graves' disease is an autoimmune, inflammatory disorder in which TSH receptor auto-antibodies bind to, and stimulate, the TSH receptor, resulting in hyperthyroidism. Graves' disease affects more women than men, with a peak incidence in the fifth decade of life.

2.5.1.1 Clinical Manifestations

In addition to the clinical features of hyperthyroidism, Graves' disease can be manifest in several characteristic eye signs, including:

- Exophthalmos. This is a process by which t-cell-mediated Ab release stimulates the proliferation of orbital adipocytes and fibroblast production of glycosaminoglycans (hydrophilic). In turn, this increases retro-orbital water content + fat deposition, which anteriorly displaces the globe.
- Chemosis-conjunctival oedema.
- Keratitis and conjunctivitis.
- Lid lag and lid retraction.

2.5.1.2 Treatment Options

There are three treatment options for Graves' disease; medication, RAI and surgery. In Australia, first-line therapy for Graves' disease consists of anti-thyroid medication. However, relapse with medical treatment occurs in about 50% of cases. RAI[131]is indicated where patients are refractory to medical management or have a contra-indication to anti-thyroid medication. Graves' ophthalmopathy may be exacerbated by RAI[131], and as such, it is a relative contra-indication. Total thyroidectomy should be considered in patients for whom medical therapy has failed, and who are unwilling or unable to tolerate RAI therapy. Surgery has a near complete cure rate for Graves' disease. However, it is the most invasive treatment option and involves more significant risks than medication or RAI.

2.5.2 Neoplastic

2.5.2.1 Toxic Multinodular Goitre (MNG)

Trophic changes due to TSH release result in hypertrophy of parts of the gland. Recurrent episodes of parenchymal involution associated with inflammation result in patchy fibrosis. The trophic effect of constant stimulation of follicular cells by TSH can result in autonomous thyroid hormone production. Management of toxic multinodular goitre is similar to management of Grave's disease.

2.5.2.2 Toxic Nodule

Toxic (papillary) thyroid adenomas are benign thyroid lesions with no malignant potential. They are typically solitary, homogenous and well-encapsulated nodules. Surgery is considered in cases refractory to medical management, for patients unable to tolerate RAI, and for large (typically >3–4 cm) or symptomatic adenomas.

2.5.3 Preparation for Surgery in Hyperthyroidism

Control and optimisation of hyperthyroidism for surgery should always be done with input from an experienced endocrinologist. Thionamides are the primary medical treatment for hyperthyroidism. Thionamides are a group of compounds that inhibit the activity of thyroid peroxidase (TPO). Although they generally have a rapid onset of action, the clinical effect takes much longer due to significant protein-bound thyroid hormone storage that can last weeks.

2.5.3.1 Methimazole

Methimazole directly inhibits TPO. It has a quick onset of action and can clinically improve hyperthyroidism within 6 weeks. It has a lower side effect profile (especially compared to propylthiouracil) and requires only a single daily dosing. Methimazole has been associated with birth defects, foetal hypothyroidism and goitre formation. Hence, it should be used cautiously in pregnancy, especially during the first trimester.

2.5.3.2 Carbimazole

In addition to its effects on TPO, carbimazole reduces the uptake of inorganic iodine by the thyroid. It is a pro-drug that is metabolised to its much more active form (methimazole) to exert its action. Carbimazole should be used cautiously in pregnancy.

2.5.3.3 Propylthiouracil (PTU)

In addition to its effects on TPO, PTU inhibits the peripheral conversion of T4 to T3. PTU may be hepatotoxic. It should be considered second-line therapy, especially for patients with liver disease. PTU requires multiple daily dosing and takes longer to achieve its clinical effect than either carbimazole or methimazole. PTU has a reasonable safety profile in pregnancy and can be used as first-line therapy for hyperthyroidism in the first trimester.

2.5.3.4 Beta-Blockade

Beta-blockers exert dual effects during hyperthyroidism. They treat the hyperthyroidism-related tachycardia and inhibit the peripheral conversion of T4 to T3, reducing thyroid hormone stores.

2.6 Thyroidectomy: Operative Steps

We describe here a simple, safe and stepwise approach to thyroidectomy. We acknowledge that there are many different approaches and techniques for thyroidectomy. However, the inherent principles should always remain the same. The aim of thyroidectomy is the safe removal of all thyroid tissue and the identification and preservation of two nerves (EBSLN and RLN) and two parathyroid glands (superior and inferior) on each side. This is achieved by *capsular dissection*: that is, dissecting and ligating the tertiary branches of blood vessels as they intersect with the capsule of the thyroid. Such dissection should thereby preserve the parathyroid glands and their vascular pedicles, as well as minimally expose the RLN and not disturb its blood supply.

2.6.1 Preparation

2.6.1.1 Vocal Cord Function

Detection of vocal cord palsy is a significant finding that can influence operative planning and surgical extent. The rate of idiopathic vocal cord palsy is 1%. It is recommended that all patients undergo a preoperative flexible nasoendoscopy or laryngoscopy to document vocal cord function, especially if they have voice symptoms.

2.6.1.2 Nerve Monitoring

Recurrent laryngeal nerve monitoring is now common practice in Australia. A NIMS (Nerve Integrity Monitoring System) comprising integrated surface electrodes within a specialised endotracheal tube is placed adjacent to the true vocal cords during intubation to monitor EMG activity. An NIMS reflects an intact circuit from the descending vagus nerve to the recurrent laryngeal nerve to the larynx. Loss of signal detection during thyroidectomy can signify a break in the circuit and nerve injury. Notably, there is now clear evidence that nerve monitoring systems can reduce the rate of nerve injury. NIMS can also aid in nerve identification, detection of a nerve injury, and be helpful in intraoperative decision making should a nerve injury be encountered.

2.6.1.3 Positioning

The patient is positioned with a head ring and shoulder roll to facilitate slight neck extension, with both arms tucked in. The operating table can be positioned in slight reverse Trendelenberg to reduce venous pressure in the neck. The patient is prepped and draped from the angles of the mandible to the mid-sternum and from shoulder to shoulder. Adherent drapes are useful around the contours of the neck to maintain a sterile field.

Always begin by operating on the most pathological side of the thyroid first.

2.6.2 Stepwise Operative Approach

2.6.2.1 Step 1: Incision and Sub-Platysmal Flaps

Stand on the contralateral side of the lobe being dissected.

A 5–6 cm transverse incision is made in a skin crease at or just below the cricoid. This incision is carried through the investing layers of cervical fascia and platysma, avoiding the anterior jugular veins which lie just deep into the platysma. Superior and inferior sub-platysmal flaps are raised by developing the avascular plane immediately deep into the platysma and pushing the anterior jugular veins down. Raise the sub-platysmal flaps cranially to the thyroid cartilage and caudally to the sternal notch.

2.6.2.2 Step 2: Separation and Mobilisation of the Strap Muscles

Divide the midline raphe (pre-tracheal fascia) longitudinally from the thyroid cartilage to the sternal notch to expose the sternohyoid (superficial) and sternothyroid (deep). Dissect the plane between the sternohyoid and sternothyroid muscles to expose the jugular vein and ansa cervicalis nerve. Assess the sternothyroid muscle for involvement in thyroid cancer, and if suspected, resect this muscle en bloc with the thyroid. The sternothyroid muscle may also be divided to facilitate exposure in very large goitres.

Develop the plane between the thyroid and the strap muscles by lifting the strap muscle anteriorly with a Kocher retractor, and dissect the fibroareolar tissue with a combination of blunt dissection and diathermy.

2.6.2.3 Step 3: Ligation of the Middle Thyroid Vein and Mobilisation of the Thyroid Lobe

Identify the middle thyroid vein at the anterolateral edge of the thyroid lobe and ligate between ligaclips. The lobe can then be retracted medially, and the lateral tissue dissected bluntly down to the carotid sheath. Open the carotid sheath along the anterior surface of the common carotid artery – once the middle thyroid has been divided, there are no other vascular structures crossing the anterior surface of the common carotid so this is a safe landmark along which to dissect. The visceral thyroid fascia is continuous with the carotid sheath, so clearing the anterior surface of the common carotid allows free retraction of the thyroid lobe up into the wound. The fibroareolar tissue medial to carotid, and above the ITA, should be spread gently to expose the pre-vertebral fascia.

2.6.2.4 Step 4: Ligation of the Superior Pole Vessels

Dissection of the superior pole of the thyroid begins in the 'space of Reeves', an avascular window between the cricothyroid muscle and the superior pole. Capsular dissection is especially important to avoid inadvertent injury to the external branch of the superior laryngeal nerve where it crosses the STA. Ligate the superior pole vessels between ligaclips with an energy device over the surface of the superior pole. Continue to ligate the branches of the superior pole vessels until the upper-pole is fully mobilised.

2.6.2.5 Step 5: Identification of the RLN

Before the inferior lobe is mobilised, identify the RLN. This is achieved by dissecting along a line made by bisecting the angle between the ITA and the trachea, starting high adjacent to the thyroid. Use a Crile forceps to gently fenestrate the fascia and expose a small portion of the nerve. Use the NIMS probe to confirm its location once visually identified.

Other reliable landmarks for orientation of the RLN include:

- Medial position to the Tubercle of Zuckerkandl. The nerve passes in a groove between the tubercle and the thyroid lobe.
- Deep to the main branch of the ITA.
- At the level of the trachea-oesophageal groove (when distal to the ITA).

Beware that in large goitres, the RLN and/or the typical anatomical landmarks can be displaced significantly. Extra care needs to be taken to safely identify the nerve before undertaking extensive dissection and ligation of structures.

2.6.2.6 Step 6: Exposure of the Trachea in the Midline at Inferior Border of Gland

The anterior trachea in this position is relatively avascular. It provides a safe landmark for depth of dissection around the inferior pole. Once the RLN and anterior trachea are identified and exposed, it is safe to proceed with the mobilisation of the inferior pole.

2.6.2.7 Step 7: Ligation of Inferior Pole Vessels

Mobilise the inferior pole from medial to lateral by capsular dissection. This is important to avoid damage to the RLN as it crosses the secondary branches of the ITA. Division of the ITA with clips and an energy device should be present on the thyroid gland (at the level of the tertiary branches) to preserve perfusion to the superior and inferior parathyroid glands and prevent RLN injury.

2.6.2.8 Step 8: Dissection of the Thyroid from RLN, Ligament of Berry and Superior Parathyroid Gland

The dissection of the final 1 cm of the RLN before it enters the larynx is the most dangerous, and it is important to slow down at this stage. Bleeding around the nerve at this point can be caused by small branches crossing over the RLN. Great care must be taken when ligating these fine vessels as bleeding here can be difficult to control without risking nerve damage. Trace the course of the RLN into the larynx to avoid inadvertent damage to an early branching nerve. Once the thyroid has been bluntly dissected away from the RLN, use an energy device to divide Berry's ligament and separate the thyroid from the trachea. Divide the thyroid isthmus with an energy device if hemithyroidectomy is being performed.

2.6.2.9 Step 9: Closure

Irrigate the surgical field with water. Perform a Valsalva manoeuvre and ensure meticulous haemostasis, although take great care with electrocautery in the vicinity of the RLN. Re-approximate the strap muscles and platysma, and close the skin with absorbable sutures. There is no evidence to support the use of drains in thyroidectomy.

2.6.3 Postoperative Care

Patients should be nursed with the head up 30 degrees and with ice packs to the neck. Patients who undergo total thyroidectomy should be commenced on a weight-based dose of thyroxine replacement.

Post-operative blood is not required for hemithyroidectomy. Following total thyroidectomy, we recommend performing postoperative serum calcium (corrected or ionised) and PTH in recovery. The half-life of PTH is only 2–3 min, so significant reductions in PTH levels reflect some degree of loss of parathyroid gland function. Patients in whom the PTH is <10 pmol/L are at greater risk of postoperative symptomatic hypocalcaemia [6].

If the PTH <10 pmol/L

- Commence patients on 4–6 g daily of calcium and synthetic vitamin D (calcitriol 0.25 μg BD).

If the PTH >10 pmol/L

- Commence all patients on calcium supplementation. This has been shown to be the safest and most cost-effective approach to post-operative calcium management. The dose range is 2–6 g daily, titrated to symptoms. In patients who develop symptoms of hypocalcaemia, the addition of calcitriol seems to provide a benefit [6].

A PTH and calcium level should be rechecked again at follow-up in 3–4 weeks. If normal, calcium supplementation can be discontinued. If persistent hypocalcaemia or hypoparathyroidism occurs, consider referral to an endocrinologist.

2.7 Thyroidectomy: Management of Complications

2.7.1 Haematoma

Post-thyroidectomy haemorrhage is a potentially life-threatening complication that occurs in 1–2% of operations in high-volume centres [7]. Clinically, the patient may manifest with neck swelling, dyspnoea (exacerbated by recumbency), stridor or frank hypoxia.

Bleeding in the thyroid bed, and subsequent expanding haematoma, cause venous compression and congestion in the central compartment. This results in laryngeal oedema and subsequent laryngospasm, which is thought to be the main cause of respiratory distress. In severe cases, mechanical displacement and compression of the trachea may occur. Releasing the haematoma by cutting surgical sutures at the skin and fascial level should take place on the ward as soon as identified because significant improvement in respiratory function can occur within minutes of doing so. A plan should then be made for an immediate return to the theatre for definitive control of bleeding.

2.7.2 RLN Injury/Neuropraxia

High-volume centres report temporary RLN neuropraxia in 3% of total thyroidectomies and permanent nerve dysfunction in 0.3% of them [8].

In a total thyroidectomy, the 'pathological' side should be operated on first. Loss of nerve signal may prompt the surgeon to perform a hemithyroidectomy instead, thus preventing potentially catastrophic bilateral nerve injury. The majority of non-transected RLN injuries recover, but this can take up to 12 months to occur. Full recovery may take several weeks to months but allows for a staged total thyroidectomy if required.

In experienced hands, if complete nerve transection is identified intraoperatively, immediate nerve reconstruction with an ansa cervicalis anastomosis or autograft can be performed.

2.7.3 Hypocalcaemia

Hypocalcaemia may be attributed to impaired perfusion to parathyroid glands, direct handling of the parathyroid glands or failure to identify glands in the resected specimen.

Temporary and permanent hypocalcaemia occurs in up to 20% and <1%, respectively, of total thyroidectomies. Permanent hypocalcaemia is defined as the persistence of hypocalcaemia that requires medication beyond 6 months.

Patients demonstrating severe hypocalcaemia (serum corrected calcium <1.9 mM) should receive intravenous calcium replacement (100 mL of 10% calcium gluconate in 1 L normal saline infused at a rate of 100 mL/h until normocalcaemia is achieved).

2.7.3.1 Clinical Manifestations

Calcium stabilises nerve–muscle function by limiting sodium entry into nerve cells, modulating the extent of depolarisation. This inhibition is mitigated in hypocalcaemia, resulting in nerve excitability (paraesthesia of lips/ fingers and toes), muscular tetany and cardiac arrhythmia.

Chvostek's sign – tapping over the region of the facial nerve results in twitching of the ipsilateral facial muscles.

Trousseau's sign – inflation of a blood pressure cuff over the arm to 30 mmHg greater than systolic blood pressure for 30 s, resulting in carpopedal spasm.

2.7.4 Surgical Site Infection (SSI)

SSIs occur in <1% of thyroidectomies. They can range from minor cellulitis to the development of frank abscesses. Independent risk factors include prolonged surgical time, obesity and return to theatre or re-exploration.

Top Five Takeaway Pearls for Thyroid

1. There are three principal questions when assessing a thyroid nodule; Is the nodule hyperfunctional, is the nodule malignant and is the nodule causing symptoms?
2. TSH level directs the appropriate first imaging modality for a thyroid nodule; If TSH is normal or elevated – ultrasound, and if it is suppressed – a functional radionuclide thyroid scan.
3. The extent of surgery (hemi vs. total ± central neck dissection) for differentiated thyroid cancer is contentious; if in doubt, present the case in an appropriate thyroid cancer MDT pre-operatively.
4. To identify the RLN, dissect along a line made by bisecting the angle between the ITA and the trachea using a Crile forceps.
5. The safest and most cost-effective approach to post-operative calcium management is to commence ALL patients on oral calcium supplements, and re-check calcium and PTH levels at 3 weeks.

References

1. Grant EG, Tessler FN, Hoang JK, Langer JE, Beland MD, Berland LL, et al. Thyroid ultrasound reporting lexicon: white paper of the ACR thyroid imaging, reporting and data system (TIRADS) committee. J Am Coll Radiol. 2015;12(12):1272–9.
2. Cibas ES, Ali SZ. The Bethesda system for reporting thyroid cytopathology. Thyroid. 2009;19(11):1159–65.
3. Alexander EK, Heering JP, Benson CB, Frates MC, Doubilet PM, Cibas ES, Marqusee E. Assessment of nondiagnostic ultrasound-guided fine needle aspirations of thyroid nodules. J Clin Endocrinol Metabol. 2002;87(11):4924–7.
4. Haugen BR, Alexander EK, Bible KC, Doherty GM, Mandel SJ, Nikiforov YE, et al. 2015 American Thyroid Association management guidelines for adult patients with thyroid nodules and differentiated thy-

roid cancer: the American Thyroid Association guidelines task force on thyroid nodules and differentiated thyroid cancer. Thyroid. 2016;26(1):1–133.
5. Wells SA Jr, Asa SL, Dralle H, Elisei R, Evans DB, Gagel RF, et al. Revised American Thyroid Association guidelines for the management of medullary thyroid carcinoma: the American Thyroid Association guidelines task force on medullary thyroid carcinoma. Thyroid. 2015;25(6):567–610.
6. Carter Y, Chen H, Sippel RS. An intact parathyroid hormone–based protocol for the prevention and treatment of symptomatic hypocalcemia after thyroidectomy. J Surg Res. 2014;186(1):23–8.
7. Zhang X, Du W, Fang Q. Risk factors for postoperative haemorrhage after total thyroidectomy: clinical results based on 2,678 patients. Sci Rep. 2017;7(1):1–5.
8. Wong KP, Mak KL, Wong CKH, Lang BHH. Systematic review and meta-analysis on intraoperative neuro-monitoring in high-risk thyroidectomy. Int J Surg. 2017;38:21–30.

3 Parathyroid

Tamara Preda, Peter Campbell, and Yeow Chun Tee

3.1 The Importance of Calcium to Life

Calcium (atomic number 20) is the fifth most abundant element in the earth's crust and the third most abundant metal. Calcium ions are essential for a range of biochemical processes including as second messengers in signal transduction, neurotransmitter release and muscle cell contraction. It is a cofactor for many enzymes and is responsible for maintaining the potential difference across excitable cell membranes.

Calcium is essential for bone formation and protein synthesis. Mammals need to both concentrate and store large quantities of calcium for their endoskeletons and keep the remainder of calcium ions within narrow bands for optimal function.

T. Preda (✉)
Department of Surgery, School of Medicine, University of Notre Dame, Sydney, NSW, Australia

P. Campbell · Y. C. Tee
Liverpool Hospital, Sydney, NSW, Australia

3.2 A Brief History of Parathyroid Surgery and Related Discoveries

In 1849, Sir Richard Owen was gifted the decaying carcass of the Indian Rhinoceros from the London Zoo. It was this animal in which parathyroids were first described: '*a small compact yellow glandular body, attached to the thyroid at the point where the veins emerge.*'

1852	Lucien Corvisart	Tetany post thyroidectomy noted
1880	Ivar Sandstrom	'*Glandulae parathyroidiae*' first described in humans
1891	Eugene Gley	Tetany in dogs after removal of parathyroids
1891	Friedrich Von Recklinghausen	Described osteitis fibrosa cystica osteoclastic - demineralisation and peri-trabecular fibrosis as the exemplar end organ manifestation of untreated populations with parathyroid disease
1904	Max Askanazy	Observed osteitis fibrosis cystica and parathyroid hyperplasia
1906	Jakob Erdheim	Identification of the role of parathyroids in calcium metabolism
1907	Jakob Erdheim	Recognised parathyroid hyperplasia/hypertrophy in autopsy studies of patients with osteomalacia

B. Ashford (ed.), *Head and Neck Surgery for General Surgeons*,
https://doi.org/10.1007/978-981-19-7900-2_3

1907	Halsted and Evans	Parathyroid blood supply described primarily from ITA
1915	Freidrich Schlagenhaufer	Parathyroid adenoma causing osteitis fibrosa cystica
1917	MaCallum and Voegtlin	Calcium—the cause and cure of tetany
1923–5	Hanson and Collip	Independently isolated parathyroid hormone
1925	Felix Mandl	First intentional parathyroidectomy for bone disease (EU)
1926	Edward D. Churchill	Parathyroidectomies captain Martell (USA)
1929	Fuller Albright	Published work on calcium and phosphate metabolism relating to hyperparathyroidism
1936	Churchill and Cope	Parathyroid clinical presentations and surgery codified. The issues of single adenoma vs. multi-gland hyperplasia had been delineated. The relationship of parathyroid disease to renal stones was understood, mediastinal tumours had been found and resected, and the clinical priorities of an asymptomatic vs. obstructive renal calculus and the metabolic effects of the parathyroid disease were understood. The size range of normal and pathological glands and the various cells seen in parathyroids as well as the phenomenon of fat depletion had been established
1937	Windaus and Bock	Vitamin D3 isolated
1948	Fuller Albright	Calcium metabolism systematised
1953	Laurentius Underdahl	14 cases of MEN-1 reported
1954	Paul Wermer	Autosomal dominant nature of MEN-1 described
1959	Rasmussen and Craig	Parathyroid hormone purified
1962	Rasmussen and Craig	Parathyroid polypeptide structure established
1963	Rolayn Yallow	Parathyroid immunoassay enables routine measurement
1982	Russell and Edis	Surgery for asymptomatic primary hyperparathyroidism established
1993	Edward M. Brown	Calcium sensing receptor (CaSR) identified

3.3 Parathyroid Embryology

During the fourth and fifth weeks of foetal development, six pharyngeal arches and pouches appear and the parathyroids arise from the endoderm of the third and fourth pharyngeal pouches as well as the migrating neural crest.

The third pharyngeal pouch divides into dorsal and ventral wings, the dorsal giving rise to the inferior parathyroid gland and the ventral forming the thymus. In the seventh week, the parathyroids and thymus descend caudally and medially from the pharynx; the inferior parathyroid disconnects from the thymus, which descends into the anterior mediastinum.

The fourth pharyngeal pouch also divides into a dorsal wing, which develops into the superior parathyroid gland, and a ventral wing, which develops into the ultimobranchial body that fuses to the posterolateral thyroid and contributes the parafollicular C-cells.

The height of the inferior parathyroid glands varies due to the longer route of descent.

Ectopic nests of parathyroid tissue can be found anywhere along their pathway of descent. These may be hyperplastic in secondary and tertiary hyperparathyroidism.

3.4 Parathyroid Anatomy

3.4.1 Macroscopic

The parathyroids are separate endocrine glands normally on the posterior aspect of the thyroid gland, within the pre-tracheal fascia.

Typically, there are paired superior and inferior glands. They exist in their own capsules, are 'London Tan' in colour and typically weigh between 25 mg and 50 mg. Shape is most commonly oval but can be bean or spherical. They may be bilobar (5%) or multilobulated (1%).

3.4.1.1 Superior ('P4') Parathyroid Glands

These are normally located on the postero-lateral surface of the thyroid at its middle to superior lobe. They typically lie posterior and lateral to the RLN, under the investing fascia of the thyroid. The tubercle of Zuckerkandl is used as a surgical landmark (inferior and lateral to the superior parathyroid gland). The inferior thyroid artery (ITA) enters the thyroid gland 1 cm inferior to the superior parathyroid gland. The superior parathyroid glands may be undescended. Other ectopic locations include the tracheoesophageal groove (45%), retropharyngeal space (20%) and posterior mediastinum (15%).

3.4.1.2 Inferior ('P3') Parathyroid Glands

The inferior parathyroid glands are usually found just above or in the anterior mediastinum. They are most commonly in the thyrothymic tract or just deep into the thyroid capsule on the inferior surface of the thyroid lobe.

They classically lie anterior and medial to the RLN, approximately 1 cm below the insertion of the ITA into the thyroid gland and within a 2 cm space between the ITA and the RLN.

Ectopic inferior glands can be anywhere along their course of descent from the base of the skull, through the carotid sheath, and into the anterior mediastinum. They can also be located within the thyroid parenchyma (1%) or thymus (9%).

About 10–15% of the population have ectopic parathyroid glands. Eighty-four per cent of patients have four glands, 13% have additional glands and <3% of the population have only three. Eighty per cent of parathyroid glands exhibit positional symmetry.

3.4.1.3 Blood Supply

Superior and inferior parathyroid glands are both supplied by end artery branches of the ITA. The superior thyroid artery may also supply the superior parathyroid. The superior, middle and inferior thyroid veins drain parathyroid outflow to the internal jugular and innominate veins. Parathyroid lymphatic drainage is to the paratracheal and deep cervical nodes.

3.4.2 Microscopic

The main parathyroid cell types are chief cells and oxyphil cells. In pathological states water clear cells may also be seen (Fig. 3.1).

Chief cells—Synthesise and secrete PTH. They stain dark purple on H&E stain with pale pink cytoplasm and have large round nuclei.

Oxyphil cells—Are poorly understood. On H&E stain, they are larger than chief cells with smaller nuclei and more eosinophilic cytoplasm.

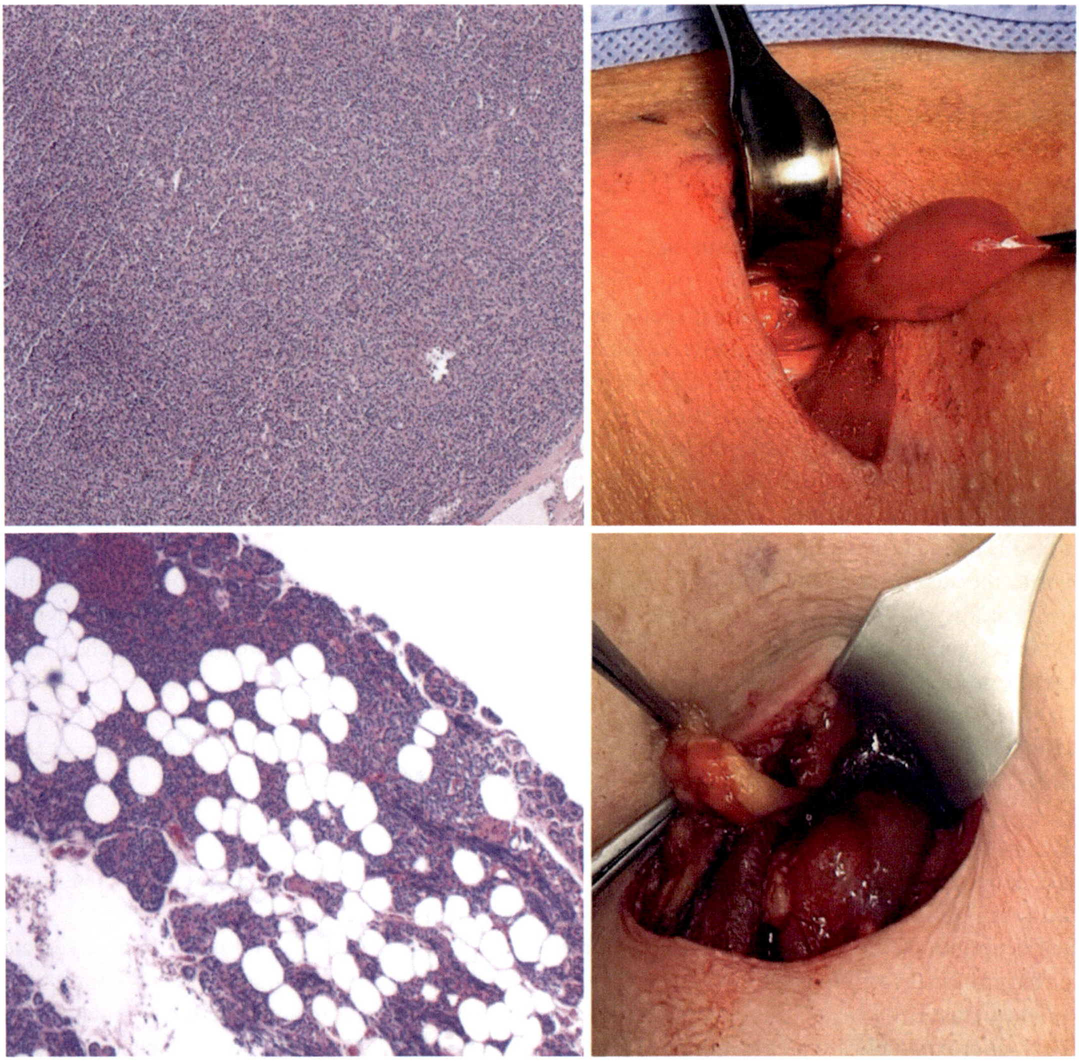

Fig. 3.1 Clockwise from top left: photomicrograph of parathyroid chief cells and fat depletion. Top right operative photograph of parathyroid adenoma lying on the recurrent laryngeal nerve. Bottom right: operative photograph of normal London Tan parathyroid embedded in thymus note contact heamorrhage. Bottom left: photomicrograph of normal parathyroid tissue with fat

3.5 Parathyroid Physiology

Parathyroid glands produce parathyroid hormone (PTH), which, in conjunction with calcitriol (1,25-dihydroxyvitamin D), modulates calcium and phosphate homeostasis. Change in serum calcium concentration is sensed by the calcium-sensing receptor (CaSR) on the parathyroid cells resulting in increased or decreased PTH secretion. There is a corresponding change in renal tubular reabsorption of calcium and phosphate. Renal activation of 1,25 dihydroxyvitamin D is increased by PTH. Parathyroid hormone indirectly stimulates osteoclastic activity in bone.

Calcitonin, a 32 amino acid hormone, serves as an antagonist to PTH and is released by the parafollicular C cells in response to rising serum calcium levels.

3.6 Parathyroid Pathophysiology

3.6.1 Primary Hyperparathyroidism (pHPT)

Primary HPT is hypercalcaemia with elevated or inappropriately normal serum PTH.

Risk factors
- Female to male ratio 2:1
- Age > 45 years
- Radiation exposure
- Genetic defects
  - e.g. MEN syndromes, familial isolated hyperparathyroidism.
- Lithium treatment

Eighty per cent are due to a single adenoma, 10–15% double adenomas and 5–10% hyperplasia.

Historically, pHPT presented with hypercalcaemic end-organ effects causing 'stones, moans, bones and groans'. In the developed world, pHPT is an asymptomatic laboratory abnormality. Non-specific symptoms of fatigue, muscle weakness, low mood and weight change can often be elicited with a minority of patients being truly asymptomatic.

Examination of a patient with pHPT commonly yields few findings as parathyroid adenomas are rarely palpable. Objective pathologies associated with pHPT are most commonly renal calculi, osteopaenia, osteoporosis and vertebral fractures.

3.6.2 Secondary Hyperparathyroidism

Secondary HPT is most commonly associated with chronic kidney disease (CKD) due to:

- Impaired renal function → decreased phosphate excretion + hyperphosphataemia. Excess phosphate binds to circulating calcium → hypocalcaemia.
- Significant hypovitaminosis D and the inability to convert vitamin D to its active form (calcitriol) decrease calcium resorption from the gut and renal tubules.

Resultant hypocalcaemia stimulates increased PTH secretion and parathyroid gland hyperplasia.

Clinical signs in secondary HPT may be present including:

- Bone remodelling due to abnormal mineralisation may cause bone pain, bone deformation and fractures seen in the chest wall, spine (kyphoscoliosis), hip joints, pelvis and lower limbs.
- Extraosseous calcium deposition—Arterial walls, viscera, skin and the cornea or conjunctiva. Calcium deposition may occur in the pericardium and cardiac valves resulting in valvular dysfunction and ventricular failure.
- Calciphylaxis—Calcification of small cutaneous arterioles resulting in ulceration and skin necrosis. It usually affects the extremities and is considered a significant indicator of mortality risk in secondary HPT.

Other causes of secondary HPT are:

- Dietary calcium and vitamin D deficiency
- Inadequate calcium absorption in gut disorders causing malnutrition
- Medications including lithium

3.6.2.1 Lithium-Induced Hyperparathyroidism

About 15–40% of patients receiving lithium develop hyperparathyroidism. The mechanism is unclear but probably lithium blocks calcium receptors within the parathyroids, preventing feedback control.

Patients present with symptoms of hypercalcaemia; however, it should be noted that psychiatric symptoms may be marked. Equal numbers of patients have been found to have adenomas and hyperplastic glands, the former being diagnosed earlier than the latter.

Cessation of lithium will usually result in normalisation of serum calcium within 4 weeks; however, patients on long-term lithium therapy (>10 years) may require surgery.

3.6.3 Tertiary Hyperparathyroidism

Tertiary hyperparathyroidism develops from secondary hyperparathyroidism in renal patients but is distinguished from it by hypercalcaemia due to the autonomous production of PTH. It occurs in approximately 8% of patients with secondary hyperparathyroidism after a successful renal transplant.

3.6.4 Normocalcaemic Hyperparathyroidism

Normocalcaemic hyperparathyroidism (NHPT) was described in 2008. It remains a controversial entity and may manifest with elevated ionised calcium and iPTH with osteoporosis and renal stones [1].

3.6.5 Hyperparathyroidism in Pregnancy

Pregnancy alters calcium homeostasis, and serum calcium levels are routinely in the low-normal range in the first trimester and the high-normal range in the second and third trimesters. PTH interestingly follows the same trend rather than the expected inverse relationship, and foetal calcium levels mirror maternal levels. Hyperparathyroidism in pregnancy has an incidence of 1%. Moderate to severe hypercalcaemia can carry significant maternal and neonatal risks so early detection and management is important. Maternal risks include hyperemesis, weight loss and anorexia, nephrolithiasis, renal impairment, pancreatitis, pre-eclampsia and cardiac arrhythmias.

Neonatal risks include neonatal tetany, PTH suppression and permanent hypoparathyroidism secondary to parathyroid aplasia, preterm delivery, IUGR, low birth weight and stillbirth and postnatal death.

Surgery should be offered as early as possible generally in the second trimester. Routine screening for phaeochromocytoma in all pHPT patients should be undertaken.

3.6.6 Parathyroid Cysts

Parathyroid cysts represent 1–3% of neck masses with the majority being non-functional.

Serum calcium and PTH levels confirm hyperfunction and ultrasound/CT scans are the imaging modalities of choice. A clue to the diagnosis is in the location of the mass, with cysts being found in the usual locations of parathyroid glands. Larger cysts can often be found in the anterior mediastinum. An FNA biopsy demonstrating elevated PTH concentration is diagnostic.

Symptomatic cysts should be excised. Asymptomatic functioning cysts follow the same management criteria as for asymptomatic pHPT. Asymptomatic non-functioning cysts often require no immediate management and should be monitored.

3.6.7 Parathyroid Carcinoma

Parathyroid malignancy is a rare cause of hyperparathyroidism. Non-parathyroid malignancies (particularly squamous tumours and renal carcinomas) that secrete PTH can masquerade as pHPT and should be considered as a differential diagnosis. Patients may be symptomatic, presenting with a neck mass, parathyroid crisis, acute pathological fracture or acute renal complications. Laboratory findings often demonstrate significantly elevated serum calcium levels (= > 3.5 mmol/L) and PTH levels 5–10 times the upper limit of normal. Imaging may demonstrate a large neck mass(usually = > 1.5 cm) adjacent to the thyroid gland. There may be a local invasion of surrounding tissues with regional nodal involvement and distant metastases. Parathyroid carcinoma may be associated with

Hyperparathyroidism-Jaw Tumour Syndrome, discussed later in this chapter. Staging is performed via CT neck/chest/abdomen and pelvis or PET nuclear imaging. Surgical resection is the mainstay of treatment. En bloc resection of the parathyroid gland and involved adjacent structures (including the ipsilateral hemithyroid) is the operation of choice.

Pre-operative vocal cord assessment is necessary, and an involved RLN may be sacrificed; the possibility of resection with nerve reconstruction should be discussed pre-operatively. Prophylactic lymph node clearance is not routinely undertaken as it is of unclear benefit. If parathyroid malignancy is diagnosed postoperatively on histopathology, revision surgery with further resection as above may be indicated. For inoperable disease, the focus is on medical control of hypercalcaemia [2].

3.6.8 Hypercalcaemic Crisis Due to Hyperparathyroidism

Parathyroid crisis, or parathyroid storm, is a rare and life threatening complication of pHPT. There is severe symptomatic hypercalcaemia (often >3.8 mmol/L) and grossly elevated PTH levels (>15 times the upper limit of normal).

Symptoms include mental state changes ranging from confusion through to loss of consciousness, neuromuscular effects (fatigue, lethargy, muscle weakness, etc.), nephrolithiasis, pancreatitis, severe unexplained abdominal pain, bony disease (including fractures) and renal/other organ calcification. The most severe manifestation is alveolar calcification with loss of oxygen exchange and acute respiratory distress.

Parathyroid crisis can complicate known pHPT or may be a sentinel event. The exact mechanism is unknown; however, precipitants are concurrent illness, marked dehydration or infarction of a parathyroid adenoma. Management involves aggressive rehydration and reduction of serum calcium levels in a monitored environment. This may include the use of bisphosphonates, calcimimetics and surgery. Medical management is a temporising measure, and definitive parathyroidectomy is required by four-gland exploration. Post operative rebound hypocalcaemia is likely.

3.7 MEN and Other Genetic Parathyroid Conditions

3.7.1 MEN Syndromes

These rare autosomal dominant disorders predispose to endocrine tumours. Mutations are on chromosome 11 in MEN-1 and the RET proto-oncogene on chromosome 10 in MEN-2 (A and B).

3.7.2 MEN-1

Nearly, 100% of MEN-1 patients present with parathyroid adenomas. They may also have pituitary adenomas, pancreatic endocrine tumours (together with parathyroid adenomas, the 'three P's) as well as gastrinomas, foregut carcinoid tumours and adrenocortical adenomas.

As multiple parathyroid adenomas are common, four gland exploration is necessary. Subtotal vs. total parathyroidectomy (± parathyroid autograft) is debatable with a view to balancing recurrent disease and postoperative hypoparathyroidism. Surgery should include thymectomy due to the presence of intra-thymic parathyroid rests and glands. MEN-1 patients may have thymic carcinoid tumours.

3.7.3 MEN-2A

Parathyroid disease affects 10–25% of patients. In contrast to MEN-1, parathyroid disease in MEN-2A is almost always multi-glandular hyperplasia. Associated endocrine tumours include phaeochromocytoma and medullary thyroid cancer, which should be diagnosed preoperatively. Four gland exploration follows the other manifestations in priority. MEN-2A parathyroid disease recurs less than in MEN-1.

MEN IIb (MEN 3) does not cause hyperparathyroidism.

MEN-4 is a rare CDKN1B 12p13 mutation characterised by multi-gland hyperparathyroidism also with pituitary adenomas, reproductive organ cancers (testicular cancer and neuroendocrine cervical carcinoma) adrenal and renal tumours.

3.7.4 Familial Hypocalciuric Hypercalcaemia (FHH)

FHH is a benign autosomal dominant inherited disorder usually due to inactivating mutations in the CaSR (calcium-sensing receptor) gene on chromosome 3, which increases renal tubular reabsorption of calcium and magnesium.

Biochemistry demonstrates

- High serum calcium levels with inappropriately normal or elevated PTH levels
- Low urinary calcium levels (typically <5 mmol/24 h)
- High normal or elevated magnesium levels

Calcium: Creatinine clearance is a more sensitive test for FHH than 24 h urinary calcium levels as it demonstrates the resorption characteristics of the renal tubules. Commonly ratios of 0.01 are seen (i.e. >99% of calcium is resorbed within the kidneys), despite high serum calcium levels. Symptoms of hypercalcaemia are rarely present. Surgery is ineffective so FHH must be distinguished from pHPT.

3.7.5 Hyperparathyroidism-Jaw Tumour Syndrome (HPT-JT)

This autosomal dominant syndrome of varying penetrance is due to the inactivation of the CDC73 gene, which encodes for parafibromin. The most common manifestation is pHPT, and 20% have parathyroid carcinoma. Other clinical manifestations include cemento-ossifying fibromas limited to the maxilla and mandible and mixed epithelial and stromal tumours of the kidney.

3.7.6 Familial Isolated Hyperparathyroidism (FIHP)

Patients have multi-gland hyperplasia affecting two or more kindred members but lacking features or mutations of MEN I, MEN IIa HPT-JT or FHH; 20% have a GCM2 gain of function mutation and may have Ashkenazy Jewish heritage.

3.8 Epidemiology

Parathyroid disorders are the third most common group of endocrine diagnoses after diabetes and thyroid disease. Familial disorders of the parathyroids account for 10–15% of all cases. When multi-channel blood analysis was introduced in 1974, the observed rate of hypercalcaemia rose from 7.4 to 129 per 100,000 person-years. Typical gender ratios female to male are 3–4:1. Mild primary hyperparathyroidism that fails to meet guidelines for surgery is progressive in about 37% observed over 15 years. Only 10% of patients with primary hyperparathyroidism undergo parathyroid surgery.

In Australia, the average number of private sector parathyroidectomies per annum in 2016–21 was 2250 distributed across the states and territories by population. Figure 3.2 shows the age and gender demographics for this group.

In Australia, 73% of private sector parathyroidectomies are performed by minimal access, 22% are four gland explorations and 6% of procedures are for re-exploration. The total number of private sector mediastinal explorations for parathyroids in the last 5 years was 24 in Australia. In NSW in 2018–21, there were 1507 parathyroidectomies performed in the public system across 16 local health districts (range 4–238).

About 1.7 million Australians have biochemical renal impairment and 5100 patients per 100,000 population are dialysed. In the USA, parathyroidectomy rates in the dialysed population ranged from 5 to 12 per 1000 patient years. Thirty per cent of renal transplant recipients develop tertiary hyperparathyroidism although 20% of those may have single or double adenomas.

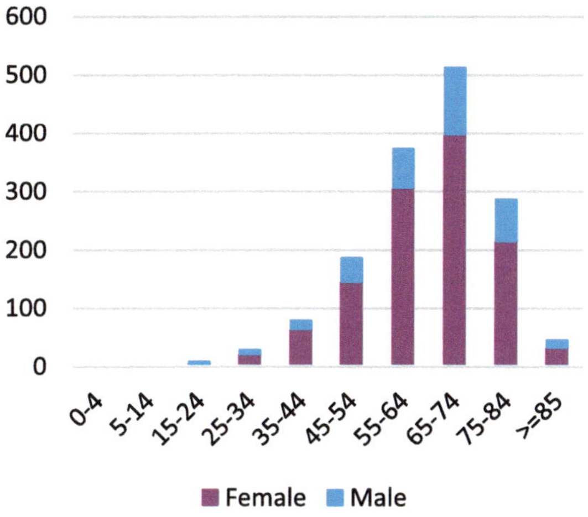

Fig. 3.2 Hyperparathyroidism in Australia by age and sex

3.9 Clinical Evaluation and Diagnostic Work Up of Hyperparathyroidism

3.9.1 Biochemistry

3.9.1.1 Serum Calcium (Ca) Corrected for Albumin

A single elevated serum Ca level should be repeated to confirm the diagnosis of pHPT prior to further investigation. Previous values should be used to establish a trend.

In secondary HPT, calcium levels are within the normal range.

3.9.1.2 Serum Parathyroid Hormone (PTH)

Approximately 90% of patients with pHPT will have an elevated PTH level. The elevation is usually modest (within two times the upper limit of normal). In 5–10% of pHPT patients, the PTH may be within the normal range (inappropriate in the setting of hypercalcaemia).

PTH in secondary hyperparathyroidism is elevated by a greater magnitude than in pHPT-typically 10+ times the upper limit of normal.

3.9.1.3 24 h Urinary Calcium Excretion

This can be used to distinguish pHPT from FHH. In asymptomatic pHPT, high levels of urinary calcium confer an increased risk of future renal complications. Calcium creatinine clearance can also be used.

3.9.1.4 Serum 1,25 Dihydroxyvitamin D

Deficiency of vitamin D is a cause of secondary HPT. The appropriate replacement may be the only intervention required in these patients to normalise serum PTH levels.

3.9.2 Parathyroid Imaging

The aim of imaging is to localise pathological parathyroid gland(s) in both normal and unusual locations. It is important to be aware of concurrent thyroid pathology (goitre, suspicious nodules and thyroiditis). CT imaging may also detect the 1% of patients with a non-recurrent RLN.

Imaging is more likely to detect parathyroid adenomas than hyperplastic glands and may facilitate a minimally invasive operation.

Interested and experienced nuclear medicine and radiology clinicians who understand parathyroid embryology/anatomy provide the best localisations. Superior gland location is less variable than for inferior glands. CT and SESTAMIBI should encompass Level I of the neck to the aorto-pulmonary window to avoid missing ectopic glands.

It is ideal to have congruous imaging results. Imaging modalities vary by location; however, neck ultrasound and Tc-99 m SESTAMIBI are generally considered the most appropriate first tests.

On ultrasound, parathyroid glands are seen as well-defined hypoechoic (relative to thyroid) round or oval structures often with a 'polar vessel'. Sensitivity is 76–80%.

Dual-phase Tc-99 m sestamibi/SPECT CT acquires images in anterior, lateral and oblique planes ± additional pinhole views (Fig. 3.3). There is characteristic retention of tracer in abnormal parathyroids compared to thyroid tissue, and this is thought to be due to high metabolic activity and mitochondrial content of abnormal parathyroid glands. Sensitivity is 84%.

4D-CT is of value for patients who do not localise an abnormal gland on primary imaging

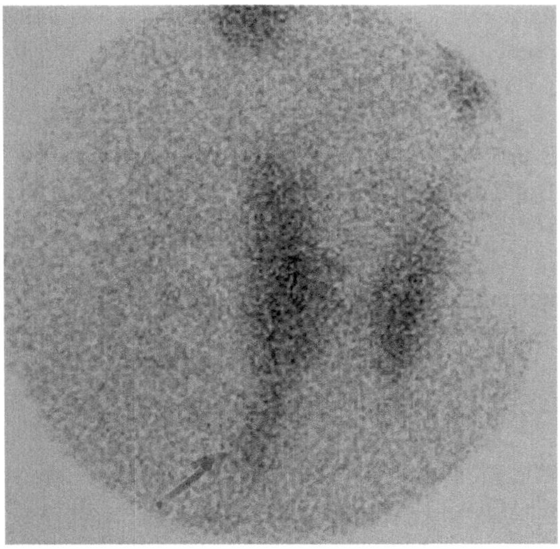

Fig. 3.3 SESTAMIBI scan showing right thyro-thymic parathyroid with helpful arrow

or who do not have concordant results. Parathyroid adenomas have avid arterial enhancement and rapid washout on the venous phase. CT radiation dose is significant. Sensitivity is 73–89%.

If no parathyroids are imaged, then the underlying pathology may be multi-gland hyperplasia, and bilateral neck exploration is necessary.

Parathyroid carcinoma is rare but should be suspected with a large parathyroid gland with indistinct margins or invasion into surrounding structures.

With recurrent or persistent hyperparathyroidism with no pathological gland seen on standard imaging, selective venous sampling should be considered. Blood is sampled bilaterally at standard sites along the parathyroid/thyroid venous drainage pathway in the neck and mediastinum to determine pathological iPTH elevation near the 'missing' adenoma.

During pregnancy, SESTAMIBI and 4D CT are both contraindicated. Localisation is by ultrasound and occasionally MRI.

3.9.3 Other Imaging Studies

DEXA-BMD—document baseline bone density (T score).

Renal tract USS to look for renal stones.

3.10 Indications for Surgery [3, 4]

Untreated hyperparathyroidism causes end-organ pathologies including osteoporosis, renal calculi, peptic ulcer and cardiovascular disease.

3.10.1 Primary Hyperparathyroidism

In pHPT, absolute indications from the 2014 NIH guidelines include:

1. Serum calcium >1 mg/dL above the upper limit of normal (>2.85 mmol/L)
2. Bone density T score < −2.5 (osteoporosis)
3. Vertebral fracture by imaging
4. Creatinine clearance <60 mL/min
5. 24-hour urine calcium >400 mg/d and increased stone risk by biochemical analysis
6. Presence of kidney stones
7. Age < 50 years

Relative AAES indications for surgery include: all patients with 'soft symptoms' such as fatigue, mood changes, poor memory/concentration, arthralgias and thirst; fragility fractures; clinical or biochemical suspicion for parathyroid carcinoma; those with neuro-cognitive or neuropsychiatric symptoms and those unable/unwilling to undertake regular surveillance.

3.10.2 Secondary Hyperparathyroidism

In HPT secondary to chronic kidney disease, clinical consequences include marked loss of bone density, fragility fractures, bone ache, pruritis, anaemia refractory to EPO treatment, generalised weakness and rarely calciphylaxis. Medical management includes high-dose vitamin D replacement, calcium-binding agents and calcimimetics (calcium-sensing receptor agonists). The use of calcimimetics is limited by accessibility, cost and side effects (vomiting, diarrohea and abdominal pain) and potential for life-threatening hypocalcaemia.

The attending nephrologist determines the patient's suitability for renal transplant and may prefer parathyroidectomy prior to renal transplantation, as this may improve renal allograft survival and function. Others rely on renal transplantation to correct secondary hyperparathyroidism with a minority developing tertiary hyperparathyroidism.

Pre-transplant parathyroidectomy is indicated when maximal medical management does not mitigate end-organ damage or symptoms.

Surgical options include total parathyroidectomy with or without auto-transplantation or subtotal parathyroidectomy with a vascularised remnant in situ. A cervical thymectomy reduces the risk of disease recurrence, particularly in non-transplant patients [5, 6].

3.10.3 Tertiary Hyperparathyroidism

Surgery is indicated for those with symptomatic hypercalcaemia; acute hypercalcaemia or asymptomatic hypercalcaemia with serum calcium >3 mmol/L for >1 year [6].

3.11 Consent for Surgery: Expected Benefits and Potential Risks

Patients and their families should be warned about rare complications such as bleeding and infection, recurrent laryngeal nerve injury and persistent or recurrent disease. Expected biochemical cure rates should be discussed. In pHPT, post-operative hypoparathyroidism may require calcium ± calcitriol supplementation until the residual parathyroid function is restored particularly for multiple gland resections. The potential for hemithyroidectomy and thymectomy for parathyroids in these locations needs to be discussed and consented. The cosmetic outcome for scars should be mentioned.

Surgery for secondary hyperparathyroidism carries significantly higher risks due to concurrent CKD and common comorbidities, such as vascular, cardiac or endocrine disorders, and the profound metabolic changes occurring after the removal of parathyroids. In the USA, a mortality rate of 2% and a 30-day re-admission rate of 24% in patients with secondary hyperparathyroidism undergoing surgery has been noted. Calciphylaxis carries a high risk.

In many units, admission to HDU/ICU is standard for monitoring and replacement of calcium and other electrolytes (phosphate, magnesium and potassium). About 27–100% of patients will experience 'Hungry Bones Syndrome' after parathyroidectomy. The abrupt fall in PTH level triggers a mismatch between osteoblast and osteoclast activity with transient or prolonged hypocalcaemia.

Improvement in presenting symptoms and biochemical parameters are to be expected following surgery for pHPT. Recurrent renal calculus formation is reduced. Most patients with pHPT have osteopaenia or osteoporosis, and this is more severe in renal hyperparathyroidism [7]. About 50–75% of patients with renal HPT show a marked reduction in bone density at the distal radius, and more than ¼ have a Z-score below −2 at other sites. An improvement in bone density particularly of the distal radius of 2–5% may be seen in the first 6–12 months after surgery in pHPT and 7–23% in those with renal hyperparathyroidism.

Whilst general energy levels frequently improve quickly, cognitive and musculoskeletal symptoms typically take months to improve. A formal questionnaire such as the Pasieka Parathyroidectomy Assessment Score (PAS) might be used to assess outcomes.

3.12 Technique for Surgical Parathyroid Exploration

The surgeon aims to discover and resect sufficient hyperfunctioning parathyroid tissue to normalise calcium metabolism whilst avoiding hypoparathyroidism and anatomical complications. The search for parathyroids on anatomical and embryological grounds is unique [8].

Frail patients can endure surgery with a cervical plexus block and local anaesthetic infiltration. Contraindications to modern general anaesthesia are rare (perhaps intractable cardiac failure). Some institutions routinely use a local anaesthetic.

The patient notes and imaging are displayed and form part of the timeout procedure. The incision and the side (for unilateral parathyroid exploration) are marked. A small shoulder roll with a modest neck extension avoids neck pain and improves access. Nerve integrity monitoring may be used.

3.12.1 Minimal Access vs. Routine Four Gland Exploration

The enthusiasm for minimal access surgery is tempered by unrecognised functionally significant multi-gland disease. In localised redo parathyroid surgery, a focussed lateral surgical approach may help.

3.12.2 Image Negative Cases

SESTAMIBI scans may be negative or ambiguous in 20% of cases. Ultrasound and CT scanning may help. An experienced surgeon performs four-gland exploration commencing on the most convenient side first. Some have adopted the approach of limiting the exploration to one side if an appropriate parathyroid is found. This may result in missed functionally significant contralateral parathyroid glands.

3.12.3 MEN-1 and Other Familial Syndromes

Patients in whom multiple glands are likely to be involved have a four-gland parathyroid exploration encompassing the usual locations and the superior anterior mediastinum.

3.12.4 Secondary Hyperparathyroidism

Renal patients should have a four-gland parathyroidectomy. They should have a cervical thymectomy to reduce the risk of disease recurrence, particularly if they are not transplant candidates. This can be a total or subtotal parathyroidectomy with or without graft. Total parathyroidectomy has the lowest recurrence rate and requires more calcium support early on.

3.12.5 Parathyroid Incidental to Thyroid Pathology and Surgery

Some conditions, such as bulky Hashimoto's glands and large benign multinodular goitre, are difficult to rotate; occasionally, a lobectomy is required to facilitate parathyroid access. There is a 5–7% risk of thyroid malignancy in patients with primary hyperparathyroidism. About half of these are more than micro cancers, so thyroid resection may be necessary.

3.12.6 General Principles

3.12.6.1 Incision Appropriate to the Circumstances

Incisions are orientated to Langer's lines, and often, there is a suitable skin crease.

The four-gland incision should span the medial borders of the sternomastoid muscle unless the thyroid is significantly enlarged.

The level of the incision in neck extension lies at least 30 mm above the jugular notch and may lie as high as the cricoid cartilage; if the jugular notch is deep, the incision should be high enough to avoid unsightly bridging scars.

Pre-operative ultrasound may be used to determine the best level for the incision.

The standard length of a minimal access incision is 25 mm but it is longer in the muscular or obese and when the parathyroid is large, caudal or posterior. This incision crosses the most medial 10 mm of the sternocleidomastoid muscle avoiding the external jugular vein and facilitates the separation of the strap muscles and ansa cervicalis from the sternocleidomastoid muscle.

3.12.6.2 Maximum Exposure

Infiltration with local anaesthetic and adrenaline and a cervical plexus block may be used. Sharp vertical incision of the dermis maximises access. Avoid thermal injury to the skin that causes locally hypertrophic scars. The platysma is incised, and a space is created on the superficial investing layer of the deep cervical fascia with blunt dissection or diathermy.

Maximal cranio-caudal mobilisation of the strap muscles and the sternomastoid provide tension-free access. Mobility of the strap muscles can be improved by a lateral release of the investing layer of the deep cervical fascia, preserving the ansa cervicalis. Some surgeons divide the strap muscles routinely; however, this may impair three-dimensional counter-traction to display the exploration zone. A single standard-sized Kocher retractor or two or three retractors of Kocher or Langenbeck type are used. Longer retractors may be useful when the target area is deep. S-retractors may assist with descended posterior mediastinal locations. Minimal access surgery is affected by retracting the strap muscles medially, and the omohyoid may be mobilised or divided for access to superior parathyroids. Care is taken with the sternomastoid branch of the superior thyroid artery, which runs at its upper border. The plane on the thyroid capsule and the lateral aspect of the thyro-thymic tract is the working space.

3.12.6.3 Bloodless and Blood Mitigating

The surgeon aims for a bloodless field and avoidance of blood-stained tissues. This may be mitigated by normal saline irrigation with pressure and suction over a Raytec, but avoidance of bleeding is the best policy.

During the raising of the strap muscles, the capsular thyroid branches from the strap muscle branch of the superior thyroid artery should be controlled with electrocautery. Division of the middle thyroid vein may facilitate access to the posterior aspect of the thyroid.

3.12.6.4 Nerves

The recurrent laryngeal nerves are at risk of temporary and permanent injury but are less vulnerable than in thyroid surgery. The recurrent laryngeal nerve lies immediately deep to the inferior parathyroid and close and medial to the upper extent of the superior parathyroid. Sometimes the recurrent laryngeal nerve (particularly a small medial motor branch) may lie bridging the superior parathyroid and is particularly at risk of being mistaken for the parathyroid blood supply.

3.12.6.5 Early Exploration Strategy

A localised parathyroid is sought first. Useful landmarks include the intersection of the recurrent laryngeal nerve and the inferior thyroid artery; most parathyroids lie within 1–2 centimetres of this point. Occasionally, the superior and inferior parathyroids are in contact with each other (kissin' cousins), and this may lead to misinterpreting the number of glands that have been found. Alternatively, the tubercle of Zuckerkandl is a good landmark and guide to the posterior extent of dissection.

3.12.6.6 Scope of Anatomical Exposure

Dissection of the deep aspect of the sternothyroid muscle extending to its lateral edge onto the common carotid artery provides the access needed to explore parathyroids. Care should be taken to sweep all the fibrofatty and lymphoid tissue from the muscle; occasionally, an inferior parathyroid may be elevated and hidden by the retractor.

3.12.6.7 Tissue Handling

Exploration involves interrogation of the surface of the thyroid and the structures between it and the common carotid artery, starting medially. Blood vessels have elastic properties, which, if stretched in slow motion, are less inclined to bleed. Older vessels are more fragile. Exploratory windows are created moving out from the typical parathyroid locations. Blood vessels are sealed with appropriate electro cautery or fine ties and clips if abutting the nerves. Some surgeons use a mosquito or Crile forceps. These have a three-to-one mechanical advantage by applying increased tension and decreased tactile feedback. The closed 'double DeBakey technique' is expeditious. These are, in effect, two small blunt bodkins for dissection. The small teeth on one DeBakey jaw can lift and displace fine fascial layers.

3.12.6.8 Parathyroid Identification and Preservation of Normal Parathyroids

Normal parathyroid tissue is London Tan coloured (**PANTONE16–1334 TCX Tan**) Adenomas are larger, brick red in colour and softer in consistency than thyroid. They have a prominent, polar blood supply with a secondary thyroid capsular supply. They may have adjacent fat and a small normal parathyroid on the surface. Other structures that may confound identification include extra thyroid nodules, brown fat, undescended thymus, intrathyroidal fat, colloid nodules, and reactive and granulomatous lymphadenopathy. Parathyroids may undergo cystic degeneration. Parathyroid carcinomas are similar in colour to parathyroid adenomas but larger, firmer and adherent, with more parasitic blood vessels from the thyroid. Secondary hyperparathyroid glands commonly weigh more than 1000 mg and are often subject to repeated haemorrhage, fibrosis and septated scarring; they may be lighter in colour as a result. Parathyroids have definite planes of separation from the thyroid and other structures. When the parathyroid is embedded in fat or thymus, its mass effect may be interrogated by ballottement with a closed DeBakey forceps showing it moving in undissected fatty tissues or the thyro-thymic tract. When searching unsuccessfully for a parathyroid adenoma, the surgeon is tempted to remove prominent normal parathyroids as an act of desperation. This is a mindset to be eschewed. Patients with mild renal impairment, or pregnancy, typically have upper range normal parathyroids. If a parathyroid adenoma is subsequently discovered, this may lead to hypoparathyroidism.

3.12.7 Use of Frozen Section

Many experienced parathyroid surgeons do not perform frozen sections routinely but may do so when the identification of a gland is a problem. Less experienced surgeons may remove structures that look like parathyroids and finish the exploration without finding the parathyroid adenoma. The routine frozen section enables experience and rapport to develop between pathologists and surgeons. The occasional chastening misidentification of a parathyroid at operation underpins this choice. Thyroid tissue and parathyroid tissue with acinar structures and eosinophilic pseudo colloid can be misidentified by frozen section analysis.

3.12.8 Visual Enhancement

The gamma probe with SESTAMIBI is used by some surgeons to assist in determining the location and completeness of parathyroidectomy and to confirm that a resected specimen is gamma particle avid. In the past, methylene blue IV was used to enhance the appearance of parathyroid glands during operation. More recently, immunofluorescent techniques have been reported as well. The cure of 96% of patients with primary hyperparathyroidism with or without the use of these techniques is dependent on surgical experience.

3.12.8.1 Mobilisation and Resection

One aims for an R0 resection of the parathyroid adenoma with the gland capsule intact. This avoids the risk of parathyromatosis, which would prevent the cure of hyperparathyroidism. The process involves dissecting the patient from the parathyroid by retracting and dissecting the tissues that surround it. Inadequate exposure can lead to risky dissection of the parathyroid under tension. Care needs to be taken with multi-fronded, cystic and bilobed parathyroids, which can lead to the retention of functionally active parathyroid tissue.

3.12.8.2 Capsular vs. wider Fat Resection

Most surgeons would perform a capsular dissection of a benign parathyroid adenoma. Careful microscopic examination of the adventitial fat around parathyroids will show small parathyroid rests of parathyroid tissue; these may give rise to persistent or recurrent disease.

3.12.8.3 Correlation with Pre-Operative Expectations

Before completion of parathyroid exploration, it is important to review the biochemistry and imaging to make sure that an appropriate parathyroid or parathyroids have been excised, which fits the clinical presentation and, particularly, the expectations from imaging. If this does not add up, then further exploration is required. One example is a high undescended parathyroid antero-inferior to the submandibular gland [9].

3.12.8.4 Rapid PTH Assay

Some surgical units rely on the intraoperative PTH assay to demonstrate biochemical cure. In some cases, this may prompt the need for further exploration. Surgeons can achieve high cure rates with or without the use of these techniques. Sometimes the rapid PTH assay can produce misleading results due to the shortcomings of the technique and its interpretation, including slow-falling PTH in the elderly and those with renal impairment. Intra-operative PTH measurement may be useful in selected cases with unusual anatomical variants. Sometimes internal jugular vein sampling may assist with the lateralisation of the missing adenoma.

3.12.8.5 Weighing the Parathyroid

Portable milligram scales have become available and inexpensive online. Either the surgeon or the pathologist should weigh glands trimmed of fat to determine their size compared to a normal parathyroid (30–60 mg). Glands weighing more than 300 mg are reassuring, but resection of smaller glands of appropriate appearance may be curative.

3.12.8.6 Parathyroid Marking

When performing sub-total parathyroidectomy and there is potential for re-exploration in the future for recurrent disease, parathyroid gland marking may assist in finding glands and can be achieved with a prolene suture at the non-vascular pole crossed by a medium LIGACLIP®.

3.12.8.7 Non-standard Location Strategy

When the parathyroid thought to be the cause of hyperparathyroidism is not discovered, there are a number of scenarios that need to be considered with a measured and stepwise series of explorations to be carried out.

3.12.8.8 Biopsy of Normal Parathyroids

The number and location of already discovered normal parathyroids must be considered. Some surgeons perform the biopsy and frozen section to confirm normal parathyroids. This can lead to hypoparathyroidism but if performed carefully is powerful evidence of correct identification by exclusion of the missing parathyroid. The technique is to excise the smallest possible amount of parathyroid tissue (not fat) from the non-vascular pole. This is less than 1 mm placed on a suture pack cardboard pledget and immediately immersed into saline solution. An experienced pathologist can cut a small section or imprint the tissue directly onto a slide for the identification of neuroendocrine cells.

3.12.8.9 One Missing Gland

If three normal parathyroids have been seen, then attention is directed to the usual and variant locations of the missing parathyroid (Fig. 3.4). Care needs to be taken to ensure that the missing parathyroid is determined to be superior or inferior. The relationship of the other parathyroid to the recurrent laryngeal nerve above and lateral (superior) and below and medial (inferior) will help. The 'Law of Symmetry' may assist by deducing the level and anatomical plane from the contralateral gland if seen. If there is no parathyroid seen in the usual locations, then variant locations for the parathyroid should be explored. For missing superior parathyroid, the upper pole should be mobilised to enable a more thorough exploration of the cervical oesophagus, Ligament of Berry and the Cave of Reeve. One unusual location is lateral to the superior thyroid artery at or just

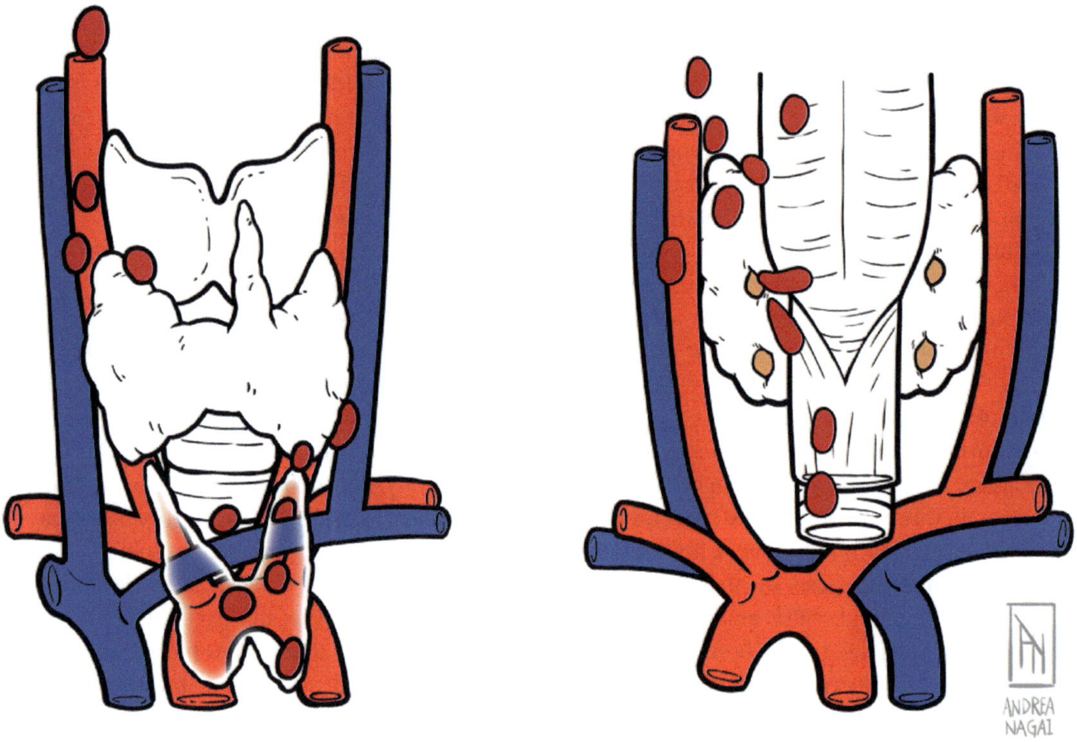

Fig. 3.4 From the left; anterior and posterior views of typical and most frequent aberrant locations of parathyroid adenomas. Illustrator: Andrea Naga

above the superior extent of the thyroid gland, and occasionally, a parathyroid may be found posterior to the superior thyroid artery proper. Parathyroids may be found deep to the recurrent laryngeal nerve and embedded in clefts at the junction of the tubercle of Zuckerkandl and the upper thyroid pole and beyond the furthest extent of a long tubercle. The retro-oesophageal space is entered on the pre-vertebral plane lateral to the recurrent nerve taking steps to avoid stretching it. This can be explored from the post hyoid level to the superior mediastinum. Rarely one might 'follow the yellow brick road' with a vascular fat pedicle leading to the medial aspect of the carotid sheath. The parathyroid may lie on the surface of the common carotid artery or within the sheath in contact with the vagus nerve. The tissue of the lateral part of lymph node level VI along the course of the recurrent laryngeal nerve may contain the parathyroid.

In the case of a missing inferior parathyroid, the surface of the thyroid from the insertion of the inferior thyroid artery to the thyro-thymic tract should be explored. The gland may lie within the medial level VI lymph node group or partly embedded in the thyroid inferior pole close to the thyro-thymic tract. Occasionally, this missing gland may lie in the superior mediastinum, deep to the subclavian artery. The thyro-thymic tract on each side should be carefully defined from the lateral and deep aspects of this lymph node group and drawn up by careful dissection and the 'hand over hand' technique, clipping inferior thyroid veins as they are encountered. The fascial envelope of the thymus is well developed in younger patients, and the fat lobulation and colour distinguish the thymus from the medial level VI lymph nodes. Care should be taken with both recurrent laryngeal nerves during this mobilisation. The thymus has a characteristic pulsatile indrawing under tension due to its pericardial attachment. When the thymus is delivered, the anterior superior mediastinum is palpated onto the manubrium to search for parathyroids in that location. The inferior parathyroids may be intra-thyroid, and this will usually necessitate a hemithyroidectomy. The lobe should be incised with a 22 blade to demonstrate the excised parathyroid.

3.12.8.10 Two Missing Glands

If there are two normal parathyroids on one side, then attention is directed to the other side using the techniques described. Diagonally missing glands need careful determination of whether the missing glands are superior or inferior to determine where to concentrate the search. Two missing inferior glands require careful mobilisation of both thyrothymic tracts paying particular attention to avoiding devascularisation of normal glands. Missing superior glands need the full mobilisation of the superior thyroid poles as detailed above for a single missing superior parathyroid.

3.12.8.11 Three Missing Glands

If only one normal parathyroid has been found, then the exposure and exploration are not adequate; surgical exposure should be improved, and the assistance of an experienced colleague sought. In this scenario even with an adequate exploration, it is occasionally the case that parathyroids are not seen by the surgeon but may be found by the pathologists at cut-up or in histological sections.

3.12.8.12 Malignant Parathyroids and Very Large Parathyroids

If there is biochemical or imaging suspicion of a very large or malignant parathyroid, consideration should be given to resection of the parathyroid and thyroid lobe 'en bloc'. This might include the level VI lymph nodes as well but the additional benefit of this has not been demonstrated.

3.12.8.13 Clearing One Side Strategy

When the parathyroid adenoma that has been excised is of modest proportions, say in the 100–200 mg range, and there is borderline enlargement of the other parathyroids, a useful strategy is complete clearance of one side, including the thyro-thymic tract and thymus. This ensures that if a re-exploration is needed, then imaging and surgery should be more limited.

3.12.8.14 Parathyroid Implantation and Cryopreservation

If normal parathyroids are inadvertently devascularised or excised, they can be morcellated and suspended in saline for injection graft into the right sternomastoid with the implantation track marked by a medium LIGACLIP®. Cryopreservation is an institutionally based process that requires infrastructure and storage, and cryopreserved parathyroid grafts have a lower success rate than normal parathyroids.

3.12.8.15 Parathyroids beyond the Scope of Neck Exploration

If the steps described have been taken, the success of surgery ranges from 96% to 98%. Multigland, syndromal surgery and re-do surgery all have lower success rates but are still in the range of 85–90%, depending on the institution. It is reasonable to halt exploration once the usual steps in the neck have been carried out. It is important to put the preservation of voice and normal parathyroids at a high priority above surgical ego. 'Calling a friend' is a mature and sensible step, bearing in mind there is always in any surgical career, at any stage, someone with more experience who might be involved during the operation or in the aftermath. The most common scenario with a thorough exploration is for an unidentified mediastinal parathyroid. Proceeding to sternotomy without localisation is unwise. Many mediastinal parathyroids may be removed thoracoscopically. In countries with a wider range of individual parathyroid caseloads, missed parathyroids are most commonly in normal positions with misinterpretation of anatomy and limited exposure being the rule rather than the exception. The learning curve for independent parathyroid practice is 100 cases and beyond. There is always much to learn from this remarkably challenging, misleadingly simple disorder.

3.13 Surgical Outcome Measures

Intra-operative findings (abnormal parathyroids) can be supplemented by biochemical tests to ensure all hyperfunctioning tissue has been correctly identified and removed. A drop in PTH level to less than 50% of the pre-incision value after the removal of the last specimen is valuable in confirming the absence of remaining hyperfunctioning parathyroid tissue. In secondary hyperparathyroidism, iPTH is slower to fall than in the primary, and iPTH <10 at 30 min is ideal with a drop to <2 expected on post-operative day 1.

Longer-term success in parathyroid surgery is defined as normocalcaemia and generally (but not always) normal serum PTH at 6 months.

Persistent disease is described as ongoing elevation of serum calcium within 6 months of surgery. Recurrent disease refers to normal serum calcium followed by recurrent elevation of calcium after 6 months from surgery has passed. Studies of recurrence rates in parathyroid surgery are limited; however, they do demonstrate that recurrence is often detected between years 5 and 10 with a significant number occurring after 10 years. Life-long annual monitoring of iPTH and serum calcium is recommended.

3.14 Multi-Disciplinary Care and Ethical Considerations

Optimal care for patients with hyperparathyroidism entails diagnosis, severity assessment, determination of peri-operative risk, localization, resection and subsequent management of calcium homeostasis.

The surgeon should view this larger picture in concert with the family doctor, endocrinologist, renal physician, anaesthetist and other relevant specialists. The patient and their family need evidence-based advice regarding perioperative risks and the expected results of surgery.

The desire and ability to perform surgery with low morbidity and mortality must be weighed against modest benefits for older co-morbid patients with limited life expectancy [10]. Expanded management guidelines may cause 'mission creep'. The real benefits of correcting hyperparathyroidism may be over-stated by a technical enthusiast but equally understated by others.

Surgical caseload impacts the results. Many surgeons do fewer than five cases per annum. Localisation studies may lead to a false sense of surgical confidence. Conversely, limiting surgery to high-volume surgical units diminishes the geographic availability of parathyroid and other surgery. General surgeons can perform parathyroid surgery well at modest volumes when suitably trained. Collaborations between urban and regional surgeons should be encouraged.

Five Takeaways

1. Parathyroid disease is the third most common endocrine disorder after diabetes and thyroid disease. Primary hyperparathyroidism is the autonomous overproduction of parathyroid hormone (iPTH). Secondary hyperparathyroidism is a physiological response to renal failure and/or low vitamin D, and when autonomy develops, it becomes tertiary hyperparathyroidism.
2. The diagnosis in primary HPT is based on the history and elevated serum iPTH and calcium. Secondary HPT is diagnosed by marked iPTH elevation responding to low active vitamin D uraemic phosphate retention and hypocalcaemia.
3. Selection of surgical candidates is guided by the presence and severity of end-organ disease or the risk of these developing together with the assessment of perioperative risk.
4. Pre-operative imaging helps to predict ectopic or multi-gland hyperplasia and co-existing thyroid disease. It informs the scope of surgery including minimal access or four gland surgery as well as thyroidectomy and thymectomy if necessary.
5. Successful surgical exploration depends on detailed embryological and anatomical knowledge and systematic patient-gentle bloodless surgery.

References

1. Zavatta G, Clarke BL. Normocalcemic hyperparathyroidism: a heterogeneous disorder often misdiagnosed? JBMR Plus. 2020;4(8):e10391.
2. Marcocci C, Cetani F, Rubin MR, Silverberg SJ, Pinchera A, Bilezikian JP. Parathyroid carcinoma. J Bone Miner Res. 2008;23(12):1869–80.
3. Bilezikian JP, Brandi ML, Eastell R, Silverberg SJ, Udelsman R, Marcocci C, Potts JT Jr. Guidelines for the management of asymptomatic primary hyperparathyroidism: summary statement from the fourth international workshop. J Clin Endocrinol Metab. 2014;99(10):3561–9. https://doi.org/10.1210/jc.2014-1413.
4. Wilhelm SM, Wang TS, Ruan DT, Lee JA, Asa SL, Duh QY, Doherty GM, Herrera MF, Pasieka JL, Perrier ND, Silverberg SJ, Solórzano CC, Sturgeon C, Tublin ME, Udelsman R, Carty SE. The American association of endocrine surgeons guidelines for definitive management of primary hyperparathyroidism. JAMA Surg. 2016;151(10):959–68. https://doi.org/10.1001/jamasurg.2016.2310.
5. Steinl G, Kuo J. Surgical Management of Secondary Hyperparathyroidism. Kidney Int Rep. 2021;6(2):254–64.
6. Ishani, et al. Clinical outcomes after parathyroidectomy in a nationwide cohort of patients on hemodialysis. Clin J Am Soc Nephrol. 2015;10(1):90–7.
7. Sankaran S, Gamble G, Bolland M, Reid I, Grey A. Skeletal effects of interventions in mild primary hyperparathyroidism: a meta-analysis. JCEM. 2010;95(4):1653–62.
8. Gilmour JR. Grocers' research scholar the gross anatomy of the parathyroid glands. J Pathol Bacteriol. 1938;46(1):133–49. https://doi.org/10.1002/path.1700460113.
9. Lee JC, Mazeh H, Serpell J, Delbridge LW, Chen H, Sidhu S. Adenomas of cervical maldescended parathyroid glands: pearls and pitfalls. ANZ J Surg. 2015;85(12):957–61. https://doi.org/10.1111/ans.12017.
10. Bilimoria KY, Liu Y, Paruch JL, Zhou L, Kmiecik TE, Ko CY, Cohen ME. Development and evaluation of the universal ACS NSQIP surgical risk calculator: a decision aid and informed consent tool for patients and surgeons. J Am Coll Surg. 2013;217(5):833–2.e1-3. https://doi.org/10.1016/j.jamcollsurg.2013.07.385. Epub 2013 Sep 18. PMID: 24055383; PMCID: PMC3805776

Parotid

4

Laurent Fradet and Jonathan R. Clark

4.1 Scope of Disease

The parotid glands are paired major salivary glands encased by the parotidomasseteric fascia. They produce predominantly serous saliva, which is watery and represents about 25% of the daily unstimulated total production of saliva [1]. Saliva has several important functions including lubrication, dental protection, antimicrobial activity, solubilisation of taste molecules, and digestion through amylase [1].

The salivary secretory units are composed of secretory cells arranged in acini and surrounded by myoepithelial cells. Their secretions drain in progressively larger ducts: intercalated, striated, excretory, and collector. The parotid also contains lymph nodes, which are mainly distributed in the superficial lobe. Thus, both benign and malignant neoplasms arising from these tissues, along with inflammatory, infectious, and congenital causes, must be considered when investigating a parotid mass (Table 4.1).

4.1.1 Benign Salivary Neoplasms

Overall, 75% of parotid neoplasms are benign [1]. Although there are 11 different benign salivary neoplasms described in the most recent edition of the World Health Organisation Classification of Head and Neck Tumours [2], pleomorphic adenomas are by far the most common, representing about 45% of all salivary neoplasia [1]. Also known as "benign mixed tumour", its name is derived from the fact that it has epithelial, myoepithelial, and chondromyxoid components. Pleomorphic adenomas have a risk of malignant transformation, which typically happens a decade after the initial diagnosis, and are estimated to be around 5–15% [3]. These tumours are thus surgically excised at the time of diagnosis unless the patient has a limited life expectancy or overwhelming comorbidities. The recurrence rate following an appropriate resection is 2.9%, but increases to 26.9% in cases of capsule disruption during the procedure, and up to 80% with gross tumour spillage [3].

The second most common benign salivary neoplasms are Warthin tumours, otherwise known as *papillary cystadenoma lymphomatosum*. They comprise 10% of parotid tumours and are typically located in the parotid tail. Approximately 10% of them will be bilateral, and they are strongly associated with smoking. If they are asymptomatic and the clinical, radiological, and cytological features all point towards this

L. Fradet (✉)
Division of Otolaryngology, Faculty of Medicine, Université de Sherbrooke, CIUSSS de l'Estrie—CHUS, Sherbrooke, QC, Canada
e-mail: Laurent.Fradet@USherbrooke.ca

J. R. Clark
Department of Head and Neck Surgery, Sydney Head and Neck Cancer Institute, Chris O'Brien Lifehouse, The University of Sydney, Sydney, NSW, Australia
e-mail: Jonathan.Clark@lh.org.au

B. Ashford (ed.), *Head and Neck Surgery for General Surgeons*,
https://doi.org/10.1007/978-981-19-7900-2_4

Table 4.1 Differential diagnosis of a parotid mass

Benign neoplasms	Malignant neoplasms	Others
Primary epithelial salivary neoplasms • Pleomorphic adenoma • Warthin tumor • Oncocytoma • Myoepithelioma • Basal cell adenoma • Canalicular adenoma • Cystadenoma • Ductal papilloma **Other neoplasms** • Hemangioma • Schwannoma • Neurofibroma • Lipoma	**Primary epithelial salivary tumours** • Mucoepidermoid carcinoma • Adenoid cystic carcinoma • Salivary duct carcinoma • Acinic cell carcinoma • Epithelial/myoepithelial carcinoma • Carcinoma ex pleomorphic adenoma • Polymorphous adenocarcinoma • Adenocarcinoma not otherwise specified • Secretory carcinoma • Lymphoepithelial carcinoma • Intraductal carcinoma • Basal cell adenocarcinoma • Clear cell adenocarcinoma • Cystadenocarcinoma • Adenosquamous carcinoma **Other tumours** • Nodal metastasis of a cutaneous primary • Lymphoma • Metastasis from another primary cancer (e.g. renal cell carcinoma) • Sarcoma	• Sialolithiasis • Acute/chronic parotitis • Juvenile recurrent parotitis • Benign lymphoepithelial cyst • Salivary duct cyst/ retention cyst • First branchial cleft cyst • Sialadenosis • Lymphovascular malformation • Reactive lymphadenopathy • Mycobacterial infection • Cat-scratch disease • Mumps • Toxoplasmosis • Actinomycosis • Sarcoidosis (uveoparotid fever) • Granulomatosis with polyangiitis • Kimura disease • Rosai-Dorfman disease • Kikuchi disease

diagnosis, Warthin tumours can be observed with serial ultrasounds. Although malignant transformation has been reported (50 cases worldwide), it is likely that these cases were misdiagnosed [3]. Warthin's tumours are part of a spectrum of diseases with oncocytosis and oncocytomas that capture technetium in a salivary scintigraphy, due to the high mitochondria content of their oncocytic cells [4].

The other benign tumours, such as myoepitheliomas and basal cell adenomas, are uncommon and do not have specific clinical characteristics. Haemangiomas must be considered in the paediatric population. Facial nerve primary neoplasms, such as schwannomas, and parotid lipomas, are rarely encountered.

Table 4.2 Primary tumour staging of major salivary gland malignancies, AJCC manual, eighth edition

T stage	Description
Tx	The primary tumour cannot be assessed
T0	No evidence of primary tumour
Tis	Carcinoma in situ
T1	Tumour 2 cm or less in greatest dimension, without extraparenchymal extension
T2	Tumour lager than 2 cm but smaller than 4 cm in greatest dimension, without extraparenchymal extension
T3	Tumour larger than 4 cm and/or with extraparenchymal extension
T4a	Tumour invading the mandible, ear canal, and/or facial skin
T4b	Tumour invading the skull base, pterygoid plates, and/or encasing the carotid artery

4.1.2 Malignant Salivary Neoplasms

Malignant salivary neoplasms are even more diverse than benign neoplasms, with 22 different carcinomas described in the WHO classification [2]. The eighth edition of the American Joint Committee on Cancer (AJCC) staging for salivary malignancies is presented in Table 4.2.

Malignant salivary neoplasms display a wide range of aggressiveness, based on their degree of differentiation. While low-grade tumours have a good prognosis after complete resection and do not typically metastasise, high-grade tumours have a poor prognosis and require more extensive surgery and post-operative radiotherapy. Adjuvant chemotherapy is rarely given for primary salivary cancers, as its benefit is unproven [4].

Mucoepidermoid carcinomas are the most common primary salivary gland cancers, accounting for 35% of cases [1]. As the name suggests, they contain mucous, intermediate, and epidermoid cells. They are graded according to their composition (solid versus cystic) and the presence of perineural invasion, necrosis, mitosis, and anaplasia [1]. The MAML2 rearrangement is present in 82% of cases and is highly specific, which is helpful for diagnosis [5].

Adenoid cystic carcinoma is the second most common salivary malignancy. It is an unencapsulated tumour with a strong tendency for perineural invasion, which accounts for the high rate of positive margins and local recurrences (15–85%) [4]. Histologically, it grows in either a tubular, a cribriform, or a solid architecture, the latter having the worst prognosis. Another key feature of this tumour is its strong tendency to produce indolent distant metastases (25–55%), most commonly pulmonary, which may present years after the initial diagnosis [4].

Salivary duct carcinoma is typically regarded as the most aggressive salivary cancer, with rates of distant metastases of up to 75% [1]. Approximately 50% of them arise in the context of a carcinoma ex pleomorphic adenoma, i.e. from a pleomorphic adenoma that undergoes malignant transformation [6]. They typically harbour androgen receptors, and about 40% of cases demonstrate ERBB2 amplification [7]. This has been targeted with Trastuzumab, with promising initial reports, but it has not translated into routine treatment [8]. In the presence of nodal disease, the five-year disease-free survival is only 19% [9].

Acinic cell carcinomas comprise about 10–15% of salivary epithelial malignancies [1]. They almost exclusively affect the parotid. Although usually slow-growing and low-grade, local recurrence rates are around 35% [6].

Secretory carcinoma, previously known as "mammary analogue secretory carcinoma" (MASC), has similar histopathologic features to the secretory carcinoma of the breast. It is low-grade and harbours the pathognomonic *ETV6-NTRK3* gene fusion [7].

As discussed earlier, there are approximately 20 lymph nodes per parotid, which are mainly distributed in the superficial lobe [1]. These are the first echelon lymph nodes draining the skin of the upper face and scalp. In countries with high UV exposure and high proportions of Fitzpatrick I–II phototypes, such as Australia, metastatic cutaneous malignancies are the most common type of cancer presenting in the salivary gland [10]. These lymph nodes can also be a site of lymphoma, particularly in patients with Sjogren's disease.

4.1.3 Infectious, Inflammatory, and Miscellaneous Pathologies

Parotid cysts are not uncommon and may be challenging to distinguish from cystic neoplasms. They typically have no solid component and hence a diagnosis is unlikely to be definitive on cytology. In all parotid tumours, it is essential to match the clinical features with imaging and cytology. Understanding the nuances of these rare and diverse lesions requires considerable experience. If there is any doubt, the patient should be referred to a head and neck specialist surgeon for assessment.

The other most common diagnoses of this category are discussed in the section "non-surgical pathologies and management".

4.2 Key Elements of History

A thorough history is the first step in investigating any head and neck pathology. The patient's age will influence the most likely diagnosis, with malignancy being more common with advanced age.

There are no definite associations between smoking or alcohol consumption and parotid cancer, however, tobacco use is associated with Warthin tumours. A history of exposure to ionising radiation increases the likelihood of primary parotid cancer, and UV solar exposure increases the risk of metastatic cutaneous squamous cell carcinoma and melanoma. The surgeon should question the patient on any prior head and neck cutaneous lesion resection, especially from the scalp, forehead, ear, and periocular areas. Patients with a history of immunosuppression, in particular solid organ transplantation, are at very high risk of cutaneous malignancy and parotid metastases compared to the general population. A history of autoimmune disease may be relevant, especially Sjogren's syndrome. This syndrome may present with a range of parotid disorders such as parotitis, severe sialectasis, benign lymphoepithelial lesions, and non-Hodgkin's lymphoma. Anticholinergic medications, radioactive iodine therapy, and recent systemic illness predispose to acute parotitis.

The history of the present illness should include a detailed chronology of the mass and associated symptoms such as pain, infection, skin involvement, associated lymphadenopathy, weight loss, and lethargy. The surgeon should specifically ask for any history of facial weakness/paralysis or sensory disturbance (pain, paraesthesia, dysesthesia, anaesthesia) in the distribution of the auriculotemporal and great auricular nerves. A relapse-remitting pattern may suggest repetitive inflammation of reactive lymphadenitis. Progressive masses are of concern for malignancy.

4.3 Clinical Examination Pearls

A full head and neck examination, including the scalp and facial skin, is warranted for every case of parotid mass. Note should be made of the patient's skin type and evidence of generalised sun damage, as up to 24% of metastatic cutaneous cancers arise from unknown primary cutaneous sites in patients with widespread actinic changes [11]. Skin examination should focus not only on current lesions but also on scars that could indicate previous excisions. Examination of the ear canal may rarely demonstrate invasion in cases of malignancy, or that in fact, the primary cancer arises from the ear canal skin with subsequent parotid invasion through the fissures of Santorini or the foramen of Huschke [1]. Examination of the pharynx may demonstrate a fullness of the peritonsillar area in cases of parapharyngeal extension of the tumour. In very rare instances, a deep lobe parotid tumour may invade the post-styloid parapharyngeal cranial nerves. Thus, it is good practice to test the integrity of cranial nerves IX, X, XI, and XII as part of the examination.

Palpation of the parotid will reveal the size of the mass, its approximate location, and its mobility. The firmness and mobility of the mass are important in raising the suspicion of malignancy. Adherence to the overlying skin is a concerning feature and important to note in surgical planning. Palpation of the neck will reveal the presence of clinically involved nodal metastases.

Examination of the facial nerve function is a key element for every case. The function of all five branches of the nerve should be routinely assessed as demonstrated in Fig. 4.1. Any weakness should be documented and is very indicative of an underlying malignant process with facial nerve invasion, which occurs in 12–15% of malignancies at presentation [4]. The House-Brackmann scale has traditionally been used to describe the degree of facial nerve palsy in the surgical literature [12]. It was however designed specifically to grade facial nerve recovery following vestibular schwannoma surgery and, thus, is not optimal to describe acute or subacute palsies. The Sunnybrook Facial Grading System describes the resting symmetry, voluntary movement symmetry, and synkinesis of different regions of the face, and is the most commonly used scale in the rehabilitation literature [13]. Similarly, the eFACE scoring system, an electronic assessment scale described in 2015, also evaluates static, dynamic, and synkinetic parameters for each region of the face [14]. It can be used as a mobile phone electronic application and has a moderately strong agreement with the Sunnybrook scale [14].

Movement	Branches	Example
Wrinkling the forehead upwards	Temporal	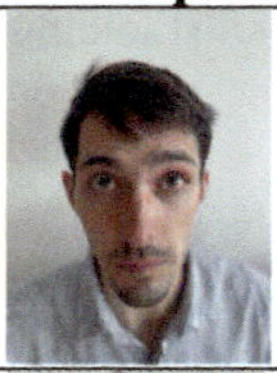
Closing the eyes forcefully	Temporal and zygomatic	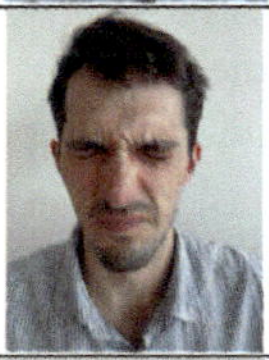
Smiling forcefully	Buccal	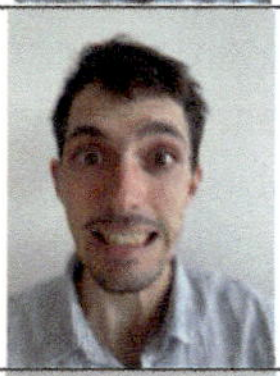
Opening the mouth widely	Buccal and marginal mandibular	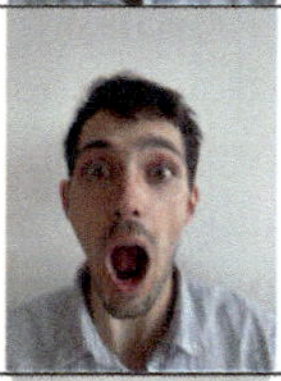
Blowing a kiss	Buccal and marginal mandibular	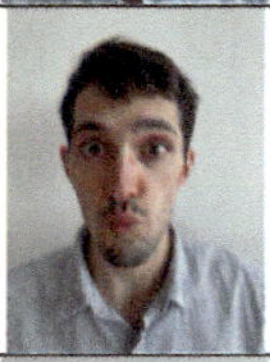
Frowning the lips down	Marginal mandibular	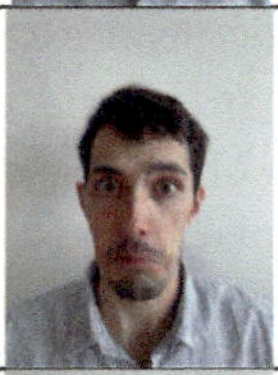
Showing the lower teeth forcefully	Marginal mandibular and cervical	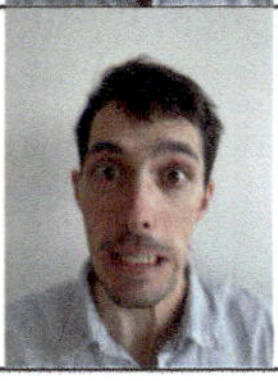

Fig. 4.1 Facial nerve function examination

4.4 Investigations and Limitations

4.4.1 Ultrasound

Ultrasound is a good first-line investigation for salivary masses. It provides excellent discrimination between the parotid tissue and most salivary gland tumours, which are typically hypoechoic to the surrounding parotid tissue. As most masses are in the superficial gland, they are easily visualised, and can be biopsied at the same time. Ultrasound is a useful adjunct to the surgeon to assess the extent and characteristics of the mass and as part of the postoperative follow-up. The drawbacks of ultrasound are the user variability and the difficulty assessing the deep parotid lobe because of shielding from the mandibular ramus.

4.4.2 CT and MRI

Cross-sectional imaging is useful in cases of suspected malignancy, extensive benign tumours, and some non-neoplastic pathologies such as sialolithiasis, for which a CT sialography with intraductal injection of contrast may be useful. Contrast-enhanced CT is a reasonable modality for metastatic skin cancers as it also allows the concurrent assessment of the cervical nodes and temporal bone. However, CT is a poor imaging modality for primary salivary gland tumours, which frequently have similar tissue radiodensity to the parotid tissue.

MRI is a superior imaging modality for salivary masses and should be used in cases of primary salivary gland malignancy. While the normal parotid parenchyma has a high T1 and a low T2 signal, pleomorphic adenomas tend to be hypointense on T1 and hyperintense on T2 weighting [1]. Most malignancies will be hypointense on T1 and T2 weighting but will enhance on post-gadolinium T1-weighted images with fat suppression [1]. The MRI is excellent for delineating the deep extension towards the parapharyngeal space and can also suggest perineural invasion of the facial or auriculotemporal nerves if abnormal contrast enhancement is present. The T1-weighted sequences are particularly useful in assessing the normal fat planes in the region of the stylomastoid foramen and the parapharyngeal fat lateral to the pharyngeal constrictor. MRI can also be used to distinguish true parapharyngeal tumours, usually accessible through a transcervical approach, from those that originate from the deep lobe of the parotid, that will require a transparotid approach.

4.4.3 Scintigraphy

Salivary technetium scintigraphy has a limited role nowadays. As mentioned previously, Warthin tumours and oncocytomas capture technetium [4].

4.4.4 Positron Emission Tomography (PET)

PET has a limited role in salivary gland tumours. Pleomorphic adenomas and Warthin tumour are frequently PET-avid, whereas many low-grade salivary malignancies may demonstrate low glucose metabolism [4].

4.4.5 Fine Needle Aspiration Biopsy

Studies suggest that salivary fine needle aspiration (FNA) biopsies have a sensitivity of 86–100% and a specificity of 90–100%, with accuracy to differentiate malignant from benign neoplasms of 81–100% [6]. They are an important part of the investigation of any salivary mass. However, since many neoplasms have overlapping cytologic features, the accuracy for diagnosing the exact subtype of malignancy is only 48–94% [6]. Cytology can be particularly unreliable in distinguishing some benign tumours from low- or intermediate-grade malignancies, such as acinic cell carcinoma and adenoid cystic carcinoma. Thus, they should always be considered in the context of the radiological and clinical features, and it is unwise to plan the extent of resection, or a concurrent neck dissection, based on cytology alone. The concept of triple assessment (clinical, radiological, and cytological) is of utmost importance. In order to optimise communication between pathologists and surgeons, the *Milan System for Reporting Salivary Gland Cytopathology* [6] should be employed (Table 4.3).

4.4.6 Core Needle Biopsy

A core needle biopsy may be helpful in cases of undiagnostic FNA as it is more sensitive (96%) and specific (100%), with only 1.6% of specimens considered non-diagnostic [4]. While FNAs may have enough material (in the cellular block) to proceed to immunohistochemical and molecular diagnostic studies, a core needle biopsy will typically provide more material to do so. The cli-

Table 4.3 Milan classification of salivary cytology (inspired by Faquin et al. 2018)

Category	Description	Risk of malignancy (%)	Typical management
I. Non-diagnostic	The material did not provide enough cells to suggest a diagnosis	25	Clinical and radiologic correlation/repeat FNA
II. Non-neoplastic	The material is suggestive of an inflammatory or another non-neoplastic pathology	10	Clinical and radiologic correlation, ± treatment of the underlying condition
III. Atypia of undetermined significance	Cytologic atypia that are not sufficient to diagnose a neoplasm, but that are suspicious for it	20	Repeat FNA or proceed to surgery
IV. Neoplasm			
IVA. Benign	The material meets the cytologic diagnostic criteria for a benign neoplasm	<5	Surgery (versus clinic follow-up with radiologic correlation)
IVB. Salivary gland neoplasm of uncertain malignant potential (SUMP)	The material is diagnostic of a neoplasm but lacks specific diagnostic features to suggest a precise diagnosis	35	Surgery
V. Suspicious for malignancy (SM)	The material is highly suggestive of a malignancy; must indicate which diagnosis is suspected or the differential diagnosis	60	Surgery
VI. Malignant	The specimen is diagnostic of a salivary malignancy; the type and the grade should be specified	90	Surgery

nician should inform the patient of the risk of facial nerve damage during this procedure. Although concerns for tumour seeding have been raised with this procedure, a systematic review of the literature has revealed only two cases of seeding along the core needle biopsy tract reported worldwide [15].

4.5 Surgical Management and Risks

As most parotid masses will require surgical resection, parotidectomy is a common head and neck procedure. Preoperative counselling must include a thorough discussion with the patient on the potential complications, as listed below.

The procedure is performed under general anaesthesia. Before prepping and draping, subdermal facial nerve integrity monitoring (NIM) electrodes are typically inserted (Fig. 4.2c). Many studies suggest that the rate and severity of temporary facial nerve palsy are reduced with its use [16]. The surgeon should test the integrity of the circuit with gentle taps on the inserted electrodes and confirm with the anaesthetist that any muscle paralysis has worn off or been reversed before the beginning of the procedure.

The parotidectomy is typically done through a modified Blair incision (Fig. 4.2a). In cases where the dissection will be more extensive, a superior hairline extension may be added (Fig. 4.2b). Alternatively, a facelift incision, with the extension of the inferior limb towards the posterior hairline rather than in a neck crease, may be employed.

Following the incision, an anterior skin flap is elevated either in the plane just deep or superficial to the superficial muscular aponeurotic system (SMAS), depending on the surgeon's preference (Fig. 4.2d). The great auricular nerve is encountered during this elevation. While the posterior branch can be preserved, the anterior branches need to be sacrificed to access the parotid bed, which account for the postoperative numbness.

The next surgical steps will vary depending on whether an antegrade, retrograde, or focused dissection approach is chosen. While the antegrade approach is the most common, the surgeon should be familiar with all of these.

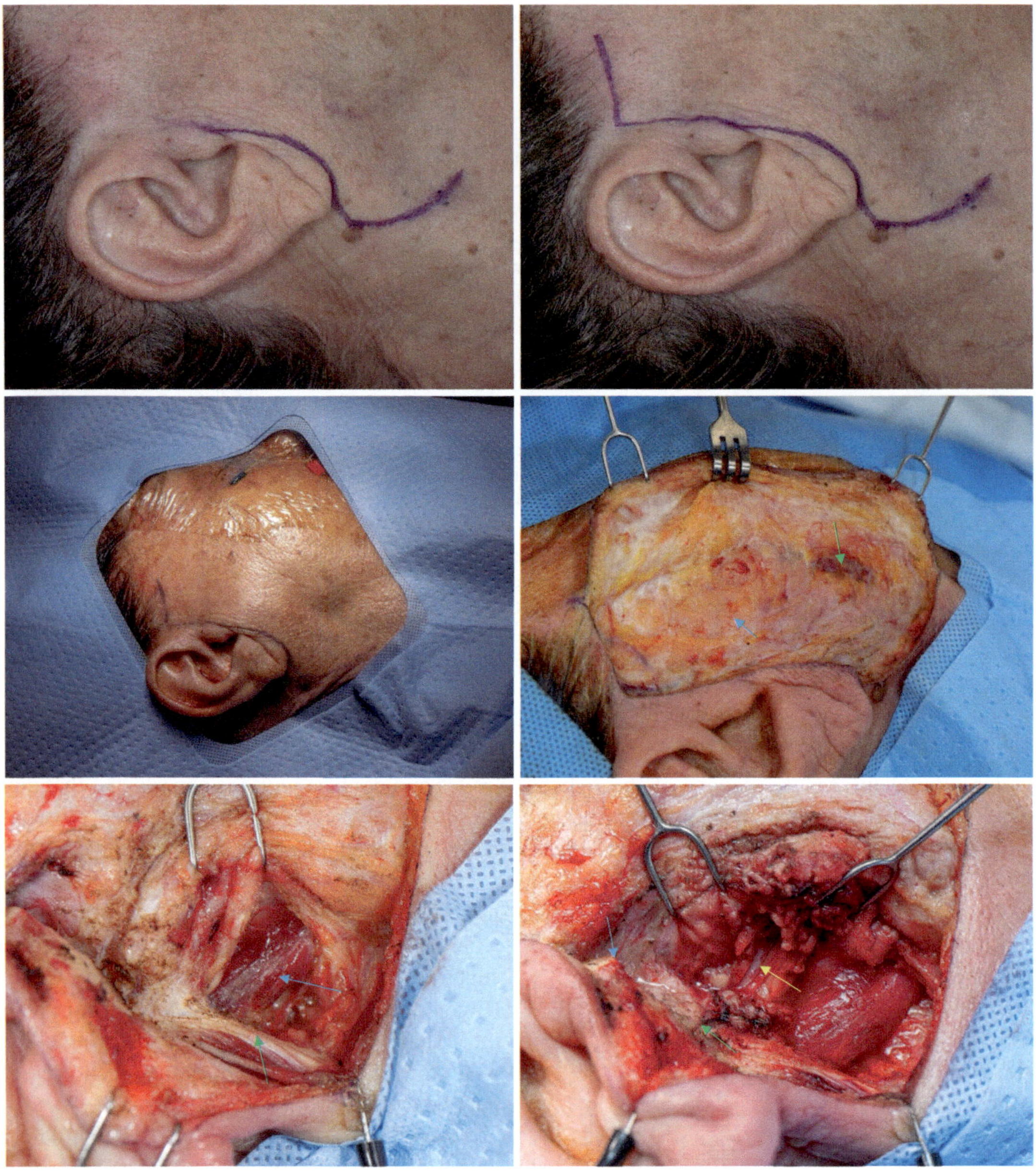

Fig. 4.2 Parotidectomy: surgical steps. (**a**) Modified Blair incision. (**b**) Optional anterior hairline extension for cases requiring a more extensive dissection. (**c**) Draping and NIM insertion. The ipsilateral face is included in the sterile field to notice any facial twitching during the procedure. (**d**) Elevation of the skin flap, either deep or superficial to the SMAS. The parotid fascia (blue arrow) and masseteric fascia (green arrow) are exposed. (**e**) Identification of posterior belly of digastric (blue arrow). The sternocleidomastoid muscle (green arrow) is retracted. (**f**) Pretragal dissection, with identification of the tragal pointer (blue arrow), tympanomastoid suture (green arrow), and facial nerve main trunk (yellow arrow). (**g**) Exposure of the *pes anserinus* (yellow arrow) and dissection of the facial nerve branches required for exposure of the tumour (in this case, the superior branches; blue arrows). (**h**) Resection of the tumour, originating from the superior portion of the deep lobe. This exposed the posterior border of the ascending ramus of the mandible (blue arrow) and required sacrifice of the external carotid artery (yellow arrow). (**i**) Dermofat graft inset. (**j**) Drain insertion and closure

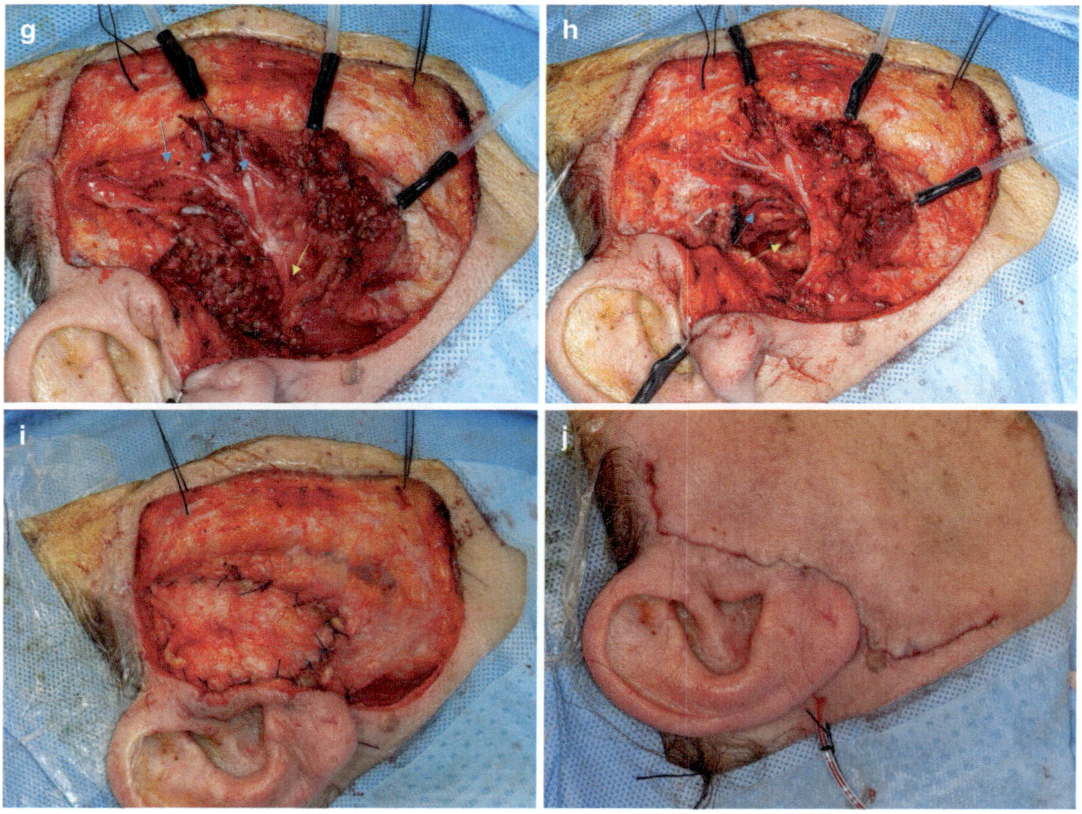

Fig. 4.2 (continued)

4.5.1 Antegrade Approach

In the antegrade approach, the facial nerve main trunk is identified proximally, and then the branches are dissected towards their distal end to the extent required for resection of the appropriate amount of tissue.

In order to safely identify the facial nerve trunk, three landmarks are typically exposed first:

- **Posterior belly of the digastric**: The fascia of the sternocleidomastoid muscle is incised and dissected anteriorly until the posterior belly of the digastric is identified (Fig. 4.2e). The main trunk of the facial nerve will be at the same depth as this landmark as it emerges from the stylomastoid foramen.
- **Tragal pointer**: The pretragal tissues are dissected layer by layer, with the use of a fine dissector and bipolar electrocautery. This exposes the tragal pointer, which is approximately 1 cm superficial and superior to the facial nerve main trunk (Fig. 4.2f).
- **Tympanomastoid suture:** The tympanomastoid suture, which corresponds to the junction of the tympanic and mastoid portions of the temporal bone, can be palpated at this stage (Fig. 4.2f). It is typically the most reliable and useful landmark, as the main trunk will be approximately 6 mm deep to it, at the same level.

The careful pretragal dissection is continued with these landmarks in view until the main trunk is identified (Fig. 4.2f). The NIM stimulation probe is helpful to confirm that the dissected structure corresponds to the main trunk, as it will result in the contraction of all the monitored branches. The dissection is carried anteriorly to the *pes anserinus*, where the main trunk splits into the superior and inferior divisions (Fig. 4.2g).

Following this, the extent of the facial nerve dissection is dictated by the location and size of the mass. Two common approaches are employed in salivary tumours located in the superficial lobe: limited parotidectomy (popularised by O'Brien) and complete superficial parotidectomy. In cases involving only the superior or inferior portions of the gland, only the associated branches need to be dissected, termed a limited parotidectomy. However, in cases where the tumour is seated more centrally in the gland, all the branches may need to be dissected. Dissection of the facial nerve should be done with a fine instrument, staying directly on the nerve, and taking care not to place unnecessary pressure on the branches (Fig. 4.2g). The feedback of the NIM may be helpful in assessing the degree of pressure put on the nerve.

Once the tumour has been excised with an appropriate circumferential margin of normal parotid parenchyma (Fig. 4.2h), hemostasis is confirmed. Depending on surgeon's preference, a dermofat graft may be harvested from the groin area to compensate for the loss of volume (Fig. 4.2i). This yields satisfactory aesthetic outcomes and reduces the risks of salivary leak, and potentially Frey's syndrome [17]. A drain is inserted, the deep layer of the skin flap is closed using a resorbable stitch such as 3–0 polyglactin, and the superficial layer reapproximated using 4–0 resorbable monofilament suture (Fig. 4.2j).

4.5.2 Retrograde Approach

The retrograde approach was described by Sistrunk in 1921, and further characterised by Richardson in 1975 [18]. In this approach, after skin flap elevation, a distal branch is identified under the parotidomasseteric fascia and dissected retrogradely towards the main trunk. The buccal branch is usually found over the masseter muscle, and the marginal mandibular, over the body of the mandible, superficial to the facial vessels [18]. Subsequent branches can be dissected as required.

Some studies suggest that the "cut-suture time" and the volume of healthy tissues dissected are lower with the retrograde approach, with comparable rates of temporary and permanent facial nerve palsies [18]. This approach is particularly useful if access to the main trunk through pretragal dissection is limited by the location of the mass, or in revision surgery, where the main trunk has already been dissected. Head and neck surgeons should thus be familiar with both the antegrade and retrograde approaches and opt for the most appropriate one for each case.

4.5.3 Focussed Approaches

Two focussed approaches have been described: the extracapsular dissection, popularised by McGurk, and the focussed tumour dissection, described by Clark. In the extracapsular approach, instead of actively finding the facial nerve and dissecting it, the parotid mass and a cuff of the surrounding normal tissue are resected [19]. In contrast, the focussed tumour dissection actively identifies the peripheral facial nerve branches in proximity to the tumour and then performs a limited dissection of the nerve to ensure an appropriate tumour margin [20]. These approaches have very low rates of facial nerve injury and other complications, such as Frey's syndrome, in experienced hands. They also avoid the need of sacrificing branches of the great auricular nerve. However, they should only be employed by surgeons with substantial experience using conventional parotidectomy approaches.

4.5.4 Deep Lobe and Parapharyngeal Surgery

The deep lobe is defined as any portion of the parotid lying deep to the facial nerve. It extends into the prestyloid parapharyngeal space. Access to this anatomical area is limited by both the facial nerve and the mandibular ramus (Fig. 4.2h).

Deep lobe parotid tumours should be distinguished from primary parapharyngeal tumours, which arise from salivary gland rests. While the former will often require a transparotid approach with dissection of the facial nerve, the latter can be approached using a purely transcervical approach in most instances. Typically, for deep lobe tumours, the superficial parotid will be elevated, and the entire facial nerve dissected and retracted to gain access to the deep lobe. A nasotracheal intubation will allow closure of the jaw and subluxation of the temporomandibular joint, thus providing better access if the mass is extending medial to the mandibular ramus. The styloid process can also be resected to improve access. In cases of malignancy, to obtain proper margins and to gain control of the full course of the carotid artery to the skull base, a mandibulotomy may be required.

4.5.5 Postoperative Course and Potential Complications

Following parotidectomy, most clinicians will recommend a short hospitalisation. However, systematic reviews of the literature suggest that ambulatory parotidectomies have the same complication rates in selected patients [21].

Patients should be counselled preoperatively of the expected postoperative anaesthesia of the great auricular nerve territory. While it typically improves postoperatively, it is not completely reversible, but generally causes minimal morbidity [22].

Facial nerve damage is the most feared complication of parotidectomy. It can either happen through neuropraxic damage because of pressure and devascularisation during dissection, in which case the damage is usually transient, or through disruption of branches, which will be permanent. The incidence of transient facial palsy following superficial parotidectomy depends on the underlying pathology and the extent of resection, and varies between 25 and 60%, whereas permanent palsy is reported in 2–6% of cases [23]. Facial nerve transection should be recognised during surgery and treated by coaptation of the nerve endings using epineural sutures. In cases where tension-free anastomosis is impossible, an interposition nerve graft, often from the great auricular nerve, can be used. If the injury results in incomplete eye closure, adequate eye care with artificial tears and lubricating ointment is paramount to prevent exposure keratitis.

Sialoceles and salivary fistulas are typically self-resolving, but persistent cases can be addressed through pressure dressing, aspirations, or intraglandular botulinum toxin injections under ultrasound guidance.

Frey's syndrome, or gustatory sweating, is defined as flushing and sudation in the surgical area during meals. It is due to aberrant reinnervation of parasympathetic fibres, normally innervating salivary tissue to stimulate salivary flow, to the postganglionic sympathetic nerves stimulating sweat production [1]. Although rarely used in clinical practice, the diagnosis can be confirmed with the Minor starch/iodine test. While its incidence is high (up to 57%), it rarely significantly affects the quality of life [4]. If so, it may be addressed with the local application of an antiperspirant or of a glycopyrrolate ointment, or with intradermal botulinum toxin injections [1].

First-bite syndrome, as its name indicates, causes pain in the parotid area with the first few bites of a meal. It is typically encountered with deep lobe and parapharyngeal surgeries rather than with superficial parotidectomies. Although its mechanism is still debated, it is believed to be due to denervation hypersensitivity of myoepithelial cells, producing a painful contraction at the beginning of each meal [1]. It is typically treated with carbamazepine.

4.6 Non-Surgical Pathologies and Management

4.6.1 Acute Parotitis

The serous parotid saliva lacks the antibacterial agents found in the mucinous saliva of the submandibular and sublingual glands (lysozyme, IgA, and sialic acid) [1]. Thus, retrograde migration of oral cavity bacteria may cause acute suppurative parotitis. Risk factors for this condition include dehydration, advanced age, diabetes, and recent surgery. Acute suppurative parotitis may also be triggered by the presence of a sialolithiasis, although these are rare, as 80% of salivary stones affect the submandibular gland [6]. The most common pathogens are *Staphylococcus aureus*, anaerobes, and streptococcus species [1]. Supportive treatment includes hydration, good oral hygiene, sialagogues, and massages. An anti-staphylococcal penicillin or first-generation cephalosporin is usually sufficient as first-line treatment for community-acquired cases, but the possibility of methicillin-resistant *Staphylococcus aureus* should be kept in mind, and treatment should be tailored to the clinical severity of the infection, the clinical response, and microbial culture and sensitivity.

Acute nonsuppurative parotitis is most commonly caused by viral infections such as mumps, mononucleosis, and cytomegalovirus (CMV), and is treated with conservative measures.

4.6.2 Juvenile Recurrent Parotitis

Juvenile recurrent parotitis is an idiopathic condition affecting children. It typically presents as a nonobstructive, nonsuppurative, and unilateral recurrent parotitis. Sialoendoscopy is both diagnostic, demonstrating narrowed ducts with blanched walls, and therapeutic, through lavage, ductal dilation, and corticosteroid irrigation [1]. This condition resolves at puberty in almost all cases.

4.6.3 Sjögren's Syndrome

Sjögren's syndrome causes xerostomia and xeropthalmia. It can be isolated (i.e. primary) or associated with rheumatologic conditions such as rheumatoid arthritis (i.e. secondary). Multiple diagnostic criteria have been published, which usually include serologic (anti-Ro/SSA antibody) or histopathologic (minor salivary gland lymphocyte focus score $\geq$ 1) evidence of underlying auto-immune disease and clinical tests. It is usually treated with a combination of artificial tears, salivary substitute, sialogogues, and referral to a rheumatologist for consideration of systemic treatment [24]. It requires long-term follow-up because of the underlying risk of lymphomatous transformation [1].

4.6.4 Benign Lymphoepithelial Cysts

These asymptomatic cystic lesions are typically caused by the human immunodeficiency virus (HIV), although they may also be seen in seronegative patients. This condition is often bilateral, and it may be the first manifestation leading to a diagnosis of HIV. Thus, any patients with clinical, radiologic, and/or histologic features suggesting this diagnosis should have a serologic HIV test as part of the investigation [25]. It typically responds to antiviral therapy but may require serial aspirations, sclerotherapy, or even parotidectomy in refractory cases [1].

4.6.5 Granulomatous Sialadenitis

Multiple infectious conditions cause salivary granulomas, such as actinomycosis, mycobacterial infection, cat-scratch disease, and toxoplasmosis [6]. Sarcoidosis may present as uveoparotid fever (Heerfordt syndrome), with the classic association of uveitis, nonsuppurative parotitis, pyrexia, and facial nerve palsy.

4.6.6 Sialadenosis

Sialadenosis, also known as sialosis, is a chronic, diffuse, bilateral swelling of parotid glands, without focal underlying masses. It is associated with multiple conditions including obesity, malnutrition, alcoholism, diabetes, hepatic disease, and certain drugs, such as antihypertensives [1].

Takeaway Points

1. While the differential diagnosis of a parotid mass is very broad, approximately 75% of them will be benign, of which pleomorphic adenomas are by far the most common.

2. Salivary malignancies can be classified as low- and high-grade, which will influence the prognosis and extent of treatment required.
3. The investigation of a parotid mass requires the integration of clinical, radiological (ideally with MRI), and cytological (Milan classification) characteristics. Most of them will require surgical resection to obtain a definitive diagnosis.
4. Superficial parotidectomy is most often accomplished through an antegrade facial nerve dissection. The typical anatomical landmarks for the facial nerve main trunk are the posterior belly of the digastric, the tragal pointer, and the tympanomastoid suture, the latter being the most reliable and useful.
5. Retrograde and focused dissections are other surgical approaches that may be of benefit in some clinical situations, and thus should be part of the armamentarium of the head and neck surgeon.

Acknowledgement The authors would like to acknowledge Dr. Murray Stokan, MBBS, BSc, FANZCA, for the photographic documentation of this chapter.

References

1. Flint PW, Haughey BH, Lund VJ, Thomas Robbins K, Regan Thomas J, Lesperance MM, et al. Cumming's otolaryngology - head and neck surgery. 7th ed. Elsevier; 2020. p. 3568.
2. El-Naggar AK, Chan JKC, Grandis JR, Takata T, Slootweg PJ. Tumours of salivary glands. In: WHO classification of head and neck tumours. 4th ed. Lyon: IARC; 2017. p. 159–202.
3. Hellquist H, Paiva-Correia A, Vander Poorten V, Quer M, Hernandez-Prera JC, Andreasen S, et al. Analysis of the clinical relevance of histological classification of benign epithelial salivary gland tumours. Adv Ther. 2019;36(8):1950–74.
4. Bradley PJ. Salivary gland neoplasms, vol. 78. 1st ed. Basel: Karger; 2016. p. 205. (Advances in otorhinolaryngology;.
5. Badlani J, Gupta R, Balasubramanian D, Smith J, Luk P, Clark J. Primary salivary gland malignancies: a review of clinicopathological evolution, molecular mechanisms and management: Primary salivary gland cancers. ANZ J Surg. 2018;88(3):152–7.
6. Faquin WC, Rossi ED, Baloch Z, Barkan GA, Foschini MP, Kurtycz DFI, et al. The Milan system for reporting salivary gland cytopathology [internet]. Cham: Springer International Publishing; 2018. [cited 2021 Nov 3]. https://doi.org/10.1007/978-3-319-71285-7.
7. Seethala RR, Stenman G. Update from the 4th edition of the World Health Organization classification of head and neck tumours: tumors of the salivary gland. Head Neck Pathol. 2017;11(1):55–67.
8. Schmitt NC, Kang H, Sharma A. Salivary duct carcinoma: an aggressive salivary gland malignancy with opportunities for targeted therapy. Oral Oncol. 2017;74:40–8.
9. Luk PP, Weston JD, Yu B, Selinger CI, Ekmejian R, Eviston TJ, et al. Salivary duct carcinoma: Clinicopathologic features, morphologic spectrum, and somatic mutations: salivary duct carcinoma. Head Neck. 2016;38(S1):E1838–47.
10. Subramaniam N, Gao K, Gupta R, Clark JR, Low T, (Hubert). Trends in parotidectomy over 30 years in an Australian tertiary care center. Head Neck. 2020;42(10):2905–11.
11. Ebrahimi A, Moncrieff MD, Clark JR, Shannon KF, Gao K, Milross CG, et al. Predicting the pattern of regional metastases from cutaneous squamous cell carcinoma of the head and neck based on location of the primary. Head Neck. 2010;32(10):1288–94.
12. House JW, Brackmann DE. Facial nerve grading system. Otolaryngol Head Neck Surg. 1985;93(2):146–7.
13. Ross BG, Fradet G, Nedzelski JM. Development of a sensitive clinical facial grading system. Otolaryngol Head Neck Surg. 1996;114(3):380–6.
14. Gaudin RA, Robinson M, Banks CA, Baiungo J, Jowett N, Hadlock TA. Emerging vs time-tested methods of facial grading among patients with facial paralysis. JAMA Facial Plast Surg. 2016;18(4):251–7.
15. Shah KSV, Ethunandan M. Tumour seeding after fine-needle aspiration and core biopsy of the head and neck - a systematic review. Br J Oral Maxillofac Surg. 2016;54(3):260–5.
16. Graciano AJ, Fischer CA, Coelho GV, Steck JH, Paschoal JR, Chone CT. Facial nerve dysfunction after superficial parotidectomy with or without continuous intraoperative electromyographic neuromonitoring: a prospective randomized pilot study. Eur Arch Otorhinolaryngol. 2018;275(11):2861–8.
17. Petrides GA, Subramaniam N, Pham M, Clark JR. Reducing the morbidity of parotidectomy for benign pathology. ANZ J Surg. 2020;90(11):2315–21.
18. Stankovic P, Wittlinger J, Timmesfeld N, Stephan SH, Georgiew R, Günzel T, et al. Antero- vs. retrograde nerve dissection in parotidectomy: a systematic review and meta-analysis. Eur Arch Otorhinolaryngol. 2018 Jun;275(6):1623–30.
19. McGurk M, Thomas BL, Renehan AG. Extracapsular dissection for clinically benign parotid lumps: reduced morbidity without oncological compromise. Br J Cancer. 2003;89(9):1610–3.
20. Petrides GA, Clark JR. Focused tumour dissection: an alternative conservative parotidectomy approach. Br J Oral Maxillofac Surg. 2021;59(2):244–6.
21. Benito DA, Pasick LJ, Bestourous D, Thakkar P, Goodman JF, Joshi AS. Outpatient vs inpatient paroti-

dectomy: systematic review and m ETA-ANALYSIS. Head Neck. 2021;43(2):668–78.
22. Ryan WR, Fee WE. Long-term great auricular nerve morbidity after sacrifice during parotidectomy: Parotidectomy and great auricular nerve. Laryngoscope. 2009;119(6):1140–6.
23. Eviston TJ, Yabe TE, Gupta R, Ebrahimi A, Clark JR. Parotidectomy: surgery in evolution. ANZ J Surg. 2016;86(3):193–9.
24. Ramos-Casals M, Brito-Zerón P, Sisó-Almirall A, Bosch X, Tzioufas AG. Topical and systemic medications for the treatment of primary Sjögren's syndrome. Nat Rev Rheumatol. 2012;8(7):399–411.
25. Zanelli M, Zizzo M, Sanguedolce F, Annessi V, Ascani S. Benign lymphoepithelial cyst of the parotid gland: mind the underlying cause. Int J Surg Pathol. 2021;29(1):78–9.

Submandibular and Sublingual Gland

5

Mirko Manojlovic-Kolarski and Timothy Eviston

5.1 Introduction

The submandibular glands are paired major salivary glands occupying the submandibular triangle (level 1B). The sublingual glands, as the name suggests, are located on the floor of the mouth in close proximity to the lingual nerve and Wharton's duct (submandibular gland duct). The two glands sit adjacent to each other and are a primary source of saliva. The submandibular gland consists of deep and superficial lobes separated by the mylohyoid muscle. The sublingual glands are wholly located above the mylohyoid muscle; however, in the setting of certain pathologies (plunging ranula) can present as neck swelling due to a deficiency in the mylohyoid. Pathology of these salivary glands is common with acute and chronic infectious/inflammatory diseases (sialadenitis), stone disease (sialolithiasis), and rarely tumors being encountered in routine clinical practice. Critically, it must be remembered that not all swellings in the submandibular triangle are salivary gland in origin and consideration must be taken to rule out malignant lymphadenopathy from the oral cavity or oropharynx primary malignancies or an underlying lymphoproliferative disorder which may masquerade as submandibular gland swelling.

5.2 Key Elements of History

Given the location of these salivary glands, it is important to identify red flag symptoms of impending airway compromise in the setting of acute disease. A history of acute onset upper neck or floor of mouth swelling, drooling, or labored breathing is of particular concern. Submandibular and sublingual abscesses can present in this way.

Ludwig's angina, a cellulitis of the floor of the mouth, and angioedema do not involve the salivary glands directly but will also cause swelling of the sublingual space and are potential airway emergencies. If these red flag symptoms are present, the airway should be secured immediately via intubation or surgical airway. Once red flag symptoms have been ruled out,a full history can be obtained.

There are several broad categories of submandibular and sublingual gland pathology. The differential diagnosis is usually guided by the patient's history. Three main categories to consider are infectious, autoimmune, and neoplastic conditions (Table 5.1). Additionally, it is important to differentiate between pathology within the salivary gland versus an adjacent lymph node.

M. Manojlovic-Kolarski
Health Sciences North, Sudbury, ON, Canada

Northern Ontario School of Medicine, Sudbury, ON, Canada
e-mail: mmanojlovickolarski@nosm.ca

T. Eviston (✉)
Mater Private Hospital, Brisbane, QLD, Australia

Department of Surgical Subspecialties, Health Sciences North, Sudbury, Canada
e-mail: Tim.Eviston@mater.org.au

B. Ashford (ed.), *Head and Neck Surgery for General Surgeons*,
https://doi.org/10.1007/978-981-19-7900-2_5

Table 5.1 Differential diagnosis of submandibular mass or swelling

Infectious	Neoplastic
• Acute bacterial Sialadenitis	Benign
• Viral (ex. mumps, HIV)	• Pleomorphic adenoma
• Tuberculosis	• Basal cell adenoma
• Actinomyces	• Oncocytoma
• Abscess	Malignant
Inflammatory	• Mucoepidermoid carcinoma
• Sjogren's disease	• Adenoid cystic carcinoma
• IgG4-related disease	• Salivary duct carcinoma
• Sarcoidosis	• Acinic cell carcinoma
Other	• Carcinoma ex-pleomorphic adenoma
• Sialolithiasis	Metastatic lymph node
• Chronic sialadenitis	• Squamous cell carcinoma
• Sialadenosis	Lymphoma

Infections can involve the salivary glands themselves or adjacent structures that spread into the submandibular and sublingual spaces. Patients will have an acute presentation with other infectious symptoms (fever, redness, pain, and swelling). Sialadenitis, an infection of the glands themselves, can be viral or bacterial. Viral infections will typically be bilateral while bacterial infections are unilateral. Mumps will typically affect the parotid gland but can affect submandibular glands as well, however, it is not commonly seen except in unvaccinated individuals. Primary HIV infection can present with salivary gland swelling as well, and should be suspected based on potential exposure to infected blood. Bacterial infections are typically secondary to saliva stasis or obstruction. Staphyloccocus aureus is the most commonly isolated bacteria. This problem is typically seen in older patients [1].

Autoimmune conditions can frequently affect the salivary glands. Specific symptoms vary by disease. When the minor salivary glands are affected xerostomia is a common presenting symptom. Secondary infections can also occur due to strictures within the submandibular duct. Sjogren's disease presents with a classic triad of xerostomia, dry eyes, and bilateral salivary gland enlargement and most commonly affects women in their 40s and 50s. IgG4-related diseases, including Kuttner's tumor and Mikulicz's disease, are a group of idiopathic immune-associated diseases causing chronic, systemic inflammation, and pseudotumor formation. Kuttner's tumor is a sclerosing sialadenitis of the submandibular glands. Mikulicz's disease is defined by symmetric enlargement of the lacrimal, parotid, submandibular, and occasionally sublingual gland [2].

Salivary gland tumors are rare, but represent among the widest variety of tumor histologies.

In the submandibular gland, there is a roughly 50% split between benign and malignant tumors. The rate of malignant tumors is higher in the sublingual gland. It is often not possible to differentiate between benign and malignant tumors on history alone. However, there are certain features that should raise the concern for malignancy. Red flag symptoms include rapid growth, changes to the overlying skin, and signs of neurological dysfunction (specifically to the lingual, hypoglossal, or marginal mandibular nerve). Typically tumors present as slow-growing masses. The most common benign tumor is a pleomorphic adenoma. These tumors have a low, but tangible risk of malignant transformation. The two other most common malignant tumors are adenoid cystic and mucoepidermoid carcinoma. Adenoid cystic carcinoma has a predilection for neural invasion and may present with neuropathy.

Another important differential consideration is level 1B lymphadenopathy. Unlike the parotid gland, there are no lymph nodes contained within the submandibular and sublingual glands; rather the lymph nodes surround the gland and are contained within the submandibular space. Patients with lymphadenopathy due to local infections in the salivary glands, teeth, or oral cavity will present acutely and with pain, whereas those with lymphadenopathy from metastasis will typically present with painless masses. The submandibular space is a common site of metastatic spread for cancers from the oral cavity and skin. Oral cavity cancers arising from the floor of the mouth, anterior tongue, buccal, and gingival mucosa can drain to this area. Skin cancers arising from anterior facial skin including lips, cheek, and nose will also drain to this area. Occasionally, regional lymphadenopathy will present after the original tumor has already been treated. It is therefore important to obtain a history of previously treated skin or oral cavity cancers. Finally, a history of B-symptoms (fever, night sweats, and weight loss) should raise the suspicion of lymphoma.

A similar approach to history taking and differential diagnosis can be applied to pediatric patients, however with some exceptions. Specific consideration should be given to congenital vascular and lymphatic malformations, which commonly present within a beard distribution.

5.3 Clinical Examination Pearls

Examination of the submandibular and sublingual glands involves examination of the oral cavity, neck, and overlying skin. Oral cavity examination should include inspection of the submandibular (Wharton's) duct, which travels along the floor of the mouth and opens beside the tongue frenulum. General notes of the mucosa and dentition should be made. Dry mucosa and gingivitis can be signs of xerostomia. Drooling and pooling of secretions in the floor of the mouth can be signs of impending airway obstruction.

In cases where malignancy is suspected, inspection should include inspection of the floor of the mouth, tongue, buccal mucosa, and gingival mucosa for primary mucosal carcinomas. The skin of the anterior face should also be inspected for primary skin cancers or scars from previous excisions. The cheek, eyelid, nose, and lips can drain into level 1B. Neck palpation for lymphadenopathy should be included as part of every physical exam.

Bimanual palpation is particularly useful in evaluating submandibular masses and differentiating between primary salivary lesions and lymph nodes. The technique is performed by placing a gloved finger along the floor of the mouth while applying pressure with the other hand along the submandibular skin. Submandibular masses can be felt within the substance of the gland which is soft and rubbery. Lymph nodes will move separately from the gland. This technique is also useful for locating salivary stones, particularly small ones, within Wharton's duct and for identifying plunging ranulas that have traversed through the mylohyoid muscle.

When there is suspicion of Wharton's duct obstruction, the gland should be massaged or bimanually palpated to express saliva through Wharton's duct. Saliva should appear clear and mucoid. Purulent discharge is seen when there is an underlying infection. A large volume of expressed saliva can be a sign of partial obstruction. While the absence of saliva is seen in complete obstruction. It is often useful to compare salivary flow to the normal contralateral side.

There are other additional exam techniques that can be considered in specific situations.

If a high-grade malignancy is suspected, a cranial nerve exam focused on lingual, hypoglossal, and marginal mandibular nerve function can determine the presence of perineural spread along these nerves. Additionally, if a dental infection is suspected, the culprit tooth can be identified by gentle tapping on suspected teeth to elicit pain.

5.4 Investigations and Their Limitations

Ultrasound is an excellent first-line imaging modality for evaluating submandibular and sublingual pathology. It provides excellent visualization of the submandibular gland and any masses. In non-neoplastic pathologies, ultrasound provides information about the general composition of the gland that may aid in diagnosis. A hyperechoic gland can be a sign of early Sjogren's disease. A hypoechoic gland can be a sign of sialadenitis, while multiple hypoechoic or anechoic areas are seen in chronic inflammation or systemic illnesses such as lymphoma or HIV.

Duct dilation is a sign of obstruction that can be seen on ultrasound along with some stones.

Masses are evaluated to determine their size, borders, internal vascularity, and composition.

Often ultrasound can help distinguish between primary salivary gland tumors and level 1B lymph nodes. The additional benefit of ultrasound is the ability to perform diagnostic fine needle aspiration at the time of imaging. This is preferable to blind biopsy as it provides real-time information about the location of the biopsy needle.

CT scan is often the next step in imaging. This scan should be ordered with contrast for additional detail. It provides useful cross-sectional information about masses and adjacent anatomic structures. It can help differentiate infection and abscess from cysts by the presence of rim enhancement and fat stranding. Compared to MRI, CT scan has a superior bony definition which is useful when evaluating the relationship to the mandibular cortex and in identifying stones. It also provides excellent resolution when evaluating regional lymphadenopathy.

MRI is a useful adjunct imaging modality when evaluating neoplasms. It provides a superior assessment of soft tissues, nerves, and bone marrow. MRI can provide additional information for certain tumors. Pleomorphic adenoma will have a characteristic appearance on MRI that is hypointense on T1 and hyperintense on T2 and enhances with gadolinium. In adenoid cystic carcinoma, MRI can demonstrate signs of perineural spread along cranial nerves.

While each imaging modality provides useful information, none will be able to definitively differentiate between neoplasms. Therefore, a biopsy should be obtained in almost all circumstances. As an initial step, fine needle aspiration is sufficient, however, core biopsy is sometimes required. If a diagnosis of lymphoma is suspected, it is appropriate to do a core biopsy as the initial biopsy.

Other imaging modalities are rarely used. Sialography can assess obstruction along the course of Wharton's duct, however, it is an invasive procedure as it requires cannulation of the duct for contrast injection. Positron emission tomography (PET) is useful in assessing for distant metastases in the setting of known malignancy. The primary site in both benign (particularly neoplasms with high mitochondrial activity such as oncocytomas) and malignant neoplasms can show increased uptake on PET.

Bloodwork can be of assistance in specific situations. Routine CBC and chemistry panels can identify signs of infection, systemic illness, and dehydration. Autoimmune panels are indicated in the correct clinical situation. Sjogren's disease is associated with antinuclear antibodies (ANA), anti-Ro (SS-A), and anti-La (SS-B). HIV screening should be considered in cases with salivary gland swelling and potential pathogen exposure.

5.5 Surgical Management Including Risks

There are two general surgical approaches to the submandibular and sublingual gland: transcervical and transoral. Transcervical approaches are standard for submandibular tumors. Transoral approaches are used for sublingual tumors and the excision of distal stones. Both approaches and their specific risks will be described in detail. The general risks common to either approach should be discussed pre-operatively. These risks include bleeding, infection, injury to the hypoglossal and lingual nerve, and salivary fistula.

5.5.1 Transcervical Approach

In addition to submandibular tumors, this approach is used when removing the submandibular gland due to chronic or recurrent infections or symptomatic proximal salivary stones. The patient is positioned supine with the head turned to the contralateral side with a shoulder roll. The procedure is done under general anesthetic. Transoral intubation can be performed and the endotracheal tube should be taped to the corner of the contralateral lip. The incision is marked a minimum of 2 cm below the inferior margin of the mandible within a skin crease if one is present. This is done to avoid injury to the marginal mandibular branch of the facial nerve (MMBFN).

Once the incision is made, subplatysmal flaps are elevated to the level of the mandible. To avoid injury to the MMBFN and devascularization of the flap, it is important to raise this flap immediately deep to the platysma muscle, but not deeper.

Next, the MMBFN is identified. The nerve lies superficial to the facial artery and vein and within 1 cm of the antegonial notch. To protect the nerve, the facial vessels can be identified inferior to the nerve, ligated, and then reflected superiorly along with the superficial fascia. If this technique is used it is critical to be right on the gland tissue and be selective with the dissection technique (e.g., bipolar cautery or sharp dissection to avoid nerve injury through thermal injury). By dissecting deep into the facial vessels the nerve remains protected. This is known as the Hayes–Martin maneuver. Once the MMBFN is protected, the gland and level 1B neck contents are separated from the inferior edge of the mandible cortex. Here the proximal nerve to mylohyoid may be encountered. In a benign disease, capsular dissection will enable the gland to be liberated through traction with an Allis or Babcock forceps, which releases the capsular attachments and preserves the encountered nerves. At this point, the posterior aspect of the gland can be separated from the neck. First, the anterior border of the sternocleidomastoid muscle and the posterior belly of the digastric are identified here. The posterior belly of the digastric marks the posterior limit of the resection. Note that the posterior belly of the digastric muscle is a safe landmark to dissect over the top as it protects deeper nerves and vessels. Only the common facial vein will cross it superficially.

The next major step is to identify the lingual nerve, hypoglossal nerve, and Wharton's duct. To do this the free posterior edge of the mylohyoid must be identified and retracted anteriorly.

Deep to the mylohyoid muscle the hypoglossal nerve will lie inferiorly surrounded by venae comitans known commonly as ranine veins. The lingual nerve is superior and attaches to the submandibular gland via the submandibular ganglion. Wharton's duct is found between these nerves. Importantly, in a transcervical approach, the duct is superficial to the lingual and hypoglossal nerves. To complete a submandibular gland excision, the submandibular ganglion and Wharton's duct must be divided. The ganglion is typically divided first, with care taken to avoid injury to the lingual nerve. Once this is done a plane is developed superficial to the hypoglossal and lingual nerves. Wharton's duct is identified here and ligated. During this maneuver, it is crucial to stay superficial to the fascia overlying the hypoglossal and lingual nerves to avoid entering the oral cavity.

Once the anterior release is completed the submandibular gland still remains attached to the neck via the facial vessels. To identify these vessels the digastric muscle is traced out. The proximal facial vein will lie superficial to the digastric muscle and facial artery. The artery takes a deep course. Both these vessels are ligated to complete the resection. Proximally, the hypoglossal nerve will run within the triangle formed by the internal jugular vein, facial vein, and posterior belly of the digastric. It is worth noting that facial vessels can be dissected through the contents of the submandibular gland and left intact. The facial artery has a variable number of branches within the submandibular gland, the main ones being the one supplying the gland itself and the submental vessels.

Postoperatively the wound is irrigated. A multilayer closure is performed. Most surgeons elect to place a surgical drain that is removed when output is less than 30 cc in 24 hours.

5.5.2 Transoral Approach

A transoral approach is indicated for the removal of sublingual tumors and distal submandibular stones. The advantages of this approach are avoiding a neck scar and the ability to preserve a functional Wharton's duct.

The procedure is usually done under general anesthetic, however local anesthetic can be considered for cooperative patients. A local anesthetic approach is appropriate for distal stones that are easily palpable on the floor of the mouth. When done under general anesthetic, a transnasal intubation is preferable as it keeps the endotracheal tube away from the field. If the patient is intubated transorally, the tube should be positioned to the contralateral side, passing via the contralateral glossotonsillar sulcus. Paralysis is required to obtain adequate mouth opening, along with a bite block or a molt mouth retractor.

For sublingual gland excision, a floor-of-mouth incision is placed over the mass with care taken to avoid Wharton's duct when possible. An elliptical excision can be used to remove redundant mucosa. The sublingual gland is located immediately deep to the floor of the mouth mucosa and is superficial to the mylohyoid muscle. The gland is lateral to Wharton's duct and the lingual nerve. To ensure the protection of the duct as it courses through the sublingual gland, a lacrimal probe is used. It is important to gently pass the probe into the duct to avoid creating a false passage. To identify the duct and lingual nerve, blunt dissection with hemostasis is performed. In cases with a mass or ranula, the entire gland should be removed. If the duct is injured, a sialodochotomy (marsupialization) can be done to maintain salivary flow through the submandibular gland. The free edge of the marsupialized duct is sutured to the edge of the floor of the mouth mucosa using a 5–0 or 6–0 absorbable suture.

For stone removal, the patient should be adequately frozen with a topical and local anesthetic. It is generally best to avoid removing stones during an acute infection. Similar to the sublingual approach, Wharton's duct should be identified at the frenulum and cannulated with lacrimal probes. The probes are gradually increased in size to dilate the duct. A small stone can be expressed through the duct after dilation with massage. For large stones, it is often necessary to make an incision overlying the stone. In this situation, the procedure is akin to that of the sublingual mass excision.

Sialoendoscopy is a newer technique that has been developed for obstructive pathology, particularly stones. The advantage of this technique compared to other transoral techniques is that it allows visualization within the lumen of Wharton's duct. In addition to stone removal, sialoendoscopy can identify strictures that would otherwise be undetected. Current iterations use rigid sialoendoscopes with working channels for baskets and laser fibers. The sialoendoscope is introduced through Wharton's duct, which is dilated using a lacrimal probe.

The success rate for stone removal depends on size, shape, and location with smaller (<5 mm), mobile, oval or rounded, and distally located stones having the highest success rate [3].

Postoperative management for transoral approaches should include antibiotic prophylaxis, regular massage of the submandibular duct to prevent stasis and obstruction, and non-alcohol-based mouth rinses.

5.5.3 Surgical Planning

Sublingual gland excisions can be approached transorally, while resections of the submandibular gland should be approached transcervically. There is debate about the best approach for plunging ranulas. A transoral approach may not achieve complete resection, while a transcervical approach is associated with increased complications [4, 5].

The extent of surgery for salivary gland neoplasms should be guided by tumor histology and grade. Generally, high-grade malignancies such as mucoepidermoid carcinoma and salivary ductal carcinoma require an elective neck dissection. A possible exception is adenoid cystic carcinoma which is generally thought to have a low risk of nodal metastases. Benign tumors and low-grade malignancies do not require elective neck dissection. Therapeutic neck dissection should be performed in those patients presenting with nodal metastases and without distant disease.

Special consideration should be given to submandibular gland biopsies that show squamous cell carcinoma (SCC). Primary SCC of major salivary glands is exceedingly rare. High-grade mucoepidermoid carcinoma can sometimes mimic squamous cell carcinoma. Mucicarmine staining can help differentiate these two pathologies. Direct invasion of oral cancers into the submandibular or sublingual glands is also a rare phenomenon. However, tumors can spread along fascial planes into the sublingual and submandibular spaces.

When SCC is identified on a biopsy from the submandibular area, the most likely scenario is a metastatic lymph node from a cutaneous or mucosal SCC. If a lesion is not readily visualized on examination, imaging and PET scan should be considered to identify the primary site.

The management of SCC and high-grade salivary gland malignancies should be discussed at a multidisciplinary tumor board. Surgery, when indicated, should include excision of the primary site with oncologic margins, and neck dissection to involved and at-risk nodal basins.

5.6 Relevant Non-Surgical Management

The majority of non-neoplastic conditions that affect the submandibular and sublingual glands are managed with systemic therapy. Chronic infections such as tuberculosis and HIV require prolonged systemic therapy and follow-up with infectious disease specialists. Autoimmune conditions should be referred to a rheumatologist.

For symptom relief, conservative management with massage and warm compress is often beneficial. Sialogogues such as lemon or sour candies can be used to stimulate saliva flow and prevent stasis. In the case of acute sialadenitis, antibiotics are indicated as well and this is often referred to as MASH (massage, antibiotics, sialogogues, and heat) protocol.

With regard to neoplasms, observation is generally appropriate for benign lesions. It is, however, important to counsel patients that there is a low risk of malignant transformation for pleomorphic adenoma.

Malignant neoplams should be discussed at multidisciplinary tumor boards.

Relevant non-surgical management includes radiation therapy and systemic therapy options. For patients who are not surgical candidates, definitive radiation therapy can be considered. The standard for radiation treatment to the head and neck is intensity-modulated radiation therapy (IMRT), which allows for confirmation of the photon beam to deliver a high dose to tumor while minimizing the dose to adjacent critical structures. Adjuvant radiation therapy is recommended in specific situations. General indications for adjuvant therapy are T3 or T4 tumors, nodal metastases (N1–3), close or positive margins, perineural invasion, lymphovascular invasion, intermediate or high-grade malignancies, and adenoid cystic carcinoma.

Systemic therapy in malignant salivary gland neoplasm is an evolving area. The standard for many years has been platinum-based chemotherapy. The general indications for this are recurrent, unresectable, or distantly metastatic tumors. Recently, new therapies have shown promise in specific tumors. These include androgen deprivation therapy for androgen receptor-positive salivary ductal carcinoma, anti-HER2 drugs for HER2+ tumors (seen in salivary ductal and mucoepidermoid carcinoma), and lenvatinib for adenoid cystic carcinoma [6].

Top Five Takeaways

1. Beware of signs of impending airway compromise with infections of the sublingual and submandibular space.
2. It is important to distinguish masses in the submandibular space arising from the submandiublar gland from those arising from level 1B lymph nodes.
3. The marginal mandibular branches of the facial nerve, lingual nerve, and hypoglossal nerve are intimately related to the submandibular gland.
4. Submandibular gland resection should be approached transcervically.
5. Sublingual pathology and distal salivary duct stones can be approached transorally.

References

1. Wilson KF, Meier JD, Ward PD. Salivary gland disorders. Am Fam Physician. 2014;89(11):882–8.
2. Kaminiski B, Blochowiak K. Mikulicz's disease and Küttner's tumor as manifestations of IgG4-related diseases: a review of the literature. Rheumatology. 2020;58(4):243–50.

3. Luers JC, Grosheva M, Stenner M, And Beutner D. Sialoendoscopy: prognostic factors for endoscopic removal of salivary stones. Arch Otolaryngol Head Neck Surg 2011;137(4):325–329.
4. Patel MR, Deal AM, Shockley WW. Oral and plunging ranulas: what is the most effective treatment? Laryngoscope. 2009;119(8):1501–9.
5. Lesperance MM. When do ranulas require a cervical approach? Laryngoscope. 2013;123(8):1826–7.
6. National Comprehensive Cancer Network. Head and Neck Cancer (Version 2.2022). https://www.nccn.org/professionals/physician_gls/pdf/head-and-neck.pdf. Accessed 1 May 2022.

6 Advanced Skin Cancer

Bruce Ashford and Matthew Beck

Skin cancer is the most common malignancy worldwide. In Australia [1] and North America, non-melanoma skin cancer (NMSC) numbers exceed those for all other cancers combined. So, while only a small percentage of cases either metastasize, recur locally in an aggressive fashion or give rise to distant disease, due to the sheer weight of numbers this represents a substantial burden on the health system.

Surgery is the mainstay of management of both routine and advanced skin cancer. The surgical assessment and management of advanced skin cancer are based on an understanding of the biology of the disease, and on routine collaboration with non-surgical specialities, including radiation and, more recently, medical oncology.

In this chapter we will review the biology of skin cancers, their surgical management, the peculiarities of high-risk cohorts and the circumstances under which adjuvant therapies are indicated. General surgeons are frequently called on to assess and manage advanced skin cancer and should be very familiar with the principles and practice of this component of practice. Due to the association of most skin cancers with ultraviolet (UV) radiation exposure, the bulk of skin cancers occur in the head and neck regions. And because the management of any surgical disease is based on a thorough grasp of the anatomy and pathology, a good working knowledge of the head and neck is required.

6.1 Skin Cancer Biology

6.1.1 NMSC

Non-melanoma skin cancers comprise mostly basal cell carcinoma and squamous cell carcinoma, but also less common skin cancers including merkel cell carcinoma. This group of cancers occur mostly in the sun-exposed skin and are related to UV radiation exposure. The molecular and genomic landscape of these cancers is dominated by a very high mutational burden, in keeping with the effect of UV radiation in causing both somatic variants and disrupting normal DNA repair mechanisms.

6.1.1.1 Basal Cell Carcinoma

BCC is the most common skin cancer. It behaves in a locally aggressive manner related to the underlying pathology. Most nodular BCC have a pushing border and are unlikely to recur with appropriate 2–3 mm margins. Aggressive

B. Ashford (✉) · M. Beck
Graduate Medicine, University of Wollongong, Wollongong, NSW, Australia
e-mail: bruceash@uow.edu.au; Matthew.Beck@health.nsw.gov.au

B. Ashford (ed.), *Head and Neck Surgery for General Surgeons*,
https://doi.org/10.1007/978-981-19-7900-2_6

subtypes, including morphoeiform or infiltrative BCCs, behave in a far more aggressive manner and require wider margins for cure. Expert pathological assessment is required to differentiate between these entities and a pathology report that does not specifically detail the type of BCC should be clarified or sent for a second opinion.

Metastasis of BCC is rare but most head and neck surgeons will have a number of cases in their log books. The assessment of metastatic skin cancer in the head and neck is based on a thorough cutaneous malignancy history (including any immunosuppression), detailed examination, high-quality imaging, and either cytology or histopathology. Most cases of metastatic BCC are managed by neck dissection to address all diseased and at-risk nodes and adjuvant radiotherapy, with the potential addition of vismodegib, a hedgehog pathway inhibitor for distant or recurrent disease.

6.1.1.2 Squamous Cell Carcinoma

Cutaneous squamous cell carcinoma (cSCC) is not the same as head and neck SCC (HNSCC). The former, while it predominantly occurs in the head and neck, is of the skin, while the latter is mucosal. This is an important distinction and is a source of confusion when exploring the literature. It is also of importance when considering metastatic SCC of unknown origin (unknown primary) as cSCC and HNSCC behave differently, are staged differently and will often require different therapies. The aetiology of cSCC is related primarily to UV radiation, whereas HNSCC is related to smoking and alcohol exposure and, particularly in the oropharynx, to human papillomavirus infection.

Once again the clinical and pathological biology of cSCC determines its treatment. Well-differentiated tumours with a pushing border and no evidence of lymphovascular invasion (LVI) or perineural infiltration (PNI) are less likely to progress and require excision with adequate (at least 2–3 mm) margins. Tumours with adverse features (poorly differentiated, infiltrative growth pattern, LVI or PNI) have a more aggressive biology and are more likely to recur and metastasize. The surgical approach to aggressive variants of cSCC needs to match this biology. Wider margins, assessment of draining lymph nodes and nearby nerves, and the consideration of adjuvant treatment are all reasonable in this context.

6.1.1.3 Merkel Cell Carcinoma

Merkel cell carcinoma (MCC) is a rare NMSC, typically seen in much older age groups and often presents with locally advanced or metastatic disease. It is a poorly differentiated neuroendocrine carcinoma in which the Merkel cell polyomavirus is implicated [2]. Immunohistochemistry is used to differentiate it from metastatic non-small cell lung cancer.

Treatment consists of wide local excision and sentinel node biopsy for clinically and radiologically node-negative patients. Radiotherapy is typically used as adjuvant treatment for any nodal positivity and for large primary lesions. There is an emerging role for immunotherapy as adjuvant therapy, particularly for distant metastatic disease.

6.1.2 Melanoma

Unlike NMSC, cutaneous melanoma is no more common in the head and neck than in the rest of the skin. Nonetheless, the general surgeon will be called on to manage primary and potentially metastatic melanoma of the head and neck.

Once the diagnosis of melanoma is made, an approach to local management is based on the clinical and pathological stage of the primary. Thin (<1 mm) and intermediate thickness (1–4 mm) melanoma should be excised with a 1 cm margin to deep fascia, while thick melanoma (>4 mm) should have a 2 cm margin where possible.

The management of melanoma is related to its pathological staging with respect to margins and nodal assessment. Melanoma Institute Australia has devised risk calculators for melanoma which are available online (https://www.melanomarisk.org.au). In particular, the sentinel node risk calculator can help guide surgeons in deciding whether sentinel node mapping and or biopsy is indicated for a given primary melanoma [3]. For non-head and neck melanoma, sentinel node biopsy is indicated for all melanomas over 1 mm Breslow thickness or with high-risk features. In the head and neck region, the same risks of lymph node metastasis apply, but given the complexity of lymphatic drainage patterns and surgical risk, a more considered approach is taken. Sentinel node/nodal biopsy information has become increasingly useful and while most patients with lymph node metastasis no longer undergo nodal dissection [4] they now have access to adjuvant immunotherapy.

Staging of stage 3 or 4 melanoma is based on PET CT. Both immunotherapy and targeted therapies (to *BRAF, NRAF, KIT* and *GNAQ/GNA11*) are increasingly used for prophylaxis and therapy in high-risk or metastatic melanoma. Access to a melanoma MDT is mandatory for surgeons treating melanoma. Access to trails is a critical component of melanoma care and the MDT provides awareness and access. Most large units encourage regional surgeons to join as required.

6.2 Surgical Problems in Local Disease

6.2.1 Local Excision Relevant to Anatomy

Management of primary cutaneous malignancy in the head and neck can be impacted by anatomical constraints. Examples include around the eye, nose and mouth and particularly in the skin overlying the branches of the facial nerve. Preoperative assessment of skin lesions of the head and neck can include imaging in the form of ultrasound, CT or even MRI to assess for local extent and likelihood of the involvement of important structures or functional units. Tissue biopsy enables an initial assessment of the likely pathology and therefore biology. Taken together, this preoperative information can enable appropriate surgery to be planned and completed without undue morbidity.

Where important structures are likely to impact appropriate margins for a primary cutaneous malignancy, options for margin control will need to be considered. Intraoperative margin assessment by frozen section can assist in achieving a clear pathological margin. Adjuvant radiotherapy can be used to control a close margin in a high-risk tumour or to manage microscopically positive margins when the achievement of a clear margin would be too morbid, for example on the facial nerve. This approach to managing microscopically involved margins can provide good oncologic outcomes [5].

Reconstruction of defects in the head and neck can be by primary closure, secondary intention, skin grafting (either split thickness or full thickness) or by the use of local, regional or free flaps. Denervation (either sensory or motor) of important structures should be considered in understanding surgical defects and, on occasions, such defects need to be overcome. The reader is directed to other chapters in this work for the specific approaches to reconstructions required for head and neck defects.

6.3 Managing Regional Lymph Node Disease and At-Risk Nodal Basins

Unlike melanoma, there are no reliable or validated predictors of metastatic potential in NMSC. Notwithstanding the propensity of MCC to metastasize, the most common skin cancer with metastatic potential is cSCC. The largest prospective trial of sentinel node biopsy in cSCC demonstrated an occult metastatic rate of 9% in high-risk but clinically N0 tumours, and the development of later non-sentinel node metastases in a further 5% [6, 7]. A combination of high-risk features, depth of invasion >5 mm and PNI increased the risk of metastasis.

Regardless of the histopathology, the assessment of at-risk nodes in all cutaneous malignancies is by clinical examination and imaging with biopsy. The pattern of lymphatic spread of skin cancers has been studied extensively [8, 9]. Patterns of spread (Fig. 6.1) from different locations of primary lesions into nodal basins can

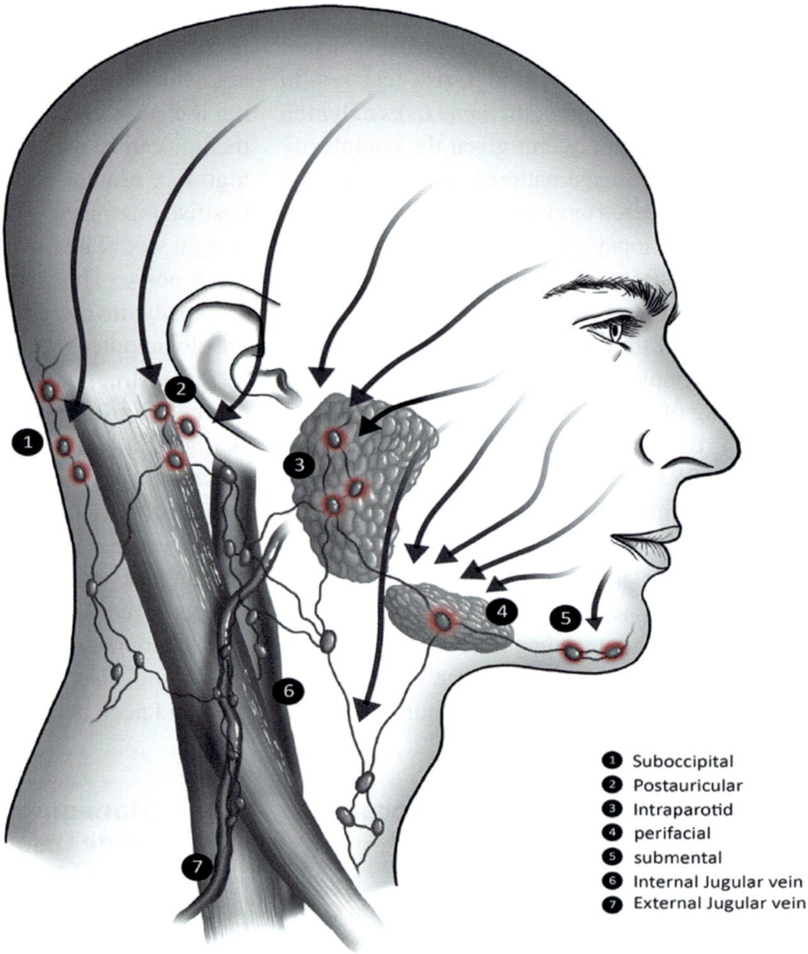

Fig. 6.1 Lymphatic drainage according to location of primary cutaneous malignancy

predict the echelons of nodal spread and also assist in planning the surgical approach to clearing nodes at risk. This pattern of spread can also assist in determining the approach to sentinel node biopsy [6, 7].

Metastasis from the temporal region and ear into the superficial parotid lymph nodes spreads further through the posterior branch of the retromandibular vein into the external jugular venous system. Further forward on the face, lymphatics directly spread to the perifacial nodes overlying the facial vessels at the margin of the mandible and then into level 1b and the deep cervical chain running alongside the internal jugular vein. Primary lesions of the posterior scalp spread to the suboccipital nodes. Blocking of lymphatics with tumour or previous surgery can disrupt precited patterns of spread to produce confounding clinical presentations.

Management of patients with locally advanced or metastatic skin cancer, whether melanoma or NMSC, should be discussed at the relevant multidisciplinary oncology team (MDT) meeting. Most teaching hospitals will have a head and neck MDT that often serves as a suitable venue for discussing cutaneous malignancy.

Despite the increasing utility of immunotherapy in metastatic skin cancer therapy, surgery remains the mainstay of contemporary management. In most cases for radiosensitive disease (particularly the NMSC), surgery is followed by adjuvant radiotherapy. The extent of ablative surgery should be dictated by the stage at presentation and may require the management of both a primary and regional nodal disease with some patients requiring concomitant reconstructive surgery.

The detailed technical discussion of both neck dissection and parotidectomy is discussed elsewhere in this book. For all cases where metastatic disease has been proven by cytology or histopathology pre-operatively, there is no place for single lymph node excision. The aim is for an oncologic dissection of lymph node levels at risk, with the preservation of critical structures. The surgeon undertaking neck dissection for metastatic skin cancer should be willing to be aggressive enough to achieve a clear microscopic margin when at all possible. This may include resecting bone of the facial skeleton or skull, sacrificing major vessels and potentially other critical structures, e.g. the eye. Obviously, the more morbid the ablative surgery, the more competent the reconstructive capability must be. Regardless of the reconstructive demands, the ablative procedure must be completed at the first operation to the most satisfactory standard possible. This is the patient's best chance at cure, and needlessly involved margins will predispose to a worse prognosis.

6.4 Surveillance of High-Risk Cancers

Surveillance for advanced skin cancer is mandatory for those patients with nodal or extensive disease who are at high risk of recurrence in the first 24 months after surgery and adjuvant treatment. Regular clinical review at 3 monthly intervals, extending to 6 monthly after 24 months is recommended. Patients who have areas of concern either in deeper structures or whose ablative defect is covered by a free tissue transfer may require cross-sectional imaging for adequate surveillance.

Clinical examination is not easy in cases who have had major operations and post-operative radiotherapy. Key components of the history should be elicited. Any evidence of major nerve embarrassment or involvement should be looked for. Eye irritation may be an early indication of facial nerve weakness signifying malignant involvement. Otalgia may indicate infiltration of the temporal bone or cervical plexus nerve roots. Any unexplained anaesthesia/paraesthesia or dysaesthesia needs to be interrogated to disprove the emergence of the perineural spread of disease. MRI is the imaging of choice for the assessment of large nerve malignant involvement.

More challenging is the approach to surveillance for pathologically aggressive excised primary tumours. As discussed earlier, the treatment needs to match the biology. Inadequate margins are best revised as soon as the pathology report is reviewed. Patients will absorb the inconvenience of further surgery if they understand the often more aggressive nature of cancer recurrences.

Where high-risk features are observed on histopathology of an excised primary, active surveillance is recommended as above. This can also be accompanied by point-of-care ultrasound to assess lymph node basins for pathological change. Lymph nodes within at-risk basins that change architecture or shape should be biopsied to exclude the emergence of metastatic disease. A change from oval to round, with loss of echogenic hilum and the observation of increased internal vascularity are all features that can be readily demonstrated in pathological lymph nodes on office ultrasound examination.

6.5 Immunosuppression and Skin Cancer

Immunosuppression impacts our defence against malignant transformation at many levels. Dysregulation of DNA repair mechanisms and the impairment of cell-based immune destruction of malignant cells promote cancer in the immunosuppressed.

Immunosuppression can be due to therapy (e.g. in solid organ transplant recipients to avoid rejection), haematologic disease (e.g. chronic lymphocytic leukaemia) or chronic disease and ageing. Regardless of causes, immune system impairment increases the risk of development of skin cancer and its severity.

Solid organ transplant recipients on formal immunosuppression are more than 60 times as likely to develop cSCC as their immunocompetent peers. This cohort has a specific problem to be addressed in the skin cancer realm. These patients have more aggressive cancers with a higher rate of both recurrence and metastasis. As always, the treatment needs to be tailored to the biology, in this case, of both the cancer and the patient. Wider margins, more aggressive use of adjuvant therapy and closer surveillance are all indicated.

Some patients with renal transplants and unresectable or metastatic cSCC can be trialled with immunotherapy. A substantial percentage of these patients may suffer transplant rejection. Obviously, the challenges for liver, lung and heart transplants in the setting of rejection are more grave, and these groups currently are not able to be managed with immunotherapy.

6.6 Role of Adjuvant Therapies

Each of the cutaneous malignancies will have different indications for both surgery and adjuvant treatment. The availability of a multidisciplinary team meeting, whether local or remote, should be sought out to discuss difficult cases.

Each individual patient and cancer will have unique indications for the consideration of adjuvant therapy for advanced skin cancer. Table 6.1 details the role of various modalities of adjuvant therapy for advanced skin cancers.

Immunotherapy has revolutionised the landscape of adjuvant therapy in melanoma. It has meant that the toxicities of other therapies, such as radiation, need to be considered as long-term survival in higher-stage melanoma has become a reality [10]. Given the predicted response to immunotherapy is related to tumour mutational burden (TMB), and the TMB of cSCC is even higher than melanoma, it is highly likely immunotherapy will be widely used in a range of settings in the management of advanced cSCC.

6.6.1 Cutaneous Squamous Cell Carcinoma Staging AJCC Eighth Edition

TX	Primary tumour cannot be assessed
T0	No evidence of primary tumour
Tis	Carcinoma in situ
T1	Tumour ≤20 mm or less in maximum dimension (this is the clinical dimension but the pathological dimension, usually macroscopic, can be used if the clinical is not available)
T2	Tumour >20 mm to ≤40 mm in maximum dimension (this is the clinical dimension but the pathological dimension, usually macroscopic, can be used if the clinical is not available)
T3	Tumour >40 mm in maximum dimension (this is the clinical dimension but the pathological dimension, usually macroscopic, can be used if the clinical is not available) pT1 or pT2 can be upstaged to pT3 by one or more high-risk clinical/pathological features including deep invasion, specifically defined perineural invasion or minor bone erosion
T4a	Tumour with gross cortical/marrow invasion
T4b	Tumour with axial skeleton/skull base/ foraminal invasion
NX	Regional lymph nodes cannot be assessed
N0	No regional lymph node metastasis
N1	Metastasis in a single ipsilateral lymph node ≤30 mm in greatest dimension, without extranodal extension
N2a	Metastasis in a single ipsilateral lymph node, more than 30 mm but not more than 60 mm in greatest dimension, without extranodal extension
N2b	Metastasis in multiple ipsilateral lymph nodes, none more than 60 mm in greatest dimension, without extranodal extension
N2c	Metastasis in bilateral or contralateral lymph nodes, none more than 60 mm in greatest dimension, without extranodal extension
N3a	Metastasis in a lymph node, more than 60 mm in greatest dimension, without extranodal extension
N3b	Metastasis in a lymph node with extranodal extension
M0	No distant metastasis
M1/ pM1	Distant metastatic disease

Table 6.1 Role of adjuvant therapies in advanced skin malignancy

	Radiotherapy	Chemotherapy	Adjuvant immunotherapy	Neoadjuvant immunotherapy
BCC	Unresectable, highly infiltrative disease with close margins	Hedgehog pathway inhibitors		
cSCC	Unresectable, highly infiltrative disease with close margins, nodal disease (extracapsular spread or multiple nodes)	No clear benefit to addition of chemotherapy to RT	Highly effective in unresectable or distant metastatic disease	Expansion of clinical trials
MCC	Routine use for MCC with nodal disease	Emerging role for targeted therapies	Emerging role	
Melanoma	Reduction in at-risk basins for N+ but toxicities may outweigh benefits	BRAF-targeted therapy for V600E + tumours at risk of metastatic disease	Either alone or in combination with BRAF-targeted therapies	Emerging/trials

6.6.2 Melanoma Staging AJCC eighth edition

T0	Primary tumour not assessed
Tis	Melanoma in situ
T1a	<0.8 mm without ulceration
T1b	<0.8 mm with ulceration or 0.8–1 mm w/o ulceration
T2a	1–2 mm without ulceration
T2b	1–2 mm with ulceration
T3a	2–4 mm without ulceration
T3b	2–4 mm with ulceration
T4a	>4 mm without ulceration
T4b	>4 mm with ulceration
N0	No nodal disease
N1a	Clinically occult node, no MSI
N1b	Clinically detected node, no MSI
N1c	0 nodes but MSI present
N2a	2–3 nodes clinically occult, no MSI
N2b	2–3 nodes clinically detected, no MSI
N2c	1 node clinically detected or occult, MSI present
N3a	>3 nodes all occult, no MSI
N3b	>3 nodes (> = 1 detected or matted) no MSI
N3c	>1 node, MSI present
M0	No distant metastasis
M1a	Metastases to the skin, subcutaneous or distant lymph nodes
M1b	Metastases to the lung
M1c	Metastases to all other visceral sites
M1d	Metastases to the brain
Any M	LDH not measured
Any M (0)	LDH normal
Any M (1)	LDH elevated

Top Five Takeaways

1. Treatment, including surgical, of cutaneous malignancy of the head and neck must match the tumour biology. The more aggressive the cancer, the more aggressive the treatment required.
2. A detailed examination of histopathology reports regarding non-melanoma skin cancers can guide appropriate therapy by highlighting high-risk features such as perineural infiltration and lymphovascular invasion.
3. Nodal metastases from primary head and neck skin cancers occur in a predictable fashion.
4. Immunosuppressed patients are at extremely high risk of developing aggressive and rapidly progressing skin cancers.
5. Immunotherapy has transformed the management of unresectable and distant metastatic cutaneous malignancies.

References

1. Wilson A, Goltsman D, Nankervis J, Clark J, Gupta R, Ashford B. Defining the incidence of cutaneous squamous cell carcinoma in coastal NSW Australia. Australas J Dermatol. 2022;63(2):213–6.
2. Harms PW, Harms KL, Moore PS, DeCaprio JA, Nghiem P, Wong MKK, Brownell I, International Workshop on Merkel Cell Carcinoma Research (IWMCC) Working Group. The biology and treatment of Merkel cell carcinoma: current understanding and research priorities. Nat Rev Clin Oncol. 2018;15(12):763–76.
3. Lo SN, Ma J, Scolyer RA, Haydu LE, Stretch JR, Saw RPM, et al. Improved risk prediction calculator for sentinel node positivity in patients with melanoma: the melanoma institute Australia nomogram. J Clin Oncol. 2020;38(24):2719–27.
4. Faries MB, Thompson JF, Cochran AJ, Andtbacka RH, Mozzillo N, Zager JS, et al. Completion dissection or observation for sentinel-node metastasis in melanoma. N Engl J Med. 2017;376(23):2211–22.
5. Iyer NG, Clark JR, Murali R, Gao K, O'Brien CJ. Outcomes following parotidectomy for metastatic squamous cell carcinoma with microscopic residual disease: implications for facial nerve preservation. Head Neck. 2009;31(1):21–7.
6. Gore SM, Shaw D, Martin RC, Kelder W, Roth K, Uren R, Gao K, Davies S, Ashford BG, Ngo Q, Shannon K, Clark JR. Prospective study of sentinel node biopsy for high-risk cutaneous squamous cell carcinoma of the head and neck. Head Neck. 2016;38(Suppl 1):E884–9.
7. Mooney CP, Martin RCW, Dirven R, et al. Sentinel node biopsy in 105 high-risk cutaneous SCCs of the head and neck: results of a multicenter prospective study. Ann Surg Oncol. 2019;26:4481–8.
8. Vauterin TJ, Veness MJ, Morgan GJ, Poulsen MG, O'Brien CJ. Patterns of lymph node spread of cutaneous squamous cell carcinoma of the head and neck. Head Neck. 2006;28(9):785–91.
9. Ebrahimi A, Moncrieff MD, Clark JR, Shannon KF, Gao K, Milross CG, et al. Predicting the pattern of regional metastases from cutaneous squamous cell

carcinoma of the head and neck based on location of the primary. Head Neck. 2010;32(10):1288–94.
10. Henderson MA, Burmeister BH, Ainslie J, Fisher R, Di Iulio J, Smithers BM, et al. Adjuvant lymph-node field radiotherapy versus observation only in patients with melanoma at high risk of further lymph-node field relapse after lymphadenectomy (ANZMTG 01.02/TROG 02.01): 6-year follow-up of a phase 3, randomised controlled trial. Lancet Oncol. 2015;16(9):1049–60.

Local Flaps of the Head and Neck

7

Tam Quinn and Sydney Ch'ng

7.1 Introduction

The degree of sun exposure to the head and neck region makes it one of the most common sites for skin cancers, in particular basal cell carcinoma (BCC), squamous cell carcinoma (SCC) and melanoma [1, 2]. It accounts for approximately 40% of BCCs and 33% of SCCs [1] and melanoma [2]. In our experience, the majority of patients will seek attention for their skin cancer when they are relatively small. Local flap reconstruction of the head and neck region is ideally suited for these lesions due to the rich vascularity of the region. They also have the advantage of optimal aesthetic outcomes due to the match in colour, texture and contour of the face, which is often different from tissue taken from other areas of the body whether in the form of grafts or regional or distant flaps.

There are a few caveats that the surgeon must be acutely conscious of when performing local flap reconstruction. Foremost is ensuring adequate oncologic margins and tumour clearance. Local flaps should be designed in a way that they are a one-to-one match for the defect in question in order to minimise the donor site morbidity. As such, there is often little room for revision and surgeons who need to re-excise a margin may come to the gut-clenching realisation that they have 'burned their bridges'. Sir Harold Gilles, the father of modern plastic surgery, extorts in his 'commandments' that one should always have a lifeboat. A surgeon can avoid finding themselves in this uncomfortable position by ensuring that they have oncological clearance prior to committing to a flap, lest one finds oneselves in one.

Ideally, tissue diagnosis is established prior to complete excision, usually in the form of a biopsy if the diagnosis is not immediately clear on clinical examination. Some tumours, such as nodular BCCs, have well-defined margins. Other forms of BCC such as the infiltrative or morpheic subtypes can be considerably more difficult to assess even if examined under magnification or dermatoscopy. If unsure, consideration of adjunctive techniques such as frozen section or delayed reconstruction after pathological examination (DRAPE)/slow Mohs can ensure that clear margins are obtained prior to definitive reconstruction. This allows the surgeon to be completely certain of the final defect before elevating a flap. If using one of the latter techniques, the wound can be covered by suturing on a moist dressing (such as a paraffin-impregnated tulle) and the patient discharged with a plan to return in a few days when the formal histopathology report is available.

T. Quinn (✉)
Peter MacCallum Cancer Centre, Melbourne, VIC, Australia

Chris O'Brien Lifehouse, Camperdown, NSW, Australia
e-mail: tam.quinn@petermac.org

S. Ch'ng
Chris O'Brien Lifehouse, University of Sydney, Camperdown, NSW, Australia
e-mail: sydney.ch'ng@lh.org.au

B. Ashford (ed.), *Head and Neck Surgery for General Surgeons*,
https://doi.org/10.1007/978-981-19-7900-2_7

Another potential pitfall is to overestimate the capabilities of your flap or to have an incomplete understanding of the blood supply. As stated earlier, the head and neck are richly supplied by numerous anastomoses between the branches of the external and internal carotid arteries. Axial pattern flaps, in which runs a known artery either mapped out by Doppler or a good understanding of the anatomy, can be planned with a three-to-one ratio (length being three times the width of the base). Random pattern flaps, on the other hand, should be limited to a one-to-one ratio, unless the flap has been delayed or its vascularity enhanced in some other way. A surgeon performing a local lap should be aware of the ways in which skin can move and understand preoperatively how much laxity is available to them. Respecting the facial aesthetic subunits is crucial in order to ensure an optimal cosmetic outcome. Additionally, the incisions should be planned in such a way that the final scar sits in or parallel to a rhytid, thus reducing the visibility of the final result.

Local flaps, while technically less difficult than their regional or distant cousins, can still prove challenging in their planning and execution. Done poorly, the subsequent defect can be far worse than the original excision, resulting in much heartache for both surgeon and patient. Done well, both flap and donor site blend almost seamlessly into the surrounding skin, earning the approval of even the most discerning colleagues and, more importantly, withstanding the scrutiny of the most aesthetically minded patients.

7.2 History and Examination

A general history of the patient's medical comorbidities and medications is, as always, an important consideration, particularly if the patient requires an operative procedure. Additionally, a history of immunosuppression and a significant family history of skin cancers can foreshadow the expected progression and prognosis of their disease.

Specific points to elicit on history are the duration the lesion has been present and its progression over time such as growth, ulceration or bleeding. Also important to know is if they have previously had treatment for either the lesion in question or any other lesions. Previous non-surgical treatments such as cryotherapy or curettage may point to a recurrent lesion. Prior surgical management can affect the planned local flap. A history of radiotherapy, either as a primary or adjuvant treatment modality, can impact the way in which the tissue handles intra-operatively and how it heals post-operatively.

A focused examination of the lesion should follow the 'look, feel, move' format as taught in medical school. An inspection of the size of the lesion and its characteristics will guide your choice of management. Is it well circumscribed or are the margins indistinct? Does it have any defining characteristics such as pearly edges and telangiectasia typical of BCCs, hyperkeratosis as seen in SCC or pigmentation and colour variegation, which could indicate melanoma? Or does it have a completely atypical appearance? Is there ulceration, suggesting that there may be tumour invading into underlying structures? Are there scars indicating previous surgery?

Palpation of the lesion can reveal surrounding induration or tenderness. In an unremarkable appearing lesion, these two features are suggestive of invasive disease. Assessing the mobility of the lesion is also important to ascertain that it is not fixed, and therefore invading into, underlying structures such as cartilage, fascia or bone. No examination of cutaneous malignancies of the head and neck is complete without palpation of the nodal basins. The location of the primary tumour can guide which lymph node group a tumour is likely to metastasise to. The lymphatic drainage of the head and neck is complex but an examination of all nodal basins is simple to perform. Cervical lymph nodes are typically divided into six levels, and all levels should be carefully palpated. Additionally, parotid and occipital nodes should not be neglected in a complete examination of the nodal basins.

Finally, for the reconstructively minded surgeon, the examination should take into account the location and direction of rhytids, skin laxity and hair-bearing skin in order to help plan incisions.

7.3 Investigations

History and examination will guide what further investigations are required. A biopsy to confirm the diagnosis is warranted in almost all circumstances. While excisional biopsies (complete excision of the lesion with a 2 mm margin) are the gold standard, it is not always feasible to do, particularly in an outpatient setting.

A punch biopsy, which should include a small rim of macroscopically normal skin, can easily be performed under local anaesthetic in the rooms and can give the pathologist the full depth of the specimen. However, there is always the possibility of a sampling error, particularly with larger lesions. If a single biopsy is unlikely to be representative of the lesion, it is recommended to take 'mapping biopsies', where several punch biopsies are taken and their locations were recorded either with a diagram or with a photograph. This technique is also useful when determining the extent of the lesion preoperatively. Generally speaking, biopsies less than 3 mm can be dressed with a haemostatic dressing (e.g. an alginate dressing), whereas larger biopsies may require sutures to close the defect.

A shave biopsy, which should include dermis, has the advantage of being able to capture the entirety of the superficial component of the lesion. However, it can lead to an underestimation of the depth of the lesion, which is critical to guiding treatment, particularly in the case of melanoma.

History, examination and tissue diagnosis will guide any imaging that may be required. Generally, for small cancers, imaging is not required and complete excision will result in cure. A lesion that is large, fixed to underlying structures or an unusual pathology (such as Merkel cell carcinoma or other adnexal carcinomas) may warrant CT or MRI to look for the involvement of underlying bony or soft tissue structures, or regional nodes. If history is suspicious for metastases or examination reveals palpable lymphadenopathy, a PET scan is indicated.

7.4 Anatomy

The anatomy of the head and neck region is, understandably, complex. A good understanding of the anatomy will increase the chances of safe and successful execution of local flaps.

7.4.1 Skin

The skin of the head and neck differs significantly from area to area and even among the various ethnicities. Generally, the skin of the eyelids is among the thinnest in the body, whereas the scalp boasts a significantly thicker dermis, rivalled only by the skin of the back. The skin over the cheeks is mobile compared to the ear where it is closely adherent to the underlying cartilage. Where there is usually significant skin laxity over the anterior neck, the skin over the forehead and scalp is relatively immobile. Caucasians generally have thinner, more mobile skin over the nasal tip and alar regions than Asians whose skin tends to be thicker and more sebaceous in this area.

Rhytids play an important role in guiding the placement of the incisions and determining the direction of skin laxity. Generally, they run perpendicular to the line of pull of the muscles of facial expression such as the nasolabial fold (zygomaticus major and minor) and the transverse brow rhytids (frontalis). Some lines of adhesion, such as the marionette lines and the tear trough, represent the attachment of facial ligaments, and their prominence with age is due to the laxity of soft tissues around these relatively immobile points. Scars are more obvious when they run perpendicular to rhytids so care should be taken, where possible, to mimic natural rhytids when planning incisions.

The amount of subcutaneous fat varies from person to person and from region to region. Additionally, the volume and distribution of fat will change with age. The appearance of youth comes from the location of facial fat pads and their retention by ligaments. Youth is characterised by rhytids obscured by the thickness of both dermis and subcutaneous fat and stronger ligaments, which retrain fat pads in their original locations. The resulting fuller cheeks and smoother face make scars more difficult to disguise. With age, the volume of skin, fat and even bone decreases and the subcutaneous fat herniates over lax ligaments and fascia. The increased prominence of rhytids and increased skin and soft tissue laxity lend flexibility to surgical planning and tissue manipulation.

7.4.2 SMAS

The superficial musculoaponeurotic system (SMAS), described by Mitz and Peyronie in 1976 [3], is a layer of fibrous tissue that invests the underlying facial muscles and connects them with the dermis, translating muscle movement into visible facial expressions. It is continuous inferiorly with the platysma, laterally with parotid fascia, in the temple region with the superficial temporal fascia and with the galea aponeurotica over the scalp. Crucially for the surgeon, it acts as a barrier between skin and the branches of the facial nerve. A surgeon who stays superficial to the SMAS is unlikely to injure this crucial structure. Tumours invading through SMAS clinically appear fixed and relatively immobile, and the excision of such lesions should not be undertaken without a sound understanding of the anatomy of the facial nerve. Equally, examination of the function of the facial nerve should be a part of the assessment of these tumours.

7.4.3 Facial Muscles

The muscles of facial expression are all supplied by the facial nerve, which runs within the substance of the parotid. With the exception of the deepest layer of facial muscles (buccinator, levator anguli oris, and mentalis), the muscles are all supplied from their deep surface. As stated earlier, the pull of the facial muscles determines the orientation of the rhytids. As such, an understanding of the location and orientation of the facial muscles will aid in determining the placement of incisions.

7.4.4 Blood Supply

There are two important concepts to understand. First is the anatomy of the major vessels of the head and neck. These vessels form a complex anastomotic network, which makes the head and neck a uniquely well-vascularised region. A sound knowledge of not only the course of the arterial supply of the head and neck, but also the layer in which it runs, is crucial to success.

The second concept is that of the angiosome, as described by Taylor et al. [4], which states that a given area of skin is supplied by a perforating vessel. When raised, a flap can capture the adjacent angiosome, and so a random pattern flap with a 2:1 length-to-width ratio can be raised with some confidence. However, if this is to be exceeded, such as in a transposition flap of the scalp, then the flap must incorporate a named vessel or be delayed to ensure complete flap survival.

Professor Taylor also described the concept of delay, which describes a technique of temporary incomplete division of a flap's blood supply, which allows vasodilation of 'choke vessels' between angiosomes, thus allowing the capture of the territory of a third angiosome [5]. Delay refers to waiting at least 72 hours, though often closer to a week, before completion of flap division to ensure that these choke vessels are completely and permanently dilated. The delay allows for a longer, larger flap to be raised when it is not possible to incorporate a named vessel within the flap.

7.4.5 Nerves

The sensory supply of the face comes from branches of the trigeminal nerve, whereas the motor supply comes from the facial nerve. An understanding of the sensory supply is extremely useful when administering local anaesthetic. Many local flap procedures can be done under local anaesthetic, with or without sedation. Not only does this allow for quick surgical turnover, it is, more importantly, a safe technique for skin cancer patients who, in general, are elderly and may have multiple comorbidities. It is possible to anaesthetise large areas of the head and neck with only a few injection sites. For example, the entire nose can be blocked with three injections – the infratrochlear nerve, the external branch of the anterior ethmoidal nerve and the infraorbital nerve.

A three-dimensional understanding of the anatomy of the facial nerve is absolutely crucial in order to avoid inadvertent injury to its many branches. The facial nerve is deep to the SMAS layer, and staying above this plane is generally safe. However, the SMAS can be surprisingly superficial in certain areas, particularly in the temple region and over the mandible where the frontal branch and the marginal mandibular branch of the facial nerve are at risk of injury. Care should also be taken not to inject long-acting anaesthetics in these areas as even a temporary facial paralysis can cause significant anxiety to both patient and surgeon.

7.5 Non-Surgical Management

Oncologically, non-surgical management should only be used for the treatment of superficial lesions such as superficial BCC or solar keratoses and in situ SCC. The choice of surgery versus non-operative management should be a joint decision between the clinician and the patient as they can be labour-intensive and potentially less effective than surgery. All lesions should be biopsied prior to non-surgical treatment in order to confirm the diagnosis. It is not unheard of that metastatic melanomas have been diagnosed with the only evidence of a primary lesion being one that had been previously treated topically by a well-meaning but misguided clinician.

7.5.1 Topical Creams

Topical therapies included 5% 5-fluorouracil (5-FU) ointment, approved for use in solar keratoses and SCC in situ, and 5% imiquimod ointment, which is used for superficial BCCs. These ointments require daily to twice daily application for up to 6 weeks.

Imiquimod stimulates innate and cell-mediated immune responses to tumour antigens, which activate cytokines such as tumour necrosis factor-alpha (TNF-a), interleukins and interferon-alpha (IFN-a). This inhibits angiogenesis and promotes apoptosis in tumour cells. 5-FU is an antimetabolite, which blocks thymidine synthesis and induces cell cycle arrest and apoptosis.

Both cause significant inflammation during the course of treatment, which improves following cessation of application. Follow-up is recommended at least 4–6 weeks after treatment is complete so that settling inflammation is not confused with residual tumour. Lesions that are resistant to topical therapy should be excised.

7.5.2 Cryotherapy

Cryotherapy can be used in similarly superficial lesions and involves the application of liquid nitrogen. It can be applied either via a cotton swab dipped in liquid nitrogen or, preferably, in spray form. Depending on the lesion, the liquid nitrogen is applied for 15–30 s and should include the lesion and an additional 1–2 mm margin. The extent of tissue injury is proportional to the rate of freezing and thawing. In some cases, a second application is recommended in which case the area should be allowed to thaw completely before liquid nitrogen is reapplied. Repeated freeze–thaw cycles produce greater tissue damage due to increased conductivity and impaired circulation of previously frozen tissue. The mechanism of damage comes from the physical damage of cellular components by ice crystals and osmotic damage during thawing. Additionally, there is immunologic stimulation due to the release of antigenic components.

Similarly, to other burn injuries, the area will become inflamed and may blister following treatment. The area then heals by secondary intention. As with topical therapies, if the lesion has not resolved by the time the area has healed, then surgical excision should be undertaken.

7.5.3 Photodynamic Therapy

Photodynamic therapy (PDT) is another option for the treatment of superficial lesions. It is especially useful in cosmetically sensitive or extensive areas of disease where other surgical or non-surgical options may not be suitable. Photosensitising agents such as methyl aminolevulinic (MAL) cream are applied to the lesion plus a 5 mm margin and an occlusive dressing is applied and the cream is left in place for three hours. The cream is then wiped clean and light is then used to activate the photosensitising agent, resulting in the formation of cytotoxic reactive oxygen species. Various light sources such as intense pulse light (IPL) or LED light can be used. Peak absorption occurs at 410–620 nm with longer wavelengths, resulting in greater tissue penetration.

7.5.4 Radiotherapy

Radiotherapy is another option, particularly for patients who are not candidates for surgical resection, either because the disease is too extensive or because their comorbidities preclude surgery. Additionally, patients who do not wish to have surgery in order to avoid scars can elect to undergo radiotherapy though the potential cosmetic outcomes such as skin discolouration and alopecia should not be underestimated.

Ionising radiation works by causing DNA damage and thus inducing cell death. Depending on the extent of the skin lesion being treated, the dose (measured in greys, Gy) and fractions (number of sessions required) are adjusted by the radiation oncologist. Side effects of radiotherapy are divided into acute and late. Acute effects include desquamation to skin or mucosal surfaces, swelling and inflammation. Later effects, which can occur months to years after treatment, include tissue fibrosis, dryness, alopecia, lymphoedema and cancer. Younger patients in particular should be counselled against radiotherapy due to the risk of additional long-term consequences such as the difficulty in surgically managing an irradiated field in the case of recurrence and radiation-induced cancers such as angiosarcoma.

7.6 Surgical Management

7.6.1 Excision

Skin cancers need to be excised with an adequate margin, which will depend on the type of malignancy. At a minimum, the full thickness of the dermis and some underlying subcutaneous tissue should be excised as a part of the specimen. Excising the lesion to the next tissue plane is oncologically indicated in most cases, and if there are any signs that the lesion is more deeply invasive, the next plane should be taken with the specimen to ensure clearance. The lesion should then be adequately oriented, conventionally with a silk suture at 12 o'clock, so that the pathologist can clearly state the margin of excision. This will make re-excision, if it is required, more targeted.

7.6.2 Direct Closure

If there is adequate skin laxity following excision, then the wound can be directly closed. The lesion should then be excised as an ellipse so that the final wound is a straight line. Alternatively, if it is uncertain whether or not the wound can be closed, the lesion can be excised with an appropriate margin and then the dog ears excised secondarily. To excise a dog ear, the edge of the wound is elevated with a skin hook, or fine forcep, and the excess, triangular piece of skin is excised in the desired direction. The final incision should lay parallel to a rhytid for the best cosmetic result.

7.6.3 Skin Grafts

Almost any defect is amenable to skin grafting, either split or full thickness. Grafts will take on any bed with the exception of bare bone, cartilage or tendon. Grafts are a good option for large defects, where local flaps are not possible or where the cosmetic results are less obvious such as in the conchal bowl or posterior ear. The main disadvantage of a skin graft is that it is cosmetically less favourable than a local flap as the colour match and the soft tissue contour are often inferior than when using skin immediately adjacent to the defect.

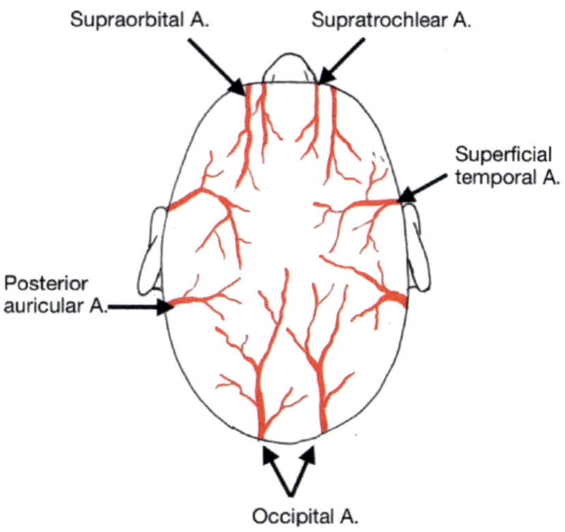

Fig. 7.1 Blood supply of scalp

7.7 Local Flaps

Local flaps can be classified depending on their patterns of blood supply, the type of movement or descriptive based on the design. For the sake of simplicity, this section will focus on the flaps based on the location on the head and neck for which they are most suited, either because of the availability of tissue laxity or because the final scar sits within, or parallel to, existing rhytids. There are myriad ways of reconstructing facial defects with local flaps, limited only by ones' imagination but more importantly by the blood supply. Described below are the most commonly used flaps for each anatomic subunit of the head and neck.

7.7.1 Scalp

The scalp has a rich blood supply (Fig. 7.1) thanks to five pairs of vessels that anastomose with each other. These vessels include the supraorbital, supratrochlear, superficial temporal, posterior auricular and occipital arteries. The galea aponeurotica is a fibrous tissue layer, which is continuous with the SMAS. Because of the density, it often acts as a good barrier to skin cancers and forms a sound oncologic plane to all but the thickest or deeply ulcerating tumours. Beneath this, the pericranium is an excellent recipient bed for grafting due to its rich blood supply. However, if the pericranium is excised as a part of the resection or if a hairless patch of skin on the scalp is cosmetically unacceptable, various local flaps should be a part of any skin cancer surgeon's reconstructive armamentarium. All local flaps of the scalp are raised deep to the galea aponeurotica in a plane, which is relatively bloodless. The underlying pericranium is left behind so that if the secondary defect is unable to be closed, it can still be grafted.

Ungraftable defects up to 3 cm can be closed with a rotation flap (Fig. 7.2). Slightly larger defects may require a second rotation flap from the opposite direction to close the defect. Rotation flaps work by redistributing the tension across a longer incision. The incisions are all closed primarily, thus preserving hair, though it may be thinned along the scar due to stretching of the skin. A back cut may be required if the tension is too great though this should be avoided due to the potential risk of compromising the blood supply. Ahuja et al. [6] described a modification of the rotation flap using the principles of the transposition flap to minimise the need for this back cut. The modification takes on some elements of a transposition flap where the tip of the flap extends beyond the edge of the defect, increasing the arc of rotation and thus further reducing the tension.

Defects up to 6 cm in size will usually require a scalp transposition flap with grafting of the

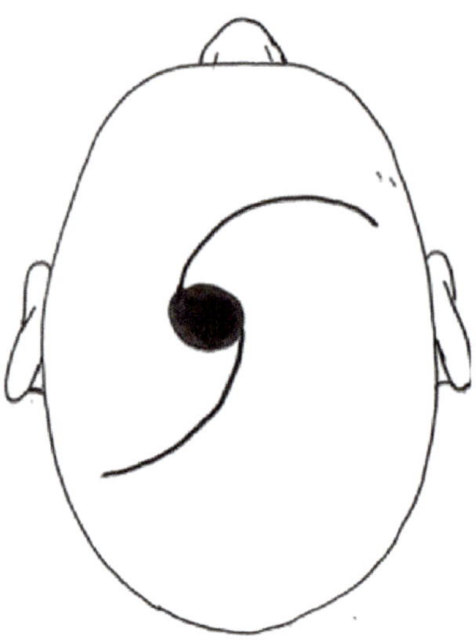

Fig. 7.2 Scalp rotation flap

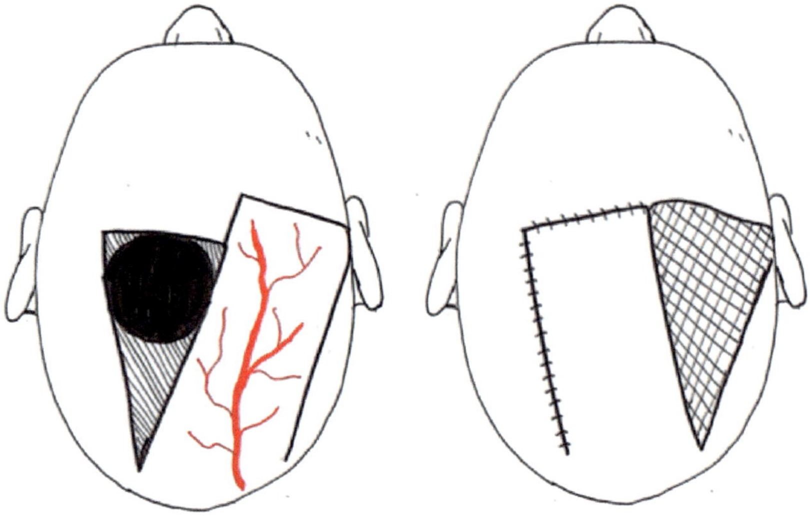

Fig. 7.3 Scalp transposition flap

secondary defect (Fig. 7.3). Because the length-to-width ratio exceeds 2:1, these need to be based on at least one of the named vessels of the scalp. To design the flap, the lesion is triangulated and this whole area is excised to minimise the resultant dog ear. The width of the flap must at least equal the size of the defect and the tip of the flap extend beyond the tip of the defect to ensure comfortable closure of the defect without undue tension.

Larger defects of the scalp will require alternative approaches such as free tissue transfer, tissue expansion or the use of acellular dermal matrixes.

7.7.2 Forehead

Advancement flaps, which have incisions parallel to the horizontally oriented rhytids of the forehead, are a good option for small defects of the forehead that cannot be directly closed. If there is insufficient laxity, then a second advancement flap from the other side of the defect, also called a H-flap due to the resulting scar, can be raised. Defects immediately above the eyebrow can be closed with an A-T flap, with the resulting horizontal limb of the scar laying parallel to the eyebrow thus preserving its shape (Fig. 7.4).

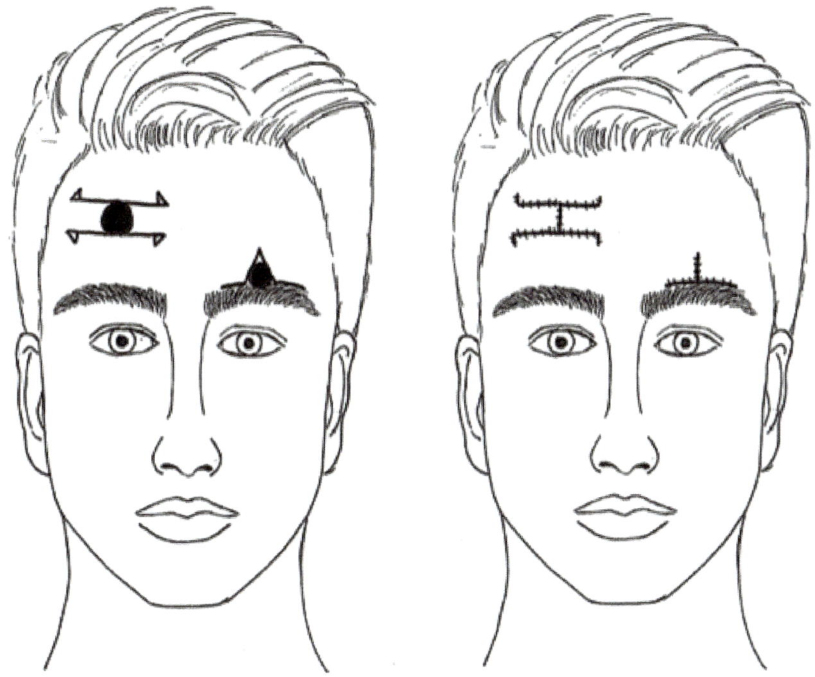

Fig. 7.4 Forehead advancement and A-T flap

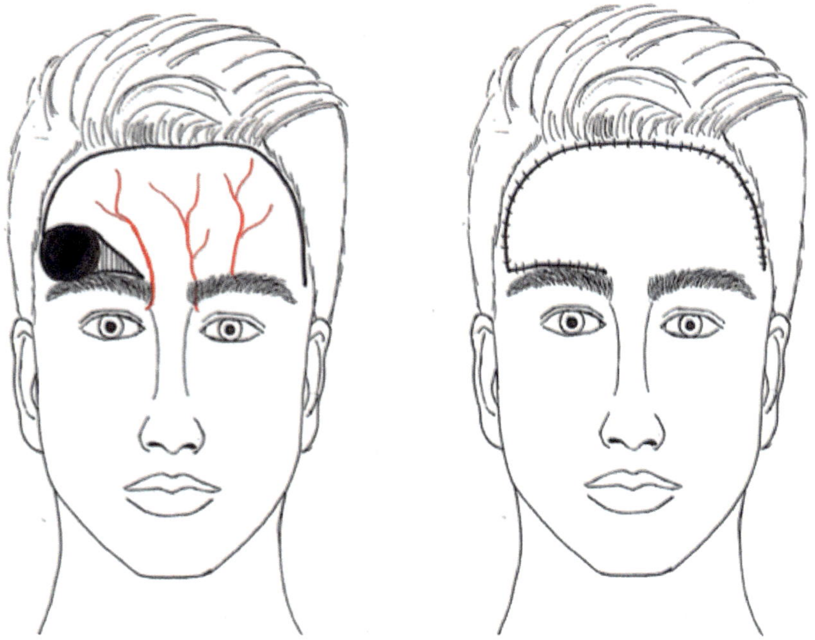

Fig. 7.5 Forehead rotation flaps 1 and 2

Larger defects can be closed with either a single large rotation flap or two rotation flaps (Fig. 7.5). These are incised along the hairline, thus preserving this important anatomical landmark. The disadvantage is that these necessarily cut the supraorbital and supratrochlear nerves, resulting in numbness of the anterior scalp (Fig. 7.6).

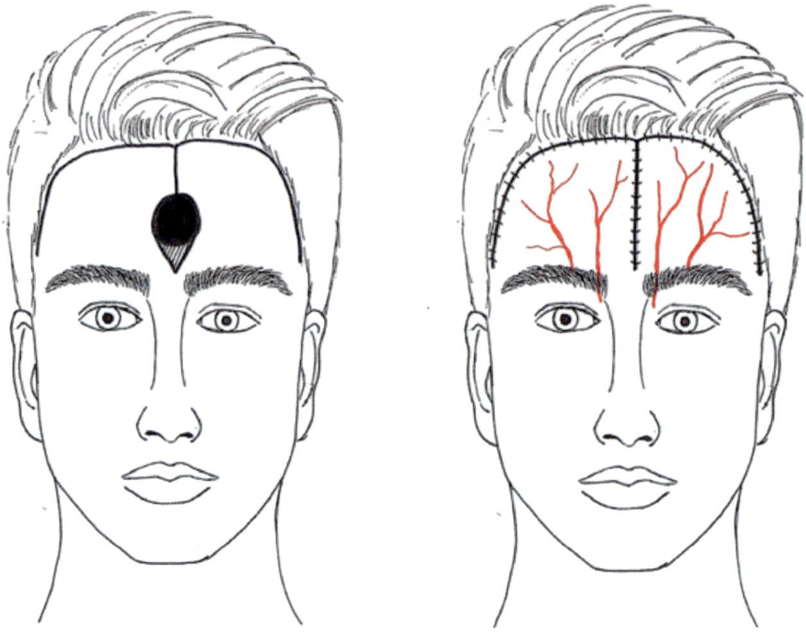

Fig. 7.6 Forehead rotation flaps 1 and 2

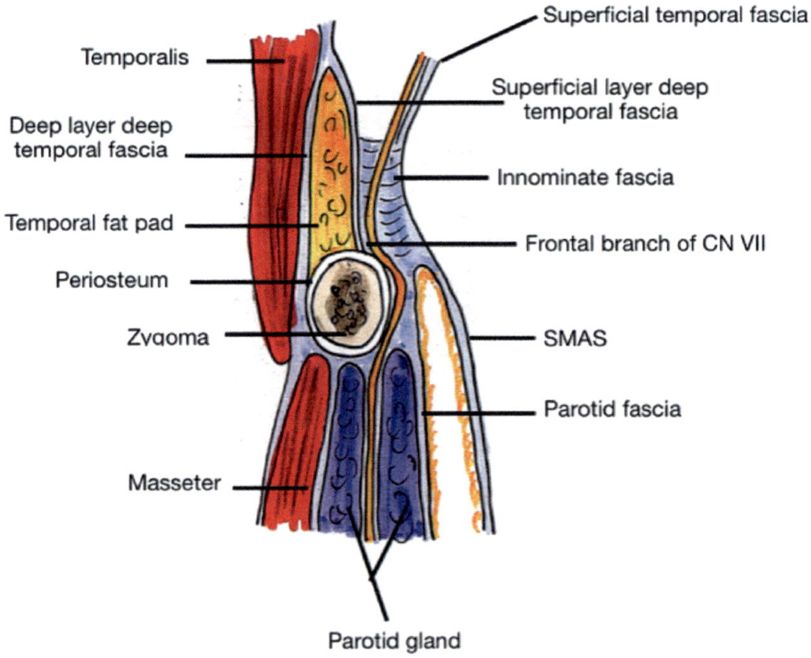

Fig. 7.7 Cross section of temporal fascia

7.7.3 Temple

When undertaking a resection of a lesion in the temple region, it is absolutely crucial to have a good understanding of the anatomy (Fig. 7.7). Pitanguy's line describes the surface landmark of the frontal branch of the facial nerve. It is a line that runs 0.5 cm below the tragus to a point 1.5 cm above and lateral to the eyebrow. However, this describes the course of the nerve in only one plane. A favourite question of examiners is to describe the fascial layers of this area and the way in which the frontal branch relates to it. In the preauricular region, the SMAS splits to encompass the parotid gland. These two layers then coalesce over the zygomatic arch, to which it is firmly adherent, to form the innominate fascia. The frontal branch is immediately deep to this fascia and superficial to the periosteum of the arch. Above the zygoma, the fascia splits into the superficial temporal fascia, also known as the temporoparietal fascia, and the deep temporal fascia, which itself has two layers, superficial and deep, which encase the temporal fat pad. These two deep temporal fascial layers then merge and become the fascia overlying the temporalis muscle. The superficial temporal fascia, being part of the SMAS, continues into the forehead as the frontalis muscle and into the scalp as the galea aponeurotica.

The frontal branch of the facial nerve lies immediately deep to the superficial temporal fascia and care should be taken not to breach this layer when resecting a tumour. If there are suspicions that the tumour invades the fascia, then the patient needs to be counselled that the nerve may need to be sacrificed in order to ensure oncological clearance, thus resulting in a brow palsy that can be corrected at a later stage with a brow lift. Even if the fascia is not breached, administration of local anaesthetic into the area can cause a temporary nerve palsy, which the patient needs to be warned about in order to minimise anxiety for the patient and phone calls/questions to the surgeon.

There is often a reasonable amount of laxity in the temple region, depending on the age and skin of the patient and lesions up to 1–1.5 cm can be closed directly. The workhorse local flap for this area is the rhomboid flap, a type of transposition flap that borrows from the relatively abundant transverse laxity to close moderately sized defects. In choosing a rhomboid flap to close the defect, the surgeon must ensure there is adequate laxity from the donor site to close primarily. If there is not, then an alternative such as a skin graft should be considered, which, in this natural hollow, can be cosmetically acceptable. With the rhomboid flap (Fig. 7.8), a transversely oriented diamond is marked around the tumour and the required margins. The obtuse angles should equal 120 degrees and the acute 60. The perpendicular line is then marked extending from point C (see diagram below), the length of which should be equal to the distance between points A and B. The flap is then raised superficial to the SMAS and transposed into the defect. The donor site is then closed primarily, resulting in a scythe-shaped scar.

7.7.4 Nose

Being centrally located within the face, the nose is particularly suited to flap reconstruction in order to preserve cosmesis. Hatchet flaps, which are a combination of rotation and V-Y advance-

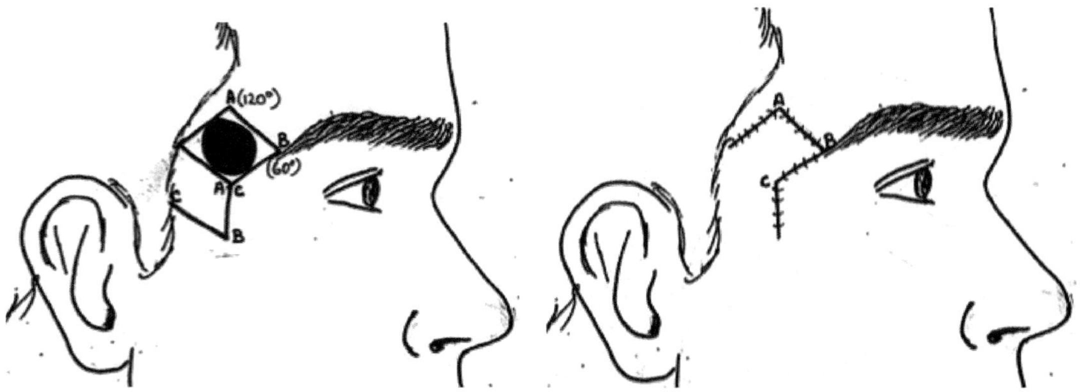

Fig. 7.8 Rhomboid flap

ment, are a good option for closure of defects of the nasal dorsum (Fig. 7.9). Bilobed flaps utilise laxity available in the nasal dorsum and sidewall to close defects of the relatively immobile nasal ala (Fig. 7.10).

Complex defects of the ala or tip may require staged reconstruction with either nasolabial or paramedian forehead flaps. The nasolabial flap (Fig. 7.11) can be superiorly or inferiorly based and rely on blood supply from the angular artery, the continuation of the facial artery. The paramedian forehead flap, the first description of which dates back to around 700 BC when it was described by the Indian physician Sushruta, is based on either the supraorbital or more commonly the supratrochlear artery (Fig. 7.12). The nasolabial flap needs to be thick enough to capture the angular artery. The paramedian forehead flap is typically raised in the subcutaneous plan in the distal third, submuscularly in the central third and subperiosteally in the proximal third to ensure that the artery is captured within the flap.

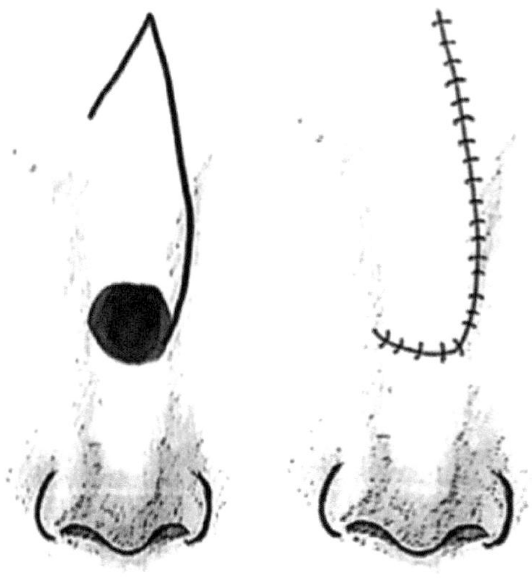

Fig. 7.9 Nose hatchet flap

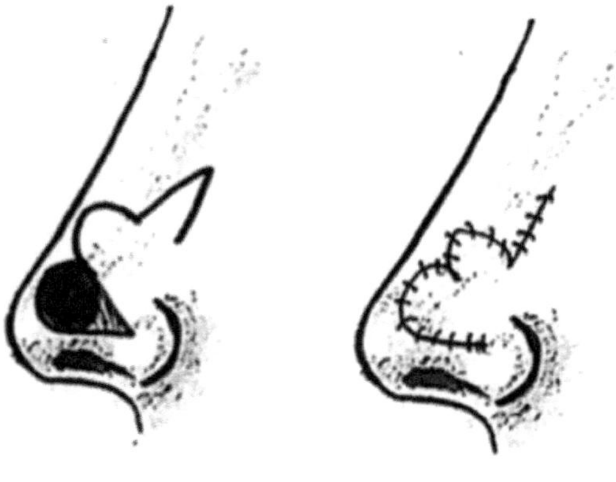

Fig. 7.10 Nose bilobed flap

Both nasolabial and paramedian forehead flaps require at least two procedures. The first stage involves raising and insetting the flaps into the defect. Once the blood supply is established at the site of the defect, the pedicle can be divided, usually 2–3 weeks after the first stage. Often, a third stage is required to thin or refine the flap prior to division, a process that is risky to do in the first stage as the already compromised blood supply can be further threatened by thinning out the tissue on which the skin depends for its survival. This intermediate stage should be at least 2–3 weeks after the first stage to maximise the blood supply. If the nasal defect is full thickness, the flap can be folded on itself or its undersurface grafted to reconstruct the mucosal surface of the nose.

7.7.5 Lip

Defects between the nose and the upper lip are usually best reconstructed with a full-thickness graft as local flaps will cross and disrupt the cosmetic subunits. Lesions involving the vermilion are best excised as a full-thickness wedge, which can be used for defects involving up to 30% of either the upper or lower lip. Defects involving up to 60% of the upper or lower lip can be reconstructed using a lip-sharing technique. The advantage of this reconstruction is that the orbicularis can be reconstituted, thus ensuring its continuity and function. For central defects, the Abbe flap (Fig. 7.13) can be based either medially or laterally. The contribution from the donor lip should be half that of the defect, ideally no more than 30% to ensure that the donor site can be primarily closed. The Abbe flap is necessarily a two-stage operation with flap division occurring 2–3 weeks after the flap is inset. During this time, mouth opening is restricted and the patient

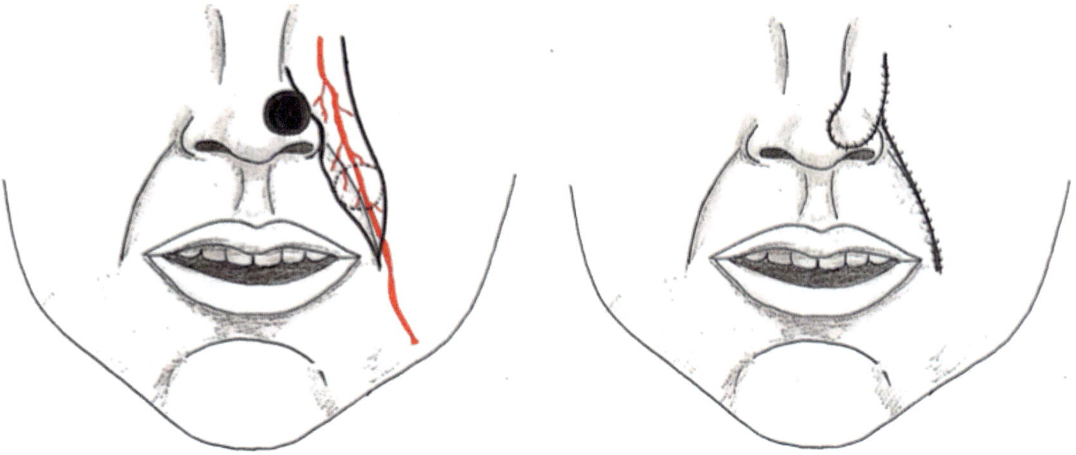

Fig. 7.11 Nasolabial flap

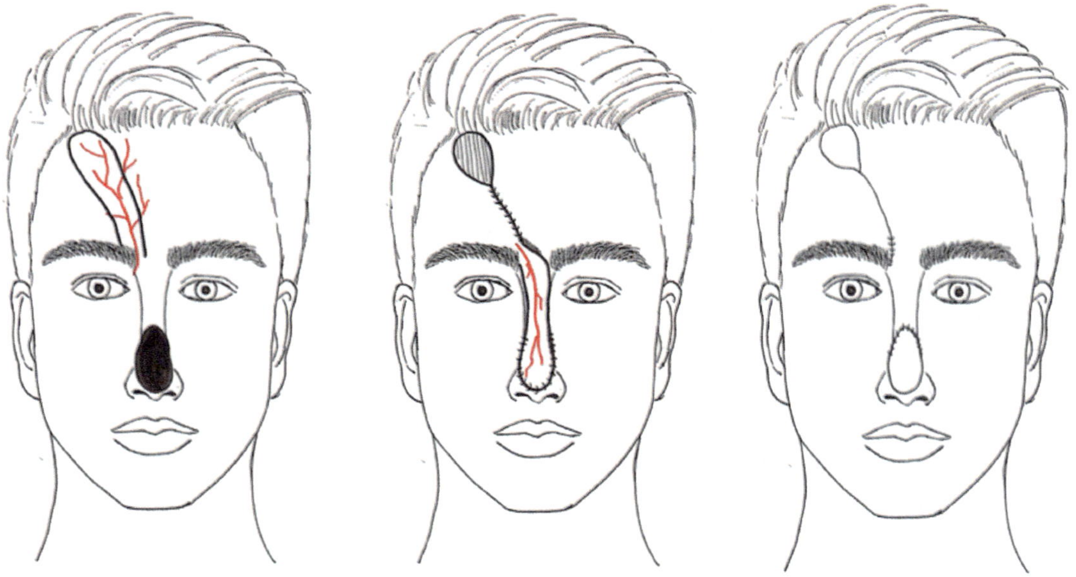

Fig. 7.12 Paramedian forehead flap

will need to be on a liquid diet so consultation with dietetics and speech therapy is crucial. The Estlander flap (Fig. 7.14) is for defects involving the commissure and is always medially based. It is theoretically a single-stage operation, but the resulting blunting of the commissure may need to be corrected with a commissuroplasty at a separate operation.

Large defects (75–100%) of the lip are challenging to reconstruct. The main issue is that of microstomia and potential loss of oral competence due to disruption of the continuity of orbicularis oris. The Karapandzic flap involves semicircular incisions extending down from the nasolabial folds, which are then rotated in to close the defect (Fig. 7.15). Care is taken to preserve the neurovascular bundle of the lip to preserve both function and sensation. The Bernard–Burrow–Webster flap uses laxity from the cheek to reconstruct up to a total lower lip defect (Fig. 7.15). Burrow's triangles are excised from the nasolabial fold to allow advancement.

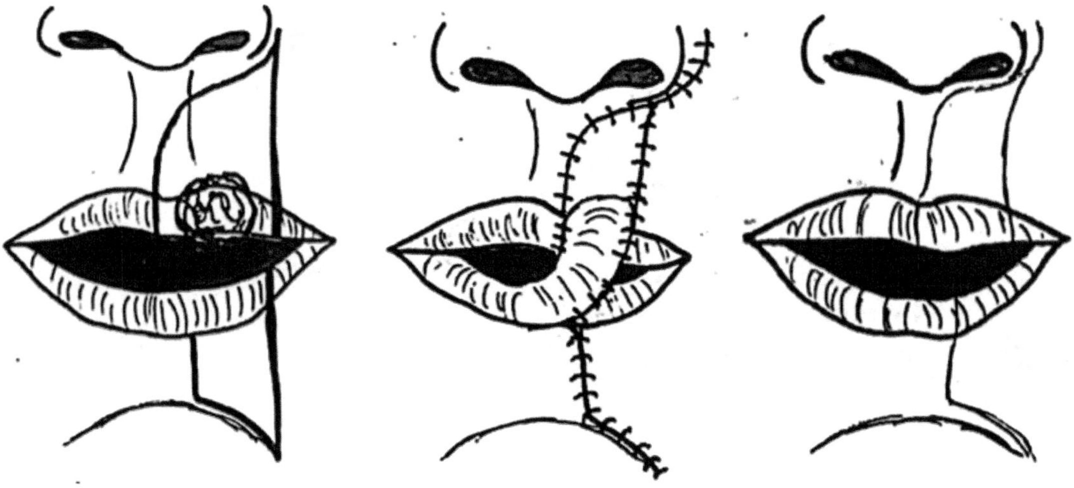

Fig. 7.13 Abbe flap

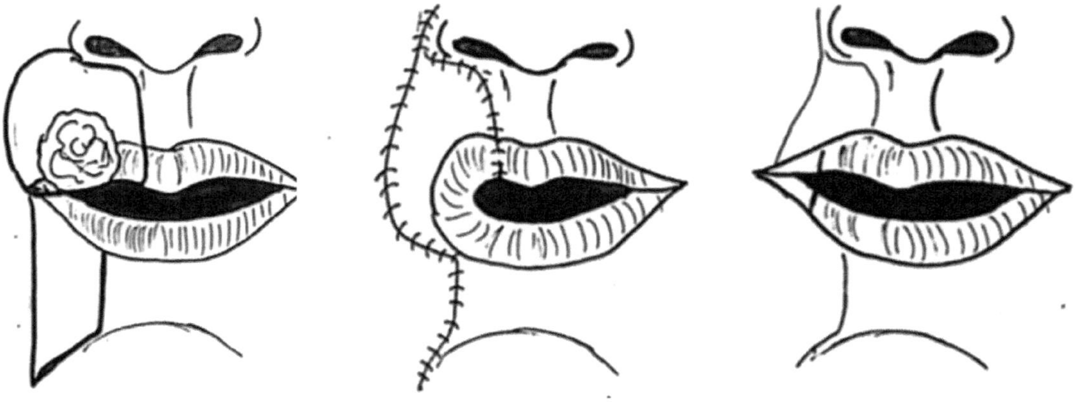

Fig. 7.14 Estlander flap

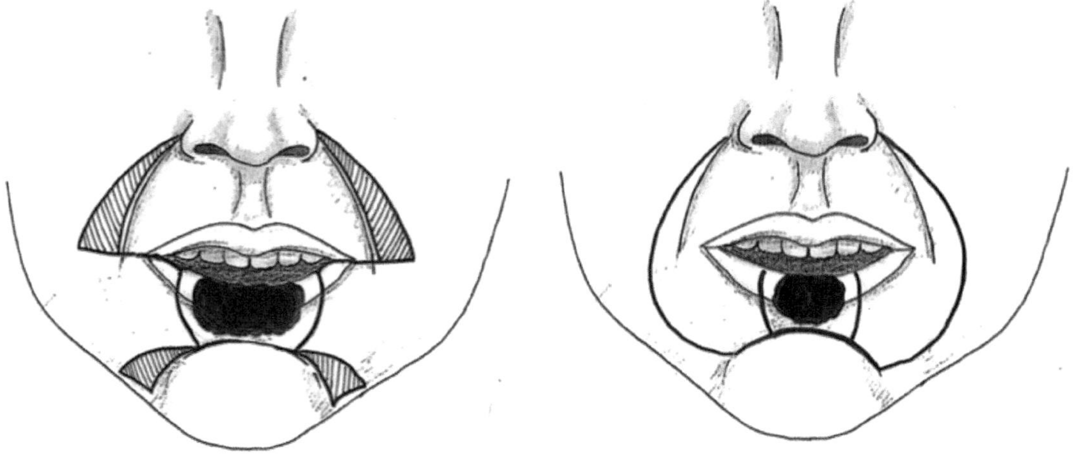

Fig. 7.15 1, Bernard–Burrow–Webster flap 2. Karapandzic flap

The buccal mucosa is incised approximately 1 cm superior to the skin incision, leaving the intervening muscle in continuity. The mucosal flap can then be advanced over the neo-lip to recreate the vermilion.

Diffuse lesions involving the vermilion may require vermilionectomy, excision of the entire red part of the lip. This can be reconstructed by a mucosal advancement flap. In this case, an island of mucosa is incised, the proximal end of which is placed in the gingival sulcus. The edge of the mucosa is sutured to the lip defect and sides are sutured with a dissolving suture such as Vicryl. The proximal part is allowed to heal by secondary intention.

7.7.6 Cheek

The key of reconstructing the cheek is to avoid downwards traction of the cheek as this can pull on the lower eyelid and cause an ectropion. Similarly, grafting the cheek is undesirable as not only is it cosmetically obvious, but secondary contraction can also cause ectropion. As such, all flaps of the cheek should be designed with this in mind so that the vector of pull is oriented transversely rather than vertically.

Medial cheek defects can be closed with V-Y advancement flaps (Fig. 7.16). In this flap, an island of skin is raised and blunt dissection is used to free soft tissues around the margins of the flap. Ideally, undermining of the flap is minimised to preserve the underlying blood supply, though often a little undermining of the leading and trailing edges of the flap is required for mobility. This V-shaped tissue is then advanced into the defect and the tail of the secondary defect is closed primarily, leaving behind a Y, hence the name.

Larger defects, particularly those more laterally under the eye, require cervicofacial flap, also known as a cheek rotation flap (Fig. 7.17), which utilises the laxity in the neck to close a cheek defect. The flap is extended lateral to the eye and up to the temple area before curving in front of and then behind the ear and down to the neck. The flap is raised in the supra-SMAS plane to prevent injury to the facial nerve while ensuring that the branches of the facial artery are maintained within the flap. Because the flap arches up to the temple, the pull of the flap occurs transversely, thus avoiding tension on the lower eyelid.

7.7.7 Ear

Skin cancers involving the ear often require excision of the underlying cartilage to ensure a clear deep margin. Because of the convolutions, grafts

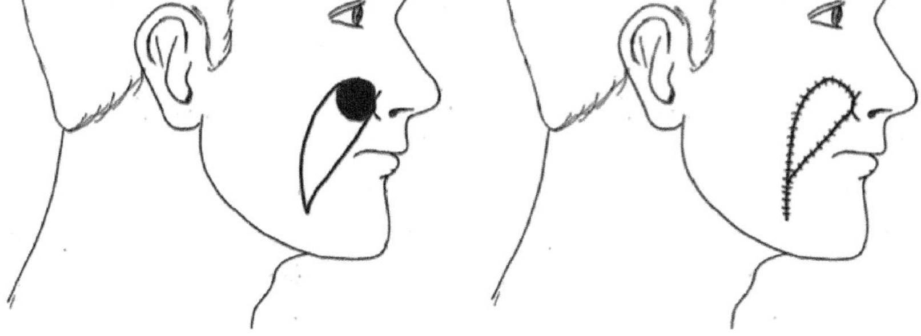

Fig. 7.16 V-Y advancement flap

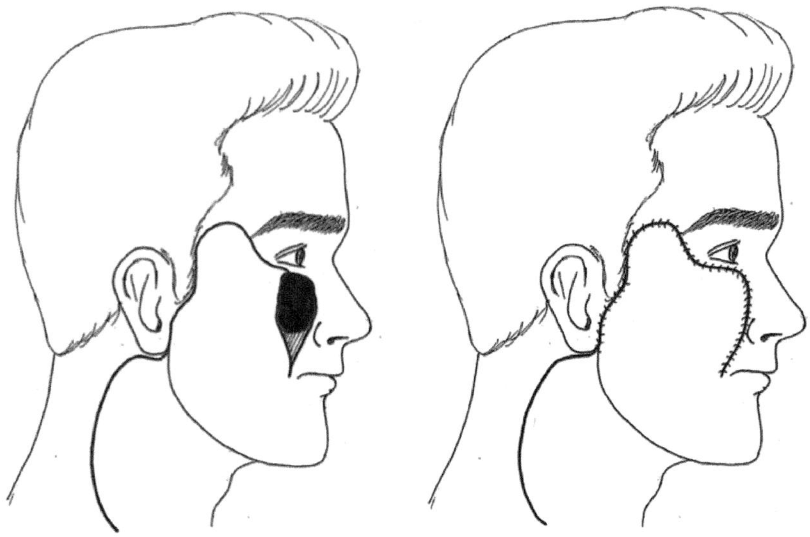

Fig. 7.17 Cheek rotation flap

to the medial portion of the ear, including the concha and even the antihelix, can be cosmetically acceptable. These grafts are secured to the underside of the underlying skin, which is often very well vascularised.

If the excision includes perichondrium, leaving behind bare cartilage, a retroauricular flap whimsically called the flip-flop-flap or more descriptively a trapdoor flap can be used. A flap of postauricular skin is raised and passed through a slit made by excising a 1–2 mm strip of cartilage. A small strip of skin is deepithelialised to allow inset into the edges of the defect, and the donor site is closed primarily or grafted in a location that is significantly less visible. The advantages of this flap include maintenance of the cartilaginous structure of the ear. However, apart from superficial lesions such as SCC in situ, it is often oncologically more sound to excise the cartilage in continuity with the skin, which is quite thin. As stated above, skin grafts are an extremely acceptable alternative to a flap in these cases.

Lesions involving the helix are often best treated with full-thickness excision and reconstruction to maintain the characteristic shape of the ear. Closure of a simple wedge excision larger than 1.5 cm can cause cupping of the ear, distorting its shape. A staggered wedge (Fig. 7.18) or an Antia–Buch flap (Fig. 7.19) should be used to

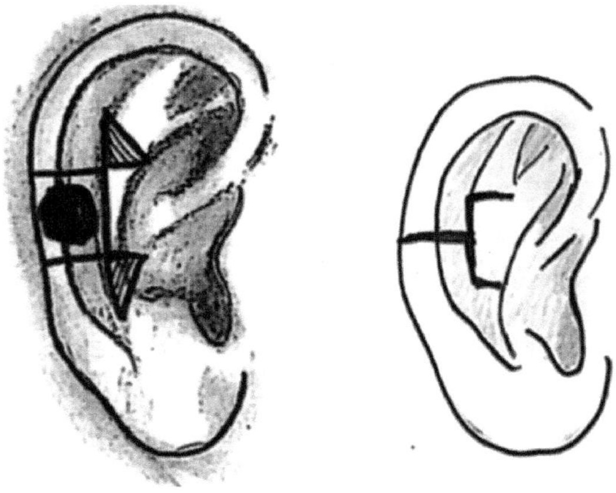

Fig. 7.18 Staggered wedge (double)

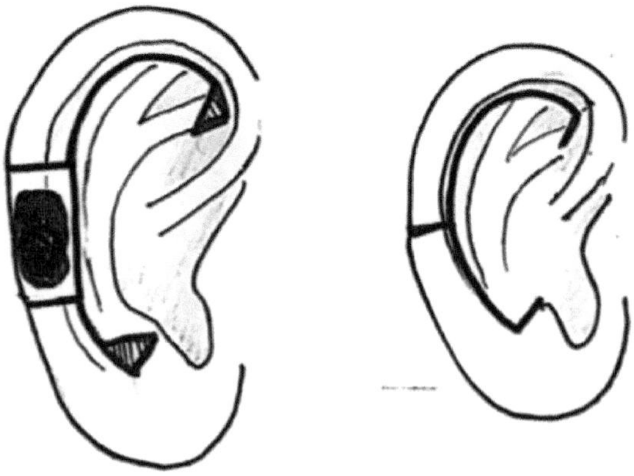

Fig. 7.19 Antia–Buch flap

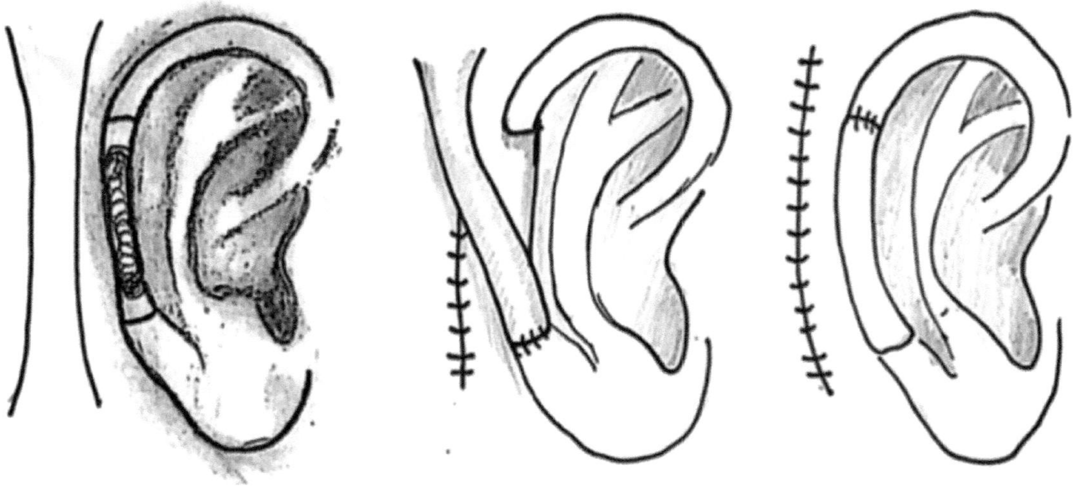

Fig. 7.20 Tubed pedicle flap

prevent this from happening. Both involve redistribution of the cartilaginous defect by excision of Burrow's triangles to allow advancement of the cartilage. The Antia–Buch flap, in addition, reduces the circumference of the cartilage of the ear, allowing redraping of the overlying skin. Both techniques will shorten the height of the ear while minimising cupping and maintaining the overall shape of the ear.

For elongated defects of the helical rim, a tubed pedicled flap of postauricular skin can be used to reconstruct the characteristic shape (Fig. 7.20). This is at least a three-stage procedure. The first stage involves incising a parallel strip of post-auricular skin, leaving the two ends intact. In the second stage a few weeks later, one of the ends of the flap is divided and inset into the corresponding end of the defect. This process is repeated with the other end of the flap at a third stage, once the blood supply is established. It is an elegant albeit rather laborious process.

Top Five Takeaways

1. Oncological Considerations

   The most important consideration of local flap reconstruction is ensuring adequate oncological clearance. It is easy to fall into the trap of compromising on the margin in favour of an easier flap raise, but the surgical oncologist must always remind themselves of the primary objective.

   Once the flap is elevated and inset, it can be difficult to ascertain where a positive margin may be, and when the deep margin is involved, scar tissue at the base of the flap can make it difficult to obtain a new margin without compromising the flap. If there are any concerns about not achieving clearance at the first excision before committing to a flap, either frozen sections or delayed reconstruction can be considered.

2. Flap Considerations

   Related to the previous point, it is important not to burn your bridges when elevating a flap. If a larger resection is required and the flap is not adequate to cover the new defect, it may not be possible to raise another local flap to cover the defect. As such, temporising measures such as skin grafts are always a good option.

3. Anatomical Considerations

   It is important to have a good understanding of the anatomy. As described above, there are a lot of structures packed into a relatively small amount of real estate. An understanding of planes will make resection and flap reconstruction safer and easier. Additionally, knowing where the blood supply is and what it is capable of doing will increase the likelihood of flap survival.

4. Aesthetic Considerations

In addition to covering ungraftable defects, the primary reason local flaps are chosen as a reconstructive option is because aesthetic outcomes are significantly better than either grafts or distant flaps. The colour and contour match are unrivalled by any other reconstructive option. As such, the surgeon should always be mindful of aesthetic subunits, rhytids and the location of hair-bearing skin in order to place scars where they will be the least noticeable once the wound has healed.

5. Patient Considerations

Local flaps are an excellent choice for patients of all ages. Many can be done under local anaesthetic with or without sedation and do not require general anaesthesia, thus making the procedure safer and the recovery faster. Having once experienced a patient gaping in shock at the size of a cervicofacial flap, a surgeon will never neglect to warn the patient in advance that, while local flap reconstruction equates to a larger incision initially, the long-term appearance, once the sutures are out and the wound has healed, is often significantly better than the alternatives.

Local flap reconstruction while fraught with potential pitfalls can be extremely satisfying to both patient and surgeon. The recommendations in this chapter will hopefully help to minimise tachycardia-inducing events and ensure safe and oncologically sound resection and reconstruction.

References

1. Subramaniam P, Olsen CM, Thompson BS, Whiteman DC, Neale RE. Anatomical distributions of basal cell carcinoma and squamous cell carcinoma in a population-based study in Queensland, Australia. JAMA Dermatol. 2017;153(2):175–82.
2. Wee E, Wolfe R, Mclean C, Kelly JW, Pan Y. The anatomic distribution of cutaneous melanoma: a detailed study of 5141 lessons. Aust J Dermatol. 2019;61(2):125–33.
3. Mitz V, Peyronie M. The superficial musculo-aponeurotic system (SMAS) in the parotid and cheek area. Plast Reconstr Surg. 1976;58(1):80–8.
4. Taylor GI, Palmer JH. The vascular territories (angiosomes) of the body: experimental study and clinical applications. Br J Plast Surg. 1987;40(2):113–41.
5. Taylor GI, Corlett RJ, Caddy CM, Zelt RG. An anatomic review of the delay phenomenon. Plast Reconstr Surg. 1992;89(3):408–16.
6. Ahuja RB. Geometric considerations in the design of rotation flaps in the scalp and forehead region. Plas Reconstr Surg. 1988;81(6):900–6.

Neck Dissection

8

Timothy Manzie and James Wykes

The performance of a neck dissection has evolved into a therapeutic and diagnostic procedure and is a crucial component in the management of head and neck malignancy. The presence of metastatic disease in the neck, from either a primary mucosal or cutaneous tumour, is the most important prognostic factor for a patient. Robbins described levels of lymph nodes in the neck into six zones (I–VI; Table 8.1), and these have become the globally accepted method of description [1]. This procedure has been refined over many years from the highly morbid radical neck dissection (RND) through to the introduction of the selective neck dissection (SND). The neck dissection has evolved from the removal of lymphatic and non-lymphatic structures (RND) to the preservation of non-lymphatic structures (modified radical neck dissection (MRND)) to the current treatment of preservation of some lymphatic structures [2]. Previous removal of the spinal accessory nerve (SAN), sternocleidomastoid (SCM) and internal jugular vein (IJV) with a RND had an increased degree of morbidity [2]. Brocca demonstrated no worsening of outcome when these structures were preserved in a MRND, and Schiff demonstrated no increased risk of recurrence when a SND was performed [2]. The aims of a neck dissection are both for diagnosis of previously undetected (occult) metastatic disease and for therapeutic reasons (removal of known tumour cells) [2]. Histopathological review of these specimens then often guides further treatment including watch and wait, radiation therapy, chemotherapy or immunotherapy.

Most commonly, a neck dissection is performed for metastatic squamous cell carcinoma (SCC) [3]. The primary site of disease is most commonly mucosal (predominantly oral cavity) or cutaneous (skin of the scalp and face) [4, 5]. If nodal disease has been confirmed prior to surgery (N+), the procedure is deemed to be a therapeutic neck dissection [5]. If neck disease is suspected, or if there is a reasonable likelihood of microscopic disease (greater than 20% in oral SCC) but not confirmed, the procedure is deemed to be an elective neck dissection of the at-risk nodal basins given the known biology of the primary lesion [6]. Given the lymphatic spread of the majority of tumours in the head and neck region, the pattern of spread for different primary tumour types and locations is based on a predictable pattern of lymphatic drainage [4, 7]. For oral cavity disease, it is uncommon for level IV to be involved unless suspected based on preoperative imaging. Metastatic disease to level V does not occur without disease being present in other levels [7]. Typically, an elective neck dissection for an oral cavity malignancy would include levels I–III [5]. For a therapeutic (known metastatic disease; N+) neck dissection related

T. Manzie (✉) · J. Wykes
Chris O'Brien Lifehouse,
Camperdown, NSW, Australia
e-mail: james.wykes@lh.org.au

B. Ashford (ed.), *Head and Neck Surgery for General Surgeons*,
https://doi.org/10.1007/978-981-19-7900-2_8

Table 8.1 Anatomical boundaries of a neck dissection [1]

	Boundary			
Level	Superior	Inferior	Anterior (medial)	Posterior (lateral)
IA	Symphysis of mandible	Body of hyoid	Anterior belly of contralateral digastric muscle	Anterior belly of ipsilateral digastric muscle
IB	Body of mandible	Posterior belly of digastric muscle	Anterior belly of digastric muscle	Stylohyoid muscle
IIA	Skull base	Horizontal plane defined by the inferior body of the hyoid bone	Stylohyoid muscle	Accessory nerve
IIB	Skull base	Horizontal plane defined by the inferior body of the hyoid bone	Accessory nerve	Lateral border of the sternocleidomastoid muscle
III	Horizontal plane defined by the inferior body of the hyoid bone	Horizontal plane defined by the inferior border of the cricoid cartilage	Lateral border of the sternohyoid muscle	Lateral border of the sternocleidomastoid muscle or sensory branches of cervical plexus
IV	Horizontal plane defined by the inferior border of the cricoid cartilage	Clavicle	Lateral border of the sternohyoid muscle	Lateral border of the sternocleidomastoid muscle or sensory branches of cervical plexus
VA	Apex of the convergence of the sternocleidomastoid and trapezius muscle	Horizontal plane defined by the inferior border of the cricoid cartilage	Posterior border of the sternocleidomastoid muscle or cervical sensory branches	Anterior border of the trapezius muscle
VB	Horizontal plane defined by the lower border of the cricoid cartilage	Clavicle	Posterior border of the sternocleidomastoid muscle or cervical sensory branches	Anterior border of the trapezius muscle
VI	Hyoid bone	Suprasternal	Common carotid artery	Common carotid artery

to an oral cavity cancer, a neck dissection would typically involve levels I–IV [5]. For a cutaneous primary lesion, the primary site provides guidance for the lymph node levels to be removed during the neck dissection and as well as a decision regarding possible surgery involving the parotid gland [4]. For lesions in the anterior face (including lips), a neck dissection including removal of levels I–III is recommended [4]. For lesions anterior to the external ear canal (EAC), a neck dissection including levels II–IV and an ipsilateral superficial parotidectomy is recommended. If the cutaenous lesion is posterior to the EAC, a neck dissection of levels II–V is recommended [4]. Lesions that are close to or involving the midline may involve the lymphatic system of each side, and treatment of both should be considered [4]. Further, staging imaging can provide additional information that may demonstrate clinically undetected disease and alter the surgical plan. As such, a good understanding of the underlying pathology and pattern of disease spread is crucial to the performance of an adequate neck dissection, which balances treating the disease with minimising the risks of the procedure.

The number of lymph nodes contained in a neck dissection is important. The American Joint Committee on Cancer (AJCC) considers a minimum yield of 10 lymph nodes for a SND and 15 for a MRND or a RND [8]. Furthermore, nodal yield is crucial as a marker of quality in a neck dissection. A neck dissection for an oral cavity cancer containing less than 18 nodes demonstrates a reduction in overall survival and disease-specific survival [9]. This represents a good rule of thumb for all neck dissections.

8.1 Key Elements of History

Involvement of the cervical lymphatic structures by a malignant process signifies an increase in disease severity and a decline in overall prognosis. The review of a patient's history is important to guide decision-making, may alter the surgical planning or if advanced/complex may suggest a non-surgical or palliative approach. Previous treatment of the neck, either surgery or radiotherapy or both, is a key component. Comorbidities such as previous cerebrovascular disease, severe cardiovascular or respiratory diseases may escalate the risk of surgical morbidity beyond benefit. Previous spinal surgery or cervical spine limitations may restrict the turning or extension of the neck and increase the surgical difficulty. Medications often need to be reviewed, with the temporary cessation and/or commencement of other 'bridging' medications such as those affecting coagulation, in the lead up to proposed treatment. Other considerations include the assessment of allergies, which may alter the peri-operative or post-operative medications, most commonly antibiotics or analgesics. It is important to consider the social history, especially nicotine/tobacco dependence and alcohol consumption. Given the elevated risk of oral and oropharyngeal cancer related to their use, it is more common in this patient population than in others. The use of nicotine replacement therapy and consideration of implementing an alcohol withdrawal scale may need to be considered pre-operatively. It is also of importance to understand the patients living conditions and supports pre-operatively as this may highlight additional services needed following discharge.

8.1.1 Underlying Disease Process

The peripheral lymphatic system, composed of lymphatic channels and lymph nodes, performs a number of functions. It is responsible for the collection and removal of the interstitial fluid, allows for the absorption of fats and facilitates the immune response [10]. Interstitial fluid is allowed to passively enter through the lining endothelial cells of the lymphatic capillaries with a local increase in fluid pressures [10]. Transport through the lymphatic system is facilitated by smooth muscle within the lining of the larger lymphatic channels allowing for contraction, gravity-dependant drainage and the pressure gradient generated by inspiration, fascial/skin movement and muscle contraction [10]. The lymph nodes feature the lymphocytes (T and B cells) that are integral for the innate immune system. These nodes can enlarge in both inflammatory conditions or secondary to either primary (lymphoma) or secondary malignant processes (such as metastatic deposits).

A number of malignancies spread via the lymphatic system primarily, namely oral, oropharyngeal and cutaneous squamous cell carcinomas. Metastasis occurs via the lymphatic system when the malignant cells are able to disseminate from the primary tumour and enter the lymphatic system. Unlike haematogenous spread, the lymphatic system allows for passive entry, offers a less hostile haemodynamic environment and has no need for extravasation at the distant site. Once tumour cells arrive at the lymphatic nodes, they require the ability to evade the host immune system and have sufficient blood supply to maintain ongoing cell division.

Involvement of the different lymph node levels may be predictable based on the location and type of the primary tumour. The risk of nodal metastasis for an oral squamous cell carcinoma varies with over 30% presenting with occult disease and up to 76% with macroscopic disease [7, 11]. The risk for cutaneous squamous cell carcinomas is approximately 5% [4]. The risk is significantly less for mucosal melanoma or sarcomas (and not considered further here). The pattern of involvement for cutaneous and oral mucosal malignancies has been studied and may guide which lymph nodes are to be removed in a selective neck dissection [7, 4]. A selective lymph node dissection balances the risk of involvement of each lymph node level against the surgical morbidity associated with dissection of that level [2]. Previous surgical treatment or radiation therapy needs to be considered as this will likely alter the pattern of nodal involvement. The spread of metastatic disease to levels beyond those or on the contralateral side needs to be considered if there has been previous treatment with clinical and radiographical examination and removal should the risk of involvement be sufficient [7, 4, 11].

8.1.1.1 Oral Cavity

The levels of lymph nodes at risk for metastatic spread are determined by a number of factors. The location, size, depth of invasion and primary tumour type are to be considered when assessing risk. The single most important factor is depth of invasion. It is important to consider whether there is macroscopic involvement of the lymph nodes (N+) or the suspicion of occult disease (N0). An elective neck dissection may be considered when the risk of occult metastasis is greater than 20% [6]. There are some guidelines that suggest that all squamous cell carcinomas of the oral cavity should undergo an elective, selective neck dissection for oral cavity squamous cell carcinomas regardless of staging; however, a depth of invasion >4 mm is commonly thought to equate to a > 20% risk of occult nodal disease and is often used to guide management decisions.

Occult Disease (N0)

Occult involvement of the cervical lymph nodes is diagnosed in oral cavity carcinomas in up to 33% of cases. It is most common to affect level I (39.7%), II (34.9%) or III (17.8%) [7]. Involvement of level IV (6.2%) and level V (1.3%) is uncommon when there is occult disease of the upper levels of the neck [7].

The risk of dissecting level IV is associated with the risk of bleeding and injury to the lymphatic system, especially on the left. The involvement of level V does not occur in isolation with a primary SCC of the oral cavity (discussed below), and thus, further adjunctive treatment, which would cover the area, would likely still occur. The risk of dissecting level V is primarily associated with the risk of injury/impairment to the accessory nerve and branchial plexus. Given the low risk of occult metastatic disease to levels IV and V, it is of limited benefit in a neck that has no detectable metastasis (N0) and is not recommended.

Macroscopic Disease (N1)

In the setting of oral SCC and macroscopic disease, the risk of metastatic spread to levels beyond I–III increases significantly. The risk of nodal metastasis to level IV and V is 10.1% and 2.2%, respectively [7]. Given the balance of surgical risk, most consider it appropriate to include level IV in a selective therapeutic neck dissection.

Level V may be considered with significant nodal disease on a case-by-case basis.

Level IIb

Level IIb provides some controversy as to the purported benefits of dissection in the setting of occult disease. The risk of dissection is additional morbidity associated with shoulder dysfunction secondary to dissection and possible iatrogenic injury to the accessory nerve. Level IIb is involved in up to 6% of cases of oral SCC with 15% of these with isolated metastatic disease to IIb [12]. As with skip lesions, there may be significant risk of failing to identify this isolated involvement of IIb should it not be dissected. On balance, it is of the authors' opinion that neck dissections for oral cavity malignancies include the dissection of IIb.

Skip Metastasis

Skip metastasis presents a treatment risk and may result in the under-staging of disease. A lack of recognition through a failure to perform a neck dissection of the affected levels, may result in the neck being staged as N0, which often negates the justification/need for additional adjunctive treatment (surgery or chemotherapy). Should disease persist beyond the dissected levels, it may represent early treatment failure and allow for disease progression to a point where cure is less likely. The benefit of performing an elective selective neck dissection is the diagnosis of occult disease, most commonly levels I–III. Thus, skip metastasis to these levels would be diagnosed with a selective neck dissection. The main risk belongs to the undetected incidence of metastatic disease to levels IV and V in the N0 neck. Thankfully, it is uncommon for 'skip metastasis' involving isolated metastasis to level IV (0.5%) and does not occur to level V without disease in other levels [7, 13].

8.1.1.2 Cutaneous Squamous Cell Disease

Cutaneous malignancies metastasise less commonly than lesions of the oral cavity (<5%) [4]. For cutaneous disease, the parotid gland also needs to be considered as a possible location for nodal metastasis and may involve intraparotid lymph nodes or soft tissue deposits in up to 75% of cases with cervical lymph nodes [4]. As such, surgical procedures addressing these lymph nodes (most commonly a superficial parotidectomy) may also be considered as part of the required surgical management. Due to the reduced risk of metastatic nodal disease in cutaneous squamous cell carcinoma, an elective neck dissection for occult disease is uncommon and not often indicated (considered for advanced T stage and other high-risk factors). A therapeutic SND, including removal of the external jugular lymph node chain, is suggested for clinically detectable macroscopic metastatic disease (N+) or radiological staging suggesting nodal involvement (N+) [4].

Parotid Positive (P+)

Metastatic cutaneous squamous cell carcinoma is the most common malignant lesion of the parotid gland in the Australian population [14]. The risk of occult cervical lymphatic metastasis with known parotid disease (P+) is up to 36% [14]. The location of cervical metastasis and therefore the subsequent levels for selective lymph node dissection vary based on the location of the primary (or presumed) cutaneous tumour [4]. The recommended treatment for the parotid gland and cervical lymph nodes is listed in Table 8.2. For primary lesions involving the external ear or anterior face, a superficial parotidectomy with a selective neck dissection of levels I–III is recommended. For lesions posterior to the external ear, a superficial parotidectomy with selective neck dissection of levels II–V should be considered.

Parotid Negative (P0)

In the instance of no macroscopic disease in either the parotid gland (P0) or cervical lymph nodes (N0), no further surgery is recommended; however, close surveillance with appropriate imaging such as ultrasound or CT should be considered. Sentinel lymph node biopsy is feasible but has not been conclusively shown to add benefit. Should there be macroscopic disease in the cervical lymph nodes of cutaneous SCC origin, a comprehensive neck dissection (I–V) with no treatment of the parotid gland is suggested.

Table 8.2 Recommended management of the parotid and levels of the neck for metastatic cutaneous squamous cell carcinoma [4]

		Recommendations for treatment	
Clinical stage	Primary site	Surgery	Adjuvant radiotherapy
P0N+	Any	CND	P and N
P+ & N0	Anterior or external ear	P and SND (I–III)	N0: P P+& N+: P and N
P+ & N0	Posterior scalp or neck	P and SND (II–V)	N0: P N+: P and N
P+ & N0	Unknown primary	P and CND	N0: P N+: P and N
P+ & N+	Any	P and CND	P and N

Key: *P* parotid, *N* neck, + positive for disease, *CND* comprehensive neck dissection (I–V), *SND* selective neck dissection

8.1.1.3 Salivary Gland Disease

The risk of cervical metastasis depends on the type of primary lesion and its grading. Overall, the risk of occult metastasis is very low compared with other malignant pathologies. The estimated incidence of occult metastasis for all types of primary malignancy salivary gland tumours is 22% [15]. Elective neck dissections for occult disease (N0) in the setting of parotid gland tumours is controversial. Metastatic lymph node involvement most commonly (73.3%) involves the intraparotid lymph nodes [16]. Indications for an elective neck dissection include advanced T stage or a high-risk histopathological diagnosis (high-grade mucoepidermoid carcinoma, salivary duct carcinoma, adenocarcinoma, SCC, oncocytic carcinoma, and adenoid cystic carcinoma) [16]. If to be performed, level II is the most common level to be involved and recommended to be included [15]. For macroscopic lymph node involvement, the surgeons' preference and underlying pathology should be considered; however, a neck dissection including levels I–IV dissection should be considered. For aggressive pathologies such as salivary duct carcinoma, a modified radical neck dissection (I–V) should be considered.

8.1.2 Previous Medical History

The patient's past medical history is an important factor to consider prior to performing a neck dissection. A targeted history regarding treatment in the head and region is discussed further. A number of medical comorbidities have systemic effects that may increase the risk of post-operative complications including infection, bleeding, fistula formation, cardiopulmonary or neurological complications. Substance misuse increases the risk of the majority of these complications so also important to consider the patient's social history [17]. A discussion with the patient and affiliated treating medical teams will help to highlight possible concerns pre-operatively. Discussion with the patient and their family should consider the impact these factors may have on the overall risk for the procedure.

There are a number of conditions that may increase the risk of infection. Diabetes mellitus (types 1 and 2) is the most common condition that will increase the risk of infection and healing through elevated circulating glucose and microvascular changes [18]. Poor nutritional status will also elevate the risk of infection and delay healing. Smoking alters the oral flora to be more pathogenic and vascular related changes [18, 19]. Excessive alcohol and a history of hepatitis may reduce the synthetic function of the liver causing an increased infection or bleeding risk and delayed healing [20].

There are a number of other conditions, which in themselves may elevate the risk of infection or secondarily through their treatment. Conditions such as lymphoma directly impair the immune response through altered lymphocyte function despite elevated circulating number of lymphocytes. Systemic inflammatory conditions and their treatments (often steroids or other immunosuppresive agents) such as the arthritidies (rheumatoid arthritis) or autoimmune conditions (systemic lupus erythematous) may increase the risk of infection or impair healing [18].

8.1.3 Previous Treatment in the Head and Neck Region

Awareness and consideration of the previous treatment in the head and neck region is important for aiding diagnosis, pre-operative assessment and planning. Patients requiring a neck dissection may initially present with no symptoms, a lump in the neck, swallowing difficulties or a known non-healing ulcer of the skin or oral cavity. A lump in the neck may have a number of differential diagnoses so it is important to take a targeted history to gather further information to guide additional investigations and suggest possible causes. There would be concerns that a regional metastasis from any previous malignancy of the head and neck may present with cervical lymphadenopathy. Focused questions regarding previous skin excisions or topical chemotherapeutics (such as imiquimod or 5-fluoruracil) may suggest regional metastatic disease from a previously treated cutaneous source. Symptoms or signs of a non-healing ulcer (skin or oral cavity) may suggest an untreated/undiagnosed primary lesion or locoregional recurrence. A lesion of the oropharynx may be suspected with symptoms of globus sensation, dysphagia, dysphonia or hoarseness. Any of these features will guide further investigations to aid in the diagnosis of an underlying causative process.

Previous surgical or radiation treatment in the head and neck region will alter or make further treatment more complex. If previously performed, these interventions increase the complexity and risks associated with any additional treatment. Further to this, studies that consider the pattern of metastatic spread via the lymph are based on non-operated and non-irradiated necks. Consideration needs to be given to include additional ipsilateral or contralateral lymphatic levels when performing a lymph node dissection in this setting [7, 4]. The review of previous surgical documentation is also important. Previously dissected structures may be present in an altered position, anatomical structures that act as surgical landmarks may have been removed and additional scar tissue will make the dissection more difficult. Radiation therapy will alter the tissue-handling characteristics and disrupt the tissue planes making dissection more difficult. Furthermore, delayed wound healing is more common and additional consideration regardining the placement of incisions and the addition of soft tissue into the region (regional or free flap) may be necessary. Patients ought to be warned of the additional surgical risk of injury to important structures such as large blood vessels resulting in bleeding, the increased risk of stroke or the sensory/motor nerves causing altered sensation or functional impairment.

To supplement the history, an examination of the head and neck will be complimentary and provide further stimuli for additional review of the patients' history. An examination of the skin for surgical scars, cranial and sensory nerve function, with thorough examination of the oral cavity, oropharynx and nasopharynx [with the assistance of flexible nasendoscopy] may provide clues to previous treatment or demonstrate new/recurrent disease.

8.1.4 Current Medications

A pending neck dissection may require the temporary withholding, cessation or commencement of new medications pending adjunctive procedures. Current medications if not withheld may increase the risk of bleeding complications, cessation of diabetic medications may elevate the risk of infection/delay healing and cessation of statin-based therapy may increase cardiovascular complications. It is important to consider the indications for treatment, and any alteration to the timing, dose or need to withhold may require discussion with the prescribing doctor prior. A single antiplatelet agent such as aspirin is likely able to be continued [18]. If dual antiplatelet therapy (DAPT) is prescribed, it is important to review the initial indication as this may no longer be required. Should DAPT continue to be indicated for a particular time duration and the procedure was elective, it may be worthwhile delaying treatment until only a single antiplatelet agent is required [18]. Alternatively, it may be possible to withhold one agent for the peri-operative period. Anticoagulants can often be temporarily withheld if being prescribed for primary prevention (i.e. no previous cerebrovascular accident) [18]. Alternatively, should there be significant risk of emboli, bridging with short-acting anticoagulants may be considered in high-risk patients. This may require a pre-surgical admission for a heparin infusion or subcutaneous low molecular weight heparin as an outpatient prior [18]. Chemo-mechanical prophylaxis for deep vein thrombosis is recommended [18]. Complex cardiac patients such as those with prosthetic valves are best discussed with the treating specialist due to the significant increased risk of an embolic event.

Long-term steroid use impairs healing, increases the risk of infection and may alter the haemodynamic haemostasis [18]. Supplemental use suppresses the hypothalamus–pituitary axis and mineralocorticoid production. This affects the ability of the body to respond to the stress caused by surgery. Consideration for an increase in dose or supplemental steroid use (commonly intravenous hydrocortisone) to replicate this stress response may be required in the days after [18]. Pre-operative discussion with the prescribing doctor or endocrinology colleagues is recommended.

Natural or herbal medications should also be considered in the patients' history. These may either alter the risk of complications such as bleeding or interact with medications that are to be prescribed during the course of admission. For example, fish oil (eicosapentaenoic acid), Japanese Honeysuckle (Lonicera japonica) and Gingko (Ginkgo biloba) can alter the function of platelets or coagulation cascade increasing the risk of bleeding both intra-operatively and post-operatively [21].

8.2 Clinical Examination Pearls

A neck swelling is the most common sign or symptom concerning for malignancy, particularly in the adult population, and likely need for neck dissection. A complete neck examination involves a targeted review of the area of the concerning swelling and further examination of the ipsilateral and contralateral levels of the neck (I–VI). A comprehensive examination should also include review of possible primary malignancy sites including an examination of the skin in the head and neck region, oral cavity, nasopharynx and oropharynx with the assistance of nasendoscopy. Swellings of the neck may either represent an enlargement of normal anatomy or a benign or malignant lesion (see Table 8.3). Malignant processes, when confirmed on tissue diagnosis, are clinically staged per the TNM classification system based on the findings of the examination. In an Australian context, metastatic cutaneous squamous cell carcinoma is the most common malignant cause, whereas there are a number of different benign lesions depending on the location of the swelling. The location and characteristic of the lesion will shorten the list of differential diagnosis and may guide further investigations.

Table 8.3 Common causes of swellings of the neck [22, 23]

Lateral neck swellings	Midline neck swellings
• Enlarged lymph node – Inflammatory Bacterial infection (local or systemic) Viral infection (local or systemic) – Neoplastic Metastatic disease Leukaemia – Autoimmune Sarcoidosis – Drugs • Branchial (lympho-epithelial) cyst • Parotid tail tumour • Pharyngeal pouch • Carotid body tumour • Cervical rib	• Thyroglossal duct cyst • Sublingual dermoid cyst • Thyroid swellings – Goitre – Grave's disease – Hashimoto's thyroiditis – Solitary adenoma – Carcinoma
Lateral or midline	
• Lipoma • Dermoid cyst • Epidermal cyst • Abscess • Lymphoma	

8.2.1 Targeted Examination

8.2.1.1 Look

Initial examination should consist of the size and location of the swelling. The overlying skin should be examined for erythema, which may suggest an infective cause or thickening which may suggest extranodal extension of a malignant process. Symmetrical swelling may be representative of a systemic process such as infection (bacterial or viral) which is more common in a younger patient or malignant process in the adult patient. The location of the swelling may provide a shortened list of differentials and often best to consider the types of structures within the region (nerves, blood vessels, muscles, lymph nodes, and organs). Centrally, swellings such as a thyroglossal duct cyst are common and would be noted to move with protrusion of the tongue. Enlargement of the thyroid gland or lesions within will move with swallowing but not tongue protrusion. A swelling in the lateral aspect of the neck may represent a lesion such as a branchial cleft cyst.

Given the risk of cutaneous disease metastasising to the cervical lymph nodes, examination should inspect for irregular crusting, ulcerative, friable or lesions that readily bleed or pigmented lesions. The presence of a punctum may suggest a benign process such as a dermoid or epidermoid cyst. Scarring may suggest previous surgical intervention if the primary lesion has already been treated. Assessment of facial nerve function (movement of the muscles of facial expression) and the trigeminal nerve (sensation to the face) is important as a small percentage of high-risk SCCs have a propensity for perineural spread. Further review or clarification of the history may provide additional clues.

When a malignant process is suspected, it is important to perform a thorough examination of the anatomical regions which would drain to the cervical lymph nodes of the head and neck region. To be comprehensive, it requires good lighting and optimal retraction, commonly with the aid of gauze to allow controlled movement of the tongue or wooden tongue depressors. Examination of the oral cavity includes review of the hard and soft tissues. Poor dentition may increase the likelihood of an infective cause, whereas the presence of an ulcerated lesion may represent a primary mucosal SCC. The examination should include all of the oral cavity including, but not limited to the tongue, buccal mucosa, floor of mouth, retromolar trigone, lips buccal sulci and hard/soft palate. The tonsils and oropharynx should be examined for asymmetry, induration, ulceration, erythema or the presence of suppuration. Nasoendocopy should be used as an adjunct to look for similar findings of the nasal cavity and nasopharynx. An examination of the skin in the head and neck region is also important. Ulcerative, heterogeneous or evolving pigmented lesions of the skin should prompt concerns for a malignant process such as a keratinocyte or non-keratinocyte-based skin cancer such as a SCC or melanoma. High-risk subsites include those in the 'H' zone including the pinna, nose and lips.

8.2.1.2 Feel

The lesion or lesions should be palpated to confirm the estimated size, number and consistency. While the number of lesions is important, it may not differentiate between a benign process such as infection or metastatic malignancy as each can have single or multiple lesions present. Tenderness of the lesion with erythema may suggest an infective cause. A non-tender lesion may be concerning for a benign or malignant disease process. A pulsatile mass may represent a vascular malformation. The consistency and texture of the lesion is also important. A soft or fluctuant lesion may represent a cystic lesion, which could be benign such as a thyroglossal cyst or an acutely inflamed lymph node or malignant lesion such as a cystic or necrotic lymph node. A firm lesion may be more likely to represent a malignant process. Given previous treatment with surgery or radiation therapy, it must be reminded that deeper structures such as the cartilages of the larynx and or hyoid may appear more prominent.

8.2.1.3 Move

The mobility of the lesion is important for both assessing the lesion and aiding the list of differential diagnoses. It should be determined if the lesion is tethered/can be moved independent of the overlying skin or deeper structures. Fontaine sign describes a lesion that can be moved anterior or posterior but not superior or inferior and historically is associated with a carotid body tumour (paraganglioma).

A lesion that is not mobile and appears to be tethered to either deep or superficial structures is concerning for a malignant disease process. Clinically, this may represent extranodal extension of a malignant process from an involved lymph node or a soft tissue deposit. Metastatic cutaneous SCC can commonly involve overlying skin and cause ulceration, and it can be difficult to determine whether the lesion is primary or metastatic.

8.2.1.4 Auscultation

There is little role for auscultation of the neck. It may be useful in the investigation of lateral neck masses. Carotid bruits may represent turbulent blood flow within the carotid vessels and are associated with stenosis or narrowing of the blood vessels. This may be associated with lesions involving the carotid body such as a paraganglioma.

8.2.2 Special Investigations

8.2.2.1 Flexible Nasal Endoscopy (FNE)

Flexible nasal endoscopy is performed at the bedside and involves the placement of a fibre-optic camera through a patient's nostril with its image displayed on a nearby screen or on the device. Topicalisation of the nasal passages and upper airways with a local anaesthetic (*Co-Phenylcaine Forte* spray) improves patient tolerance and compliance. It allows for examination of the nasopharynx, oropharynx and supraglottic structures. Asymmetry, ulceration or mucosal abnormalities may suggest a malignancy of the upper airways and prompt further investigation.

8.2.2.2 Image-Guided Biopsies

With the use of imaging modalities, a biopsy such as a fine-needle aspirate (FNA) or core biopsy can be performed. Should an infection or ranula be suspected, it may be possible to perform an aspiration to help guide further treatment. Depending on the suspected differential diagnosis, the samples can be sent for microscopy with culture and histopathology. In the setting of metastatic disease, immunohistochemistry can be performed to help identify the primary lesion. The elevated presence of p63 may suggest a cutaneous squamous cell carcinoma as the primary lesion, whereas an elevated p16 may represent a human papillomavirus (HPV)-related oropharyngeal malignancy. Core biopsies have an improved specificity compared with FNA. The risk of seeding in the head and neck region is estimated to be <0.001% [24]. The decision to pick one modality over the other may come down to the accessibility of each, given the relative ease and improved patient comfort, it may be reasonable to perform a FNA and core biopsy should it be unsuccessful.

Fine-Needle Aspirate (FNA)

A FNA involves the multiple passings of a needle under negative pressure into a lesion of interest. It provides an unoriented sample of cells for histopathological diagnosis. A FNA is typically well tolerated and if the lesion is palpable may be performed without adjunctive imaging. Compared with a core biopsy, it may be readily available and requires less training. If sufficient material is obtained, the sampled tissue may be able to have additional tests performed such as immunohistochemical staining (such as p16) to help differentiate between the oncological origin of a malignant lymph node.

Core Biopsy

A core biopsy is performed with the use of adjunctive imaging such as an ultrasound scan (USS) or computed tomography (CT). It provides an orientated core/column of tissue with increased number of cells compared with a FNA. It is more painful for the patient and requires a small incision in the overlying skin. The increased cell content allows for additional testing compared with an FNA and provides additional architecture, which may be useful in the diagnosis of lymphoma.

p16 Status
p16 is a cyclin-dependant kinase and is present and considered positive when present in elevated numbers in a number of conditions. It is positive in branchial cleft cysts, metastatic cutaneous SCC or human papilloma virus (HPV) related oropharyngeal SCC. It is demonstrated with immunohistochemistry and considered positive with the assessment of blocks of 10–20 cells. p16 is an indirect surrogate measure of HPV-related disease but is not specific for the diagnosis. The HPV strains of −16 and −18 are associated with oropharyngeal SCC and typically present with a small primary tumour with early nodal metastasis and a better prognosis than non-HPV-associated oropharyngeal SCC. For improved specificity, it is possible to confirm the association of HPV by the presence of HPV-related proto-oncogenes (E6 and E7). This is not routinely performed due to additional cost and is less readily available.

8.3 Investigations and their Limitations

Investigations performed of a lump in the neck aim to reduce the possible list of differential diagnosis and/or aid in the diagnosis of a primary lesion should metastatic disease be suspected. Imaging can delineate the size and structure of the lesion(s). It can also demonstrate associations with surrounding anatomical structures and suggest a possible organ of origin. For malignant lesions, pre-operative imaging is essential for staging. The use of magnetic resonance imaging (MRI), computed tomography (CT) or positron-emission tomography (PET) may identify a primary lesion should the neck mass represent a metastatic malignant lesion. Metastatic deposits under 5 mm are difficult to detect on any imaging modality [25].

8.3.1 Imaging

8.3.1.1 Ultrasound

Ultrasound is a non-invasive imaging modality that is based on the Doppler effect. Through the use of soundwaves, a live greyscale image is produced. With Doppler flow, it can demonstrate the direction of flow within blood vessels. It has a number of advantages including its ready accessibility, ease of use and ability to perform simultaneous procedures (such as fine-needle aspiration/core biopsy or placement of intravascular lines). It has the advantage of no radiation exposure, so is safe in the at-risk population (children/young adults or pregnancy). Its use is limited to superficial structures, requires additional training and may be difficult to interpret given limited saved still images. If a malignant process is suspected, and an unknown primary lesion the use of ultrasound is unlikely to be beneficial in its identification and another modality will be required. Ultrasound is commonly used to facilitate biopsies of neck masses for an FNA or core biopsy. For metastatic disease of the cervical lymph nodes, ultrasound has demonstrated 80% and 98% sensitivity and specificity, respectively [26]. It is particularly useful in the surveillance of at-risk nodal basins over time.

8.3.1.2 Computed Tomography (CT)

Computed tomography is a non-invasive imaging modality, which is based on the production of radiation energy to produce detailed internal images of the body. Captured in a spiralled, axial pattern, it provides cross-sectional imaging in axial, sagittal and coronal views without limitation of depth. With the addition of intravascular contrast at varying timing intervals, it can be used to highlight the arterial or venous system. It has the advantage of demonstrating a complete cross section of the area of interest and provides images that can be manipulated through modification of the viewing ‘window’ following image capture. Imaging can be exported and be used for virtual surgical planning. Compared with MRI, it has a shorter acquisition time and is better at detecting distant metastatic disease [26]. For detecting metastatic disease of the cervical lymph nodes, CT imaging demonstrates a sensitivity of 81% and specificity of 76% [26].

8.3.1.3 Magnetic Resonance Imaging (MRI)

Magnetic resonance imaging is a non-invasive imaging modality that uses a magnetic field to create detailed images of the soft tissues of the body. The use of MRI uses a number of sequences to capture imaging. T1-weighted imaging demonstrates adipose (appears more white), whereas T2-weighted imaging demonstrates H_2O molecules (appears more white) [27]. Diffusion-weighted imaging (DWI) assesses the mobility of H_2O molecules with increased signal (restricted diffusion) demonstrated by tumours [27]. Magnetic resonance imaging provides the greatest detail for soft tissue structures such as muscles, neural structures and bone marrow. The addition of contrast can also be used to identify the arterial and venous system. It produces no radiation and therefore useful in the at-risk population. Compared with CT, it is less affected by scatter caused by dental amalgam [26]. Its use may be limited in some individuals given its prolonged time for acquisition, the need to lie still and narrow chamber making it difficult in patients with claustrophobia. Patients with implantable ferromagnetic prosthesis or a history of corneal injury secondary to metallic foreign body may also be excluded [26]. For the detection of metastatic disease involving the cervical lymph nodes, MRI demonstrates a sensitivity of 76% and specificity of 86%, equivalent to USS or CT [26].

8.3.1.4 Positron-Emission Tomography (PET)

Positron-emission tomography is a non-invasive nuclear medicine imaging modality. A PET scan is an investigation used for the identification of a primary malignant lesion or to identify regional or metastatic disease. It involves the use of a radioactive nucleotide contrast agent such as fluorodeoxyglucose-18 (FDG-18; most common). Cells that are consuming an increased amount of the labelled isotope (such as glucose) take up the tracer in an increased amount compared with the neighbouring tissue. With the consumption of the tracer, two protons are produced in opposite directions, which is captured by a gamma camera. Inflammation, infection or malignancy may be demonstrated but are not able to be differentiated. The captured image is often overlayed with a CT or MRI to allow for easier interpretation. It is more accurate at diagnosing cervical metastasis than an MRI [25]. Sensitivity for detection of cervical nodes is 80.3% and specificity is 92.8%; these can be increased when combined with a CT (PET/CT) with 91.8% sensitivity and 98.9% specificity [25].

8.3.1.5 Lymphoscintigraphy

Lymphoscintigraphy is an invasive nuclear medicine imaging modality. It is used in the setting of a malignant lesion to identify the sentinel or echelon lymph node(s). It requires an injection of a radioactive tracer such as technitium-99 around the primary lesion. The tracer is taken up by the surrounding lymphatic channels and drains to the sentinel lymph node or nodes. With decay of the tracer, it causes the production of a single photon, which is captured by a gamma camera. In the setting of a sentinel node biopsy, it may prevent the need for a neck dissection or identify the sentinel nodes for targeted monitoring following management of the primary lesion [11]. The captured image is often overlayed with a CT to allow for easier interpretation.

8.3.2 Sentinel Node Biopsy

A sentinel node biopsy is an operative procedure involving the removal of the sentinel or echelon lymph node to allow for detailed histopathological assessment [11]. In the head and neck region, it may be indicated for cutaneous melanoma and small oral cavity squamous cell carcinomas (T1/T2) [11]. Lymphoscintigraphy is used to identify the sentinel node(s) with removal under local or general anaesthesia. A blue dye, such as patent blue, may be injected just prior to commencement of the procedure to cause a colour change in the targeted lymph node(s). The purpose of a sentinel lymph node biopsy is to exclude occult disease. For cutaneous melanoma, a sentinel lymph node biopsy allows for staging, prognostication and may avoid the need for a neck dissection for occult disease. In small oral cavity carcinomas with no known regional nodal disease, there may be no survival benefit compared with a selective neck dissection. There are a number of contraindications including previous surgery or radiation therapy to the region or in cases where a neck dissection may be indicated regardless of the size of the lesion (i.e. defect requiring free flap reconstruction) [11]. Previously, lesions of the anterior floor of mouth were excluded due to the proximity of the primary lesion and sentinel lymph node(s); however, new tracers may have provided more rapid clearance from the primary site. There are a number of advantages for performing a sentinel lymph node biopsy including smaller incisions, avoiding the need for neck dissection, decreased hospitalisation length and the possibility for treatment to be performed under local anaesthesia. Sentinel lymph node biopsies may be prohibitive based on the need for additional training and increased cost [11]. Its utility remains a topic for further investigation outside of melanoma in an Australian context.

8.4 Surgical Management

A neck dissection involves the removal of the lymphatic structures of the targeted levels of the neck [2]. There has been significant evolution in the approach to the neck dissection. A comprehensive neck dissection, modified radical neck dissection (MRND) and selective neck dissection (SND) have been described earlier. Based on the location of the known primary lesion or pre-operative pattern of disease, it may be possible to preserve some lymphatic and/or non-lymphatic structures.

8.4.1 Setup

The procedure is performed under a general anaesthetic with the patient in the supine position. The choice of airway is likely to depend on the source of the primary lesion if being addressed during the same procedure and the chosen reconstruction. Surgery not involving the oral cavity is feasible with an oral endotracheal tube. Surgery requiring access to the oral cavity is often best accessed with the use of a nasal endotracheal tube or placement of a tracheostomy. Optimally, the neck can be extended with either placement of a shoulder roll/bolster or extension of the head of the bed, and the head resting on a head ring.

Given a neck dissection is not often performed in isolation, other adjuncts may also be required and considered on a case-by-case basis. The placement of an indwelling urinary catheter may be required for cases expected to last greater than 4 hours. Invasive blood pressure monitoring may be needed for prolonged or medically complex patients. Patients may require post-operative enteral feeding if surgery involves the oral cavity and may require the placement of a nasogastric tube or percutaneous endoscopically placed gastrostomy (PEG) tube.

An isolated neck dissection is considered a clean procedure, and perioperative antibiotics have not been shown to decrease the risk of infection [20, 28]. Combined with an oral cavity procedure, it is considered a clean-contaminated procedure and most guidelines support the use of perioperative antibiotics covering aerobic and anaerobic organisms such as cefazolin and metronidazole [20]. Without antibiotics, the incidence of infection can be up to 80% [20].

A nerve integrity monitor may be useful, particularly if the neck dissection is performed in conjunction with a parotidectomy or if level V is dissected. The use of advanced electrocautery devices aids in minimising blood loss and maximising vision of critical structures.

8.4.1.1 Performing a Selective Neck Dissection Levels I–III

A collar incision in an appropriate skin crease is made from the midline to the mastoid tip. A subplatysmal flap is raised superiorly to the inferior border of the mandible, with care taken to avoid injury to the marginal mandibular nerve by staying on the undersurface of the platysma. A flap can be raised inferiorly in a subplatysmal plane, with care to avoid injuring the external jugular vein and great auricular nerve superiorly and exposing the omohyoid inferiorly.

The marginal mandibular nerve is then identified and dissected free of the tissue inferiorly to create the superior extent of dissection, and a guide to its location is its proximity to the facial artery and vein where they cross over the mandible. The facial artery and vein can be divided and retracted over the marginal mandibular nerve to protect it. Once safely preserved, the inferior border of the mandible is dissected anteriorly. Level IA, boarded by the anterior belly of the the digastric muscle bilaterally can then be dissected. The inferior boarder of IA is the hyoid bone, and the depth of dissection is carried down to the geniohyoid musculature. Level IB can then be dissected from anterior to posterior, with exposure of the mylohyoid and ligation of the perforating submental vessels. Once exposed, the mylohyoid is retracted anteriorly to reveal the deep lobe of the submandibular gland. Retraction of the gland inferiorly and superficially will reveal the lingual nerve, and division of the submandibular ganglion and submandibular duct will release the lingual nerve and allow it to retract superiorly. The hypoglossal nerve is deep to the fascia of hyoglossus but is close to the plane of dissection at this point. Clearance of the rest of level IB is possible now, boarded posteriorly by the posterior belly of the digastric muscle. The last structure to be divided is the proximal facial artery, which emerges from the submandibular triangle. The posterior belly of the digastric can be followed to the mastoid tip at this point. The only structure to cross the posterior belly of digastric superficially is the common facial vein, which can be retracted posteriorly along with the contents of level IB.

At this point, the fascia overlying sternomastoid is incised from the approximate position of the omohyoid inferiorly to the external jugular vein superiorly. From this superior aspect, the tail of parotid can be divided to join with the previously dissected level IB. The sternomastoid can then be unwrapped and retracted laterally, as the dissection follows the surface of the sternomastoid laterally and deep over a wide plane. This will allow identification and preservation of the insertion of the accessory nerve into sternomastoid. Once identified, the accessory nerve can be followed anteriorly to the posterior belly digastric. The tissue lateral and superior to the nerve is level IIB and can be dissected at this point, with the prevertebral musculature (splenius capitis and levator scapulae) forming the floor of dissection.

Levels IIA and III can now be dissected. Following the sternomastoid dissection inferiorly until the cervical plexus nerves are identified, the cervical plexus nerve roots can then be followed anteriorly to define the floor of the resection, and dissecting over a broad front, with the omohyoid as the inferior border of dissection, mobilises level IIA and III until the carotid sheath is identified. The dissection is carried anteriorly and superficially over first the carotid, then vagus and jugular vein, with care taken superiorly to protect and preserve the accessory nerve. From this point, the neck dissection is completed by dissecting anteriorly and superficially to the descendens hypoglossi (Fig. 8.1) and superior thyroid vascular pedicle to complete the neck dissection.

8.4.1.2 Performing a Level II–IV Neck Dissection

A level II–IV neck dissection can be performed by unwrapping the fascia overlying SCM as described above, with the lower limit of dissection being the clavicle rather than the omohyoid. The dissection is carried anteriorly and deep as described above; however, the omohyoid can be divided inferiorly and deep to access the complete level IV. In addition to the cervical plexus nerves, the floor of dissection inferiorly is defined by the transverse cervical vessels, which also overly and thus protect the phrenic nerve that is at risk of injury in level IV. Dissection can then be carried anteriorly and superficially and stops at the posterior belly of digastric and submandibular gland superiorly and the infrahyoid strap muscles inferiorly.

8.4.1.3 Level V Neck Dissection

A level V neck dissection requires a subplatysmal flap to be raised inferiorly to the clavicle and laterally to the trapezius muscle. The key to dissection of level V is identification of the accessory nerve. It typically enters the trapezius 4 cm superior to the insertion of trapezius from the clavicle and can be reliably encountered at this point. Once identified, it can be dissected medi-

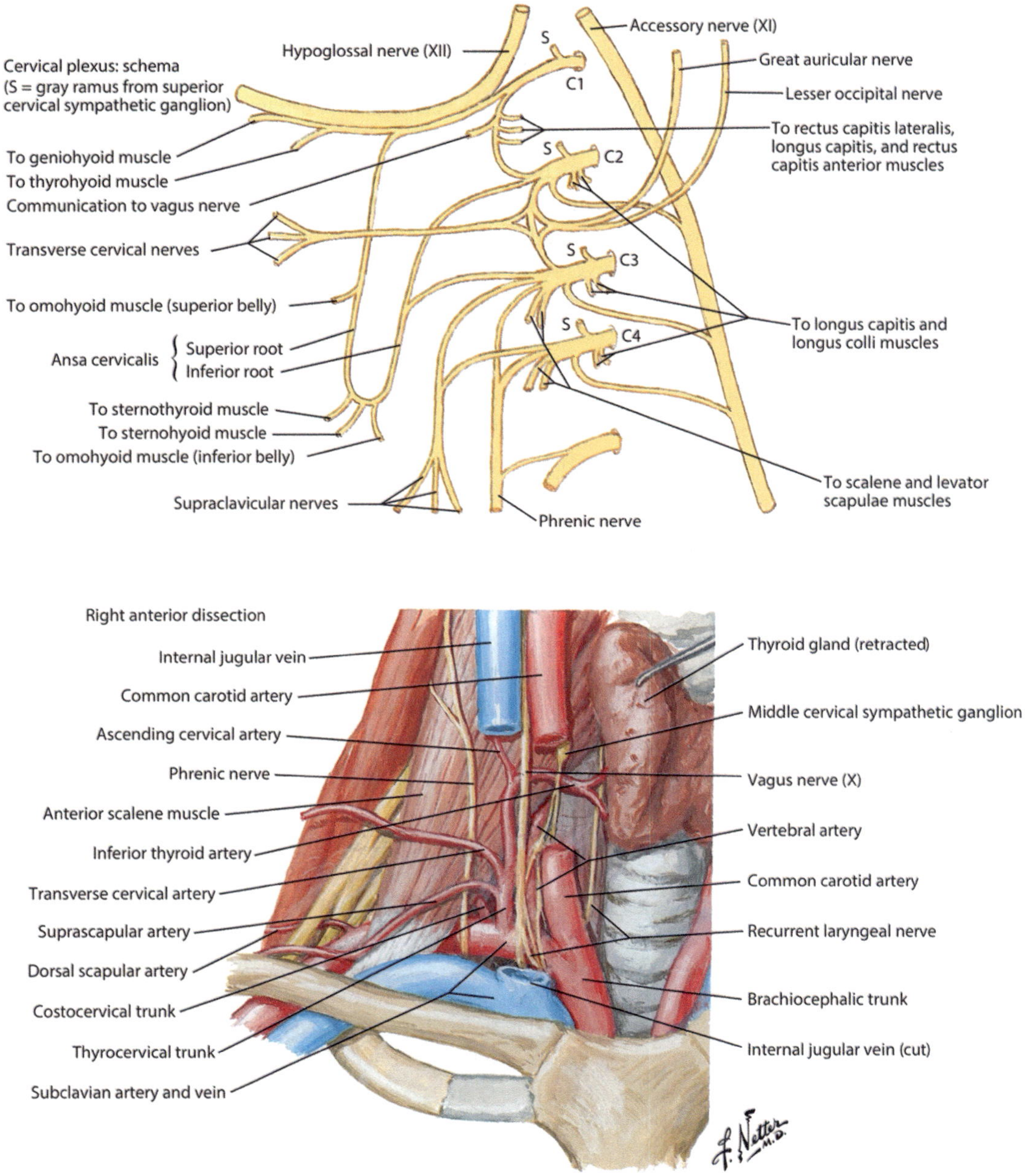

Fig. 8.1 Nerves of the neck (Netter medical illustration used with permission of Elsevier. All rights reserved.)

ally to the SCM. The tissue superior to the nerve can be dissected free of the prevertebral musculature. The tissue inferior to the nerve can similarly be freed from the prevertebral muscles with care taken to remain superficial to the roots of the brachial plexus. On the left side of the neck, the thoracic duct is at risk of injury in levels IV and V.

There are a number of risks and complications of performing a neck dissection. These may be related to iatrogenic injury or removal due to proximity or association with a malignant lesion.

8.4.2 General Surgical Complications

8.4.2.1 Blood Loss

Blood loss is possible due to the length of operation and presence of large calibre vessels within most levels of the neck. Careful surgical technique, appropriate ligation of vessels and reduced surgical time can reduce the overall risk of blood loss significantly. Historically, the average amount of blood loss associated with a radical neck dissection is 762 mL with up to 11% of patients requiring a blood transfusion following the procedure [29, 30]. With modern surgical techniques and haemostatic devices including monopolar, bipolar, advanced bipolar and ultrasonic dissection tools, blood loss should be limited to 100 mL or less.

A carotid blow-out is a rare, morbid complication with a mortality of 50%. The risk of occurrence increases with previous radiation therapy or salivary leak. Emergency ligation has significant risk of causing an ischaemia cerebrovascular incident [3]. If common carotid resection is required due to oncological reasons, a carotid occlusion test can be performed prior to surgery to determine if sufficient contralateral flow from an intact Circle of Willis could reduce the risk of a cerebrovascular event in this case.

8.4.2.2 Infection

Post-operative infection following a neck dissection is uncommon (<1%) [31]. The risk is increased if associated with a combined oral defect/procedure. Management of a post-operative infection may involve the use of post-operative antibiotics with or without surgical drainage if a collection is present.

8.4.2.3 Pain

Pain is not a common post-operative complaint. Due to the loss of cervical sensory nerves as a consequence of surgery, there are commonly cutaneous areas of permanent anaesthesia. This often encompasses the field of dissection but can be more expansive if the great auricular nerve is divided or supraclavicular nerves are sacrificed in a level V dissection. Chronic shoulder pain may be attributable to accessory nerve injury and is the most common chronic pain-related issue [3]. Acute post-operative pain is often managed with oral analgesia including regular paracetamol, non-steroidal anti-inflammatory drugs and opioid analgesia as required. Chronic pain may be managed or improved with the involvement of physiotherapy and consideration of nerve-targeted therapies such as pregabalin or amitriptyline.

8.4.2.4 Lymphoedema

Lymphoedema is the accumulation of lymphatic fluid within the interstitium. With removal of the cervical lymphatic system, lymphoedema occurs in all patients. It presents with non-tender and non-erythematous pitting oedema above the level of the neck incision. Massage and physiotherapy may be useful in diverting excessive lymphatic tissue to non-disturbed surgical regions. With time, lymphoedema often improves without further intervention.

8.4.2.5 Chyle

Chyle is a milk-like bodily fluid consisting of lymphatic fluid, emulsified fats and free fatty acids [10]. Chyle is composed of fats absorbed via the gastrointestinal tract and extracellular fluid being returned to the venous system via the right lymphatic duct and thoracic duct in the left neck [10]. These ducts are located in the inferior most aspect of the neck (level IV) but can be found superior to the thyroid cartilage [10]. The left side is largest and drains the left upper limb and body below the level of the diaphragm. Each side may drain into the venous system via the internal jugular or subclavian vein. Intra-operative injury of either the right or left duct may cause leakage of chyle fluid, a clear or milky substance when operating in the lower aspect of the neck. Post-operatively, it may be identified by a high volume of drain output of a milk-like consistency. This may be less obvious in a fasting patient but could be suspected with persistent, high volume drain outputs. Chyle leaks may be considered low (<500 mL) or high volume (>500 mL) based on a 24-h period [10].

There are a number of suggested management strategies for chyle leak. If identified intra-operatively, attempts to identify and ligate the injured duct are preferred. The duct is best located and ligated posterior to the carotid sheath. Placement of a muscle patch (sternocleidomastoid or omohyoid) has also been advocated. Conservative measures and medical management is suggested for post-operative identification or persistence of a previously identified intra-operative chyle leak. The conservative measures include bed rest, elevation of the bed head and avoidance of straining with the use of regular aperients. The use of no-fat, low-fat or medium-chain fatty acids reduces chyle flow. Octreotide, a long-acting analogue of somatostatin delivered via subcutaneous injection may reduce gastrointestinal secretions and therefore chyle production. Doses may start with 100 micrograms twice daily and can be increased to up to 200 micrograms three times per day. Common complications include nausea, vomiting and diarrhoea. Less common complications include hypoglycaemia, cholecystitis, gastrointestinal bleeding and anaphylaxis. It may not be suitable in patients with pre-existing cardiovascular or hepatic disease. Conservative management is reasonable for patients with <200 mL/day volume. Further surgical intervention may be considered should a chyle leak persist despite conservative or medical measures or a high volume leak occurs. Alternatively, sclerosing agents (OK-432 or tetracycline) injected via the existing drains or percutaneous injection to induce fibrosis have also been described. This approach may make any further surgical interventions difficult or injure structures within the wound bed. Surgical re-exploration is the preferred approach by many. To improve the chance of identifying the injured duct, pre-operative consumption of a fatty diet, Trendelenburg positioning and use of the Cernea manoeuvre may be of benefit. As described earlier, muscle flaps and ligation of the source duct are suggested. Should further re-exploration not be successful, more proximal management of the lymphatic system may be required. This can occur either through a transthoracic approach with ligation or embolisation with coils and/or tissue adhesive via a transabdominal approach [10].

8.4.3 Nerve-Related Complications

The cranial nerves are at risk of injury during a neck dissection. Overall, the risk of injury is low (<2%) [3]. Cranial nerves may need to be purposefully sacrificed to maintain an oncological margin and may not be predictable pre-operatively.

8.4.3.1 Cervical Branch of the Facial Nerve

The cervical branch of the facial nerve is the most inferior division of the facial nerve. It innervates the platysma and is found within the superficial layer of the investing fascia. The cervical division is often divided during the surgical approach with little cosmetic effects.

8.4.3.2 Marginal Mandibular Nerve

The marginal mandibular nerve is the second lowest division of the facial nerve. It is a motor nerve, innervating the depressor anguli oris, depressor labii inferioris and mentalis. Loss of innervation to these muscles results in asymmetry of smile with the lower lip appearing more superior with the loss of the pulling effect of the aforementioned muscles.

The marginal mandibular nerve is found on or within the superficial layer of the investing fascia of the neck. It may be one nerve or more commonly have multiple branches. Previous studies have described its location within the neck. Fifty-three per cent of marginal mandibular nerves extend below the level of the mandible and extend up to 1.2 cm below the lower border of the mandible [32]. The majority of these nerves have more than one branch. Six per cent extend beyond the facial vessels below the level of the mandible for a short distance [32].

8.4.3.3 Accessory Nerve

The accessory nerve is a motor nerve supplying the sternocleidomastoid (SCM) and trapezius muscles. Loss of innervation to these muscles results in shoulder weakness with difficulty raising the affected arm above the level of the shoulder or shrugging. The accessory nerve ascends into the base of skull via the foramen magnum, exits the base of skull via the jugular foramen and travels within the carotid sheath before entering the neck deep to the posterior belly of digastric muscle. It penetrates the SCM and travels out posteriorly approximately 1 cm inferior from its point of entry. On the posterior aspect, it may be identified superiorly to Erb's point by 1 cm. At the lateral aspect (level V), the accessory nerve travels superficially to enter the trapezius approximately 4 cm above the level of the clavicle. There is a number of anatomical variations of the nerve including an additional cervical contribution. The relationship to the internal jugular vein may be variable with 96% located lateral, 3% medial and 1% causing bifurcation and passing through [33]. Despite efforts to preserve the accessory nerve, up to 40% of patients with complaints regarding shoulder issues post-operatively [12]. A significant palsy will restrict abduction of the shoulder between 90 and 120 °.

8.4.3.4 Lingual Nerve

The lingual nerve is a mixed nerve with sensory and parasympathetic fibres. Loss of innervation of this nerve causes loss of sensation and taste to the ipsilateral tongue and loss of function submandibular gland (which will have no effect if concurrent removal during the neck dissection). The lingual nerve is a branch of the posterior division of the of the mandibular division of the trigeminal nerve (V3). The chorda tympani, a branch of the nervus intermedius, supplies the parasympathetic and taste fibres and joins the lingual nerve approximately 2 cm below the base of skull. The lingual nerve is located on the medial aspect of the submandibular gland and is identified with anterior retraction of the mylohyoid muscle. It is the most superior nerve structure and often described as having a ribbon appearance.

8.4.3.5 Hypoglossal Nerve

The hypoglossal nerve is a motor nerve supplying the intrinsic muscles and extrinsic muscles (excluding palatoglossus) of the tongue. Loss of innervation of this nerve results in loss of tongue movement with resulting dysarthria and swallowing difficulties. The nerve exits the base of skull via the hypoglossal canal and travels within the carotid sheath. It can be identified looping anterior and inferior to the occipital artery. It continues to travel anteriorly in a plane between the internal jugular vein and carotid artery. The hypoglossal nerve has a descending branch that forms the superior loop of the ansa cervicalis. The hypoglossal nerve is identified at a number of stages of a neck dissection. It can be identified on the medial aspect of the submandibular gland with anterior retraction of the mylohyoid muscle at or just above the digastric tendon. Further posteriorly, it is located inferior to the posterior belly of digastric muscle.

8.4.3.6 Vagus Nerve

The vagus nerve is a mixed motor, sensory nerve providing parasympathetic supply to the abdomen. It has a number of critical functions in the head and neck region and beyond. It supplies motor sensation to muscles of the larynx (including vocal cords), soft palate and sensation below the vocal cords. Loss of function may result in a large number of changes including dysphonia, dysphagia and elevated risk of aspiration. The vagus nerve leaves the base of skull via the jugular foramen and travels on the posterior aspect and in close approximation to the IJV/carotid artery within the carotid sheath.

8.4.3.7 Phrenic Nerve

The phrenic nerve is a motor and sensory nerve. It supplies the ipsilateral diaphragm and sensation to the pericardium and mediastinal pleura. It is formed from contributions of the cervical plexus (C3, C4 and C5). Loss of innervation results in elevation of the diaphragm and decline in respiratory function. The phrenic nerve can be located posterior to the carotid sheath lying deep to the middle layer of the investing fascia and superficial to the anterior scalene muscles. As the nerve descends in the neck, it travels from lateral to medial to enter the superior thoracic aperture between the subclavian vein and artery.

8.4.3.8 Branchial Plexus

The brachial plexus is a conglomerate of nerves from the cervical roots and provides motor and sensation to the upper limbs. Loss of innervation results in loss of movement to the upper limb and associated loss of sensation. The branchial plexus is within the lower aspect of level V below the fascial layer.

8.5 Post-Operative Management

8.5.1 Analgesia

Analgesic requirements following a neck dissection are typically managed with oral analgesia. In combination with additional procedures, patient-controlled analgesia may be considered. Unless otherwise contraindicated, patients can be commenced on paracetamol, a non-steroidal anti-inflammatory drug (such as celecoxib), and opioid analgesia as required. There are a number of liquid formulations that may be suitable if the patient is to remain nil by mouth or reliant on nasogastric feeds.

8.5.2 Antibiotics

The role of antibiotics in a neck dissection is determined by concurrent procedures. Antibiotics may be considered for up to 24 h post-operatively but demonstrate no benefit beyond this. Consideration for extending antibiotics beyond this may be suggested in the setting of concurrent microvascular anastomosis for free flap reconstruction [20]. For clean procedures, aerobic cover with an antibiotic such as cefazolin with the addition of metronidazole for anaerobic cover should be classified as clean-contaminated.

8.5.3 Diet

The diet following neck dissection is mostly dependent on the concurrent surgical procedures. If performed in isolation, there should be no restriction to the post-operative diet. A soft diet may be considered if the patient has elevated post-operative pain. Alternatively, should there be concerns of a chyle leak, a no-fat, low-fat or diet with medium-chain fatty acids should be considered.

8.5.4 Drains

The placement of surgical drains may reduce the risk of haematoma or seroma. The number of drains placed is often surgeon's preference. Active drains (negative pressure) have demonstrated improvement in healing and reduced post-operative complication rates [34]. Drains are monitored for the volume and contents to monitor for ongoing bleeding and presence of chyle (milk-like). As a drain matures, the volume should decrease with the contents becoming more haemoserous with time. An excessive or persistent volume in a fasting patient may be suggestive of chyle leak even if not appear clinically so.

Top Five Takeaways

1. The presence of nodal metastatic disease is the most important predictor of recurrence and inferior survival. Appropriate identification and treatment of cervical disease are therefore vital.
2. Determining the extent of neck dissection is critical and depends on the aetiology and biology of the primary lesion and the purpose of the neck dissection as either therapeutic or elective.
3. Appropriate pre-operative imaging and biopsy are crucial for surgical planning.
4. Comprehensive dissection of lymphatic structures with careful preservation of vessels, nerves and muscles is the hallmark of quality surgery. A nodal yield of 18 nodes allows for accurate determination of metastatic disease.
5. Post-operative management is crucial to aid in a complete recovery for the patient and return to near-normal function.

References

1. Robbins KT, Shaha AR, Medina JE, Califano JA, Wolf GT, Ferlito A, Som PM, Day TA. Consensus statement on the classification and terminology of neck dissection. Arch Otolaryngol Head Neck Surg. 2008;134:536–8.
2. Nikolarakos D, Bell RB. Management of the node-positive neck in oral cancer. Oral Maxillofac Surg Clin North Am. 2008;20:499–511.

3. Kerawala CJ, Heliotos M. Prevention of complications in neck dissection. Head Neck Oncol. 2009;1:35.
4. Ebrahimi A, Moncrieff MD, Clark JR, Shannon KF, Gao K, Milross CG, O'Brien CJ. Predicting the pattern of regional metastases from cutaneous squamous cell carcinoma of the head and neck based on location of the primary. Head Neck. 2010;32:1288–94.
5. D'Cruz AK, Vaish R, Kapre N, et al. Elective versus therapeutic neck dissection in node-negative oral cancer. N Engl J Med. 2015;373:521–9.
6. Weiss MH, Harrison LB, Isaacs R. Use of decision analysis in planning a management strategy for the stage N0 neck. Arch Otolaryngol Head Neck Surg. 1994;120:699–702.
7. Shah JP. Patterns of cervical lymph node metastasis from squamous carcinomas of the upper aerodigestive tract. Am J Surg. 1990;160:405–9.
8. Amin MB, Edge S, Greene F, Byrd DR, Brookland RK, Washington MK, Gershenwald JE, Compton CC, Hess KR. AJCC cancer staging manual. 8th ed. New York: Springer; 2017.
9. Ebrahimi A, Clark JR, Amit M, et al. Minimum nodal yield in oral squamous cell carcinoma: defining the standard of care in a multicenter international pooled validation study. Ann Surg Oncol. 2014;21:3049–55.
10. Delaney SW, Shi H, Shokrani A, Sinha UK. Management of chyle leak after head and neck surgery: review of current treatment strategies. Int J Otolaryngol. 2017, 2017, 2017:8362874. https://doi.org/10.1155/2017/8362874.
11. Schilling C, Stoeckli SJ, Haerle SK, et al. Sentinel European node trial (SENT): 3-year results of sentinel node biopsy in oral cancer. Eur J Cancer. 2015;51:2777–84.
12. Lea J, Bachar G, Sawka AM, Lakra DC, Gilbert RW, Irish JC, Brown DH, Gullane PJ, Goldstein DP. Metastases to level IIb in squamous cell carcinoma of the oral cavity: a systematic review and meta-analysis. Head Neck. 2010;32:184–90.
13. Woolgar JA. Pathology of the N0 neck. Br J Oral Maxillofac Surg. 1999;37:205–9.
14. O'Brien CJ. The parotid gland as a metastatic basin for cutaneous cancer. Arch Otolaryngol Head Neck Surg. 2005;131:551–5.
15. Borsetto D, Iocca O, De Virgilio A, Boscolo-Rizzo P, Phillips V, Nicolai P, Spriano G, Fussey J, Di Maio P. Elective neck dissection in primary parotid carcinomas: a systematic review and meta-analysis. J Oral Pathol Med. 2021;50:136–44.
16. Green B, Rahimi S, Brennan PA. Current management of the neck in salivary gland carcinomas. J Oral Pathol Med. 2017;46:161–6.
17. Peters TTA, Van Dijk BAC, Roodenburg JLN, Van Der Laan BFAM, Halmos GB. Relation between age, comorbidity, and complications in patients undergoing major surgery for head and neck cancer. Ann Surg Oncol. 2014;21:963–70.
18. Robson A, Sturman J, Williamson P, Conboy P, Penney S, Wood H. Pre-treatment clinical assessment in head and neck cancer: United Kingdom national multidisciplinary guidelines. J Laryngol Otol. 2016;130:S13–22.
19. Healy DW, Cloyd BH, Straker T, et al. Expert consensus statement on the perioperative management of adult patients undergoing head and neck surgery and free tissue reconstruction from the Society for Head and Neck Anesthesia. Anesth Analg. 2021;133:274–83.
20. Blatt S, Al-Nawas B. A systematic review of latest evidence for antibiotic prophylaxis and therapy in oral and maxillofacial surgery. Infection. 2019;47:519. https://doi.org/10.1007/s15010-019-01303-8.
21. Wong WW, Gabriel A, Maxwell GP, Gupta SC. Bleeding risks of herbal, homeopathic, and dietary supplements: a hidden nightmare for plastic surgeons? Aesthet Surg J. 2012;32:332–46.
22. Hugo F, Edward N-C, James W-S. Oxford cases in medicine and surgery. Oxford: Oxford University Press; 2010.
23. Newlands C, Kerawala C. Oral and maxillofacial surgery. 2nd ed. Oxford: Oxford University Press; 2014.
24. Shah KSV, Ethunandan M. Tumour seeding after fine-needle aspiration and core biopsy of the head and neck - a systematic review. Br J Oral Maxillofac Surg. 2016;54:260–5.
25. Ahuja AT, Ying M, Ho SY, Antonio G, Lee YP, King AD, Wong KT. Ultrasound of malignant cervical lymph nodes. Cancer Imaging. 2008;8:48–56.
26. Bradley P, Beasley N, Au-Yong I. Imaging of neck lumps. BMJ (Online). 2014;349:1–5.
27. Ganeshalingam S, Koh DM. Nodal staging. Cancer Imaging. 2009;9:104–11.
28. Dort JC, Farwell DG, Findlay M, et al. Optimal perioperative care in major head and neck cancer surgery with free flap reconstruction: a consensus review and recommendations from the enhanced recovery after surgery society. JAMA Otolaryngol Head Neck Surg. 2017;143:292–303.
29. Azmy MC, Pinto J, Patel NM, Govindan A, Kalyoussef E. Risk factors for blood transfusion with neck dissection. Otolaryngol Head Neck Surg (United States). 2019;161:922–8.
30. Babu MJ, Neema PK, Reazaul Karim HM, Dey S, Arora R. Effect of two different tranexamic acid doses on blood loss in head and neck cancer surgery: a randomized, double-blind, controlled study, vol. 13. Cureus; 2021. p. e20190. https://doi.org/10.7759/cureus.20190.

31. Man L-X, Beswick DM, Johnson JT. Antibiotic prophylaxis in uncontaminated neck dissection. Laryngoscope. 2011;121:1473–7.
32. Ziarah HA, Atkinson ME. The surgical anatomy of the cervical distribution of the facial nerve. Br J Oral Surg. 1981;19:171–9.
33. Hinsley ML, Hartig GK. Anatomic relationship between the spinal accessory nerve and internal jugular vein in the upper neck. Otolaryngol Head Neck Surg. 2010;143:239–41.
34. Batstone MD, Lowe D, Shaw RJ, Brown JS, Vaughan ED, Rogers SN. Passive versus active drainage following neck dissection: a non-randomised prospective study. Eur Arch Otorhinolaryngol. 2009;266:121–4.

Neck Cysts

9

Rajith Mendis and Bruce Ashford

Cystic masses of the neck are common general surgical presentations, and there are a variety of differential diagnoses to consider. The nature of the cyst can often be predicted by the history and examination and supported with imaging. The aetiology of these cysts is important to understand as each has a unique surgical approach to minimise the risk of recurrence. In this chapter, we cover benign (thyroglossal duct cysts, branchial cleft cysts and ranula) and malignant cystic neck masses and review their differing aetiologies, presentations and key management points.

At the outset, it should be noted that a significant proportion of neck cysts will not be benign. A suspicion of malignancy should be entertained in any new neck cyst in an adult. In particular, branchial cleft cysts, a common radiological diagnosis, are in fact not that common in adults. Active measures to exclude malignancy should be included in the diagnostic workup of any neck cyst in an adult.

R. Mendis
Illawarra Shoalhaven Local Health District, Wollongong, NSW, Australia
e-mail: rajith.mendis@health.nsw.gov.au

B. Ashford (✉)
Graduate Medicine, University of Wollongong, Wollongong, NSW, Australia
e-mail: bruceash@uow.edu.au

9.1 Thyroglossal Duct Cysts

Thyroglossal duct cysts are the most common congenital cysts in the neck, with an prevalence of approximately 7% [1]. Approximately half are present by 20 years of age, with the remainder presenting during adulthood [2].

Embryologically, the thyroid develops from the fourth week of gestation as an invagination in the developing pharyngeal epithelium [2]. As the embryo elongates, the thyroid descends into the neck forming the thyroglossal duct, which subsequently involutes around the 8th–10th week of gestation. As this descent occurs before the development of the hyoid, it may pass through, posterior to or surround the bone [3]. If this involution does not occur, epithelial remnants from the duct persist and can result in a thyroglossal duct or cyst [4]. Approximately two-thirds of these remnants contain ectopic thyroid tissue.

9.1.1 Clinical Presentation

Thyroglossal duct cysts commonly present as an asymptomatic palpable central upper neck mass and may become inflamed or infected in about one-third of cases causing pain, a discharging cutaneous fistula and rarely dysphagia or odynophagia [5]. Clinically, they are located in the midline; however, as they increase in size they may expand laterally, more commonly onto the left

B. Ashford (ed.), *Head and Neck Surgery for General Surgeons*,
https://doi.org/10.1007/978-981-19-7900-2_9

side [2, 6]. The cyst moves both on swallowing and uniquely with protrusion of the tongue due to attachment to the foramen caecum at the base of the tongue, which can help differentiate the lesion from a thyroid nodule. It is also important to examine the thyroid gland and the cervical nodal basin, as a thyroglossal duct cyst can occasionally harbour malignancy.

9.1.2 Imaging

9.1.2.1 Ultrasound

Ultrasound provides non-invasive, rapid images, which can be used to confirm cystic characteristics and can also assess the thyroid gland. The appearance can vary from an anechoic, well-circumscribed lesion if it is a simple thyroglossal duct cyst, to a pseudo-solid appearance if it contains mucous or other proteinaceous fluid, and may have a heterogeneous pattern if there has been a previous infection [4]. An irregular appearance should be further evaluated for a potential malignancy with a biopsy.

9.1.2.2 Cross-Sectional Imaging

Computed tomography (CT) provides accurate information about the position and size of the cyst. The cyst is most typically a non-enhancing, low-density lesion, and there may be some rim enhancement, especially if infected [3]. Magnetic resonance imaging (MRI) provides more soft tissue detail and can be useful to identify and delineate a fistula tract, particularly in the setting of recurrent cysts, which may assist with surgical planning [4] (Fig. 9.1).

9.1.3 Management

The most common complication of a thyroglossal cyst is infection, and this can be treated with antibiotics. If the infection is not resolving, needle aspiration may be required; however, it is rare to need acute surgical intervention and our preference is to avoid this if possible as incision and drainage are associated with a higher recurrence rate after definitive excision [5, 7].

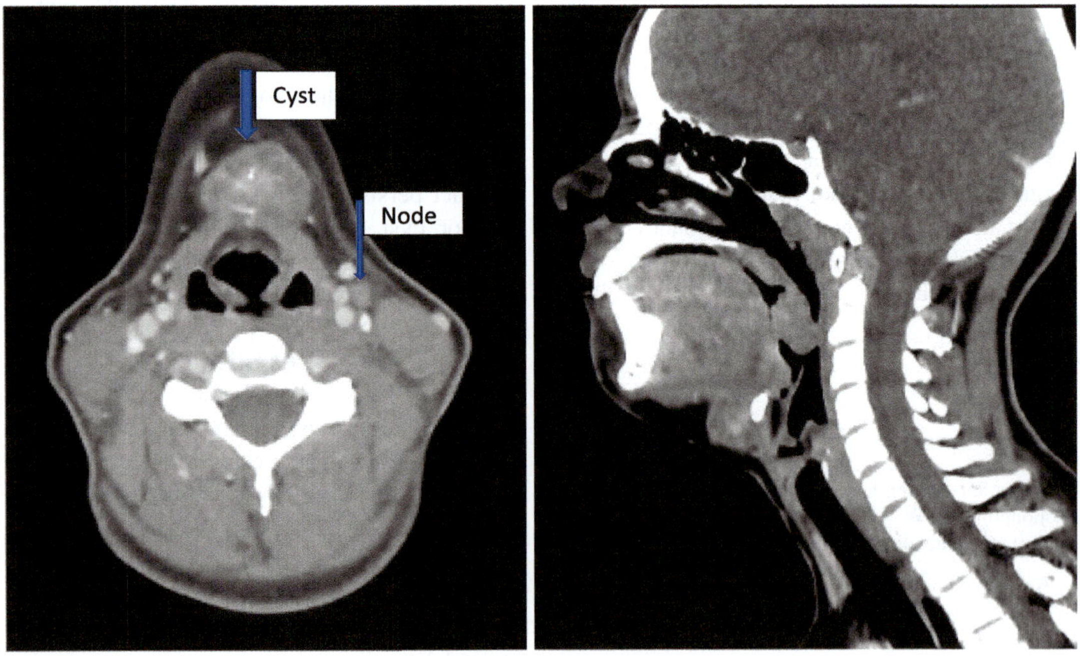

Fig. 9.1 Axial and sagittal CT scans demonstrating a malignant thyroglossal duct cyst with solid transformation and a prominent left level 2a node

Indications for excision of a thyroglossal duct cyst include malignancy, infection, pressure symptoms or cosmetic concerns.

Traditionally, surgical excision of the cyst alone was associated with a high recurrence rate; however, this has decreased significantly to approximately 5% since the description in 1920 by Sistrunk, which detailed resection of the cyst in continuity with the remnant suprahyoid thyroglossal tract and the central portion of the hyoid bone [5, 8].

9.1.3.1 Surgical Procedure

The Sistrunk procedure is performed under a general anaesthetic with the patient in a supine position with the neck in extension. A skin crease incision is made overlying the cyst, and subplatysmal flaps are raised. Often, the cyst lies deep to the sternohyoid and sternothyroid muscles although they may be separated in the midline due to the size of the cyst. A capsular dissection of the cyst is performed, commencing on the inferior aspect of the cyst, which may be attached to the pyramidal lobe. As the dissection is carried superiorly, the remnant thyroglossal duct is dissected to the hyoid bone. At this point, the muscular attachments at the lateral aspect of the body of the hyoid are released with diathermy, leaving a central portion of the hyoid intact of approximately 1 cm. The bone is cut on each side with bone cutters, and the suprahyoid dissection is carried superiorly into the region of the base of tongue where the residual tract is ligated and divided. Sistrunk described the suprahyoid extension of the procedure to completely resect this component and reduce recurrence.

9.1.3.2 Malignant Risk

Rarely, a thyroglossal cyst may harbour a malignancy, most commonly being a papillary thyroid carcinoma. This risk is low at approximately 1–2%, although higher rates of 6.5–7% have been reported [6, 9]. Two theories related to the origin of the malignancy exist: (1) malignant transformation of thyroid follicles existing within the cyst and (2) metastasis from an occult primary in the thyroid gland [6]. When managing these rare patients, the management of the thyroid gland is unclear and there are no consensus guidelines. A practical approach would be to assess the thyroid gland for any suspicious nodules and the neck for any concerning lymphadenopathy. If these are both normal, then performing a Sistrunk procedure and assessing the histopathology of the carcinoma within a multidisciplinary meeting for any high-risk features such as size >10 mm or extension beyond the cyst, in which case a total thyroidectomy with or without selective neck dissection and adjuvant radioactive iodine ablation should be considered.

9.2 Branchial Cleft Cyst

Branchial cleft cysts are among the most frequently encountered congenital lesions of the head and neck among children but may also present in adults. They arise from a failure of a branchial cleft to obliterate during development and may result in cysts, sinuses or fistulae [10]. While this remains the prevailing consensus, there are other theories associated with the persistence of the vestiges of the precervical sinus, thymopharyngeal ductal origin and cystic lymph node origin [11].

Embryologically, the branchial apparatus develops from the fourth week of gestation between the brain and heart, with six pairs of arches, clefts and pouches [12]. Of the branchial clefts, only the first branchial cleft persists as an adult structure as the epithelium of the external acoustic meatus. The other branchial clefts obliterate as the neck develops. If this does not obliterate, a branchial cyst can result, and the location allows it to be classified according to the pouch or cleft of origin.

9.2.1 First Branchial Anomaly

First branchial cleft cysts are rare, accounting for approximately 7% of branchial cysts [12].

The first branchial apparatus gives rise to the maxilla, mandible, eustachian tube, external auditory canal and some middle ear structures. As the parotid gland and facial nerve form later in development, first branch anomalies can have a variable relationship between these structures, can extend anterior or posterior to the pinna and may even extend below the angle of the mandible [13].

9.2.2 Second Branchial Anomaly

The most common of the branchial cleft anomalies, accounting for approximately 90% of all branchial cleft-associated neck masses, often present in the second to fourth decades of life [10].

The external opening if present is usually along the anterior border of the sternocleidomastoid muscle along the middle and lower third. It then travels medially to pass between the internal and external carotid arteries and courses above the hypoglossal and glossopharyngeal nerves, extending superiorly to end near the tonsillar fossa [13].

9.2.3 Third Branchial Anomaly

A third branchial cyst may have a superficial location similar to a second branchial fistula, but as it courses medially it passes deep to the carotid vessels but anterior to the vagus nerve. It then passes above the hypoglossal nerve but below the glossopharyngeal nerve and opens into the pyriform sinus by piercing the thyrohyoid membrane [13].

9.2.4 Fourth Branchial Anomaly

A fourth branchial cleft cyst is very rare with only few reported cases in the literature. The tract of a fistula arises from the apex of the pyriform sinus and passes inferior to the superior laryngeal nerve but superior to the recurrent laryngeal nerve and then courses down to the chest and around the aortic arch on the left and subclavian artery on the right [13, 14].

9.2.5 Clinical Presentation

Presentations of branchial cleft anomalies can vary from a long-standing asymptomatic cyst or fistula tract to an acute presentation with pain and swelling due to secondary infection or rupture [10]. There may be a history of a long-standing asymptomatic swelling or prior episodes of swelling or infection. Previous excision may indicate a recurrent lesion. The assessment should also include risk factors and signs or symptoms of malignancy, particularly in older patients as occasionally metastatic nodal deposits can present as a cystic lateral neck mass. This may include either squamous cell carcinoma or papillary thyroid carcinoma.

The examination should include the assessment of the mass including any overlying skin changes, presence of a punctum or fistula opening and size, borders, consistency, fixation to adjacent structures and superior and inferior extension. The examination should also include a general head and neck examination including any concerning skin lesions, assessment of the thyroid gland and the cervical lymph nodes and an oral examination including the tongue, tongue base, tonsils and nasoendoscopy.

9.2.6 Imaging

9.2.6.1 Ultrasound

This is a non-invasive and rapid imaging modality, which can also be performed by the bedside to obtain immediate additional information.

Branchial cleft cysts are hypoechoic or anechoic and compressible with well-defined margins and thin walls, and there may be posterior wall enhancement. If infected, the contents may become heterogeneous [10].

9.2.6.2 Cross-Sectional Imaging

CT imaging provides cross-sectional imaging with information both about the lesion and the relationship with important surrounding structures. Branchial cleft cysts appear as a uniformly hypodense, well-circumscribed lesion with thin walls, often with posteromedial displacement of the carotid sheath and anterior displacement of the submandibular gland if the cyst is large [10] (Fig. 9.2).

MRI provides detailed information with a better definition of the deep extent of the cyst and can more accurately identify the tract, while also

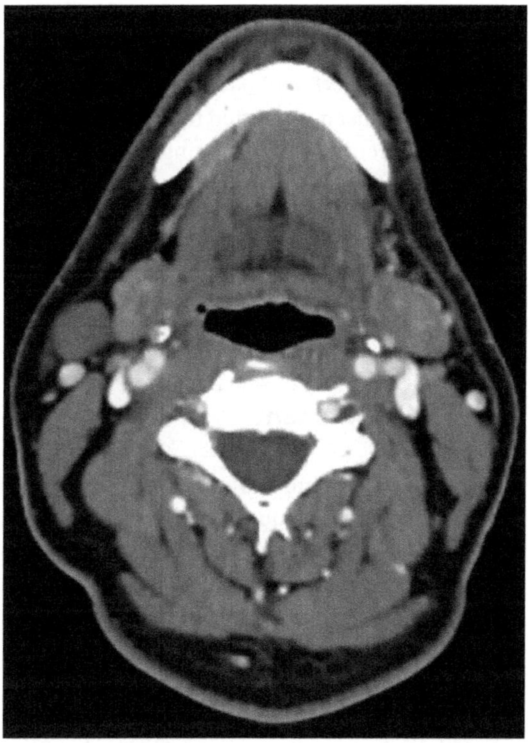

Fig. 9.2 Axial CT scan with contrast demonstrating a right-sided second branchial cleft cyst lying deep to platysma and along the anterior border of the sternocleidomastoid muscle

providing information relating to the anatomical position and relationship with adjacent structures. The cyst contents are often hypo- or isointense in T1-weighted sequences and hyperintense in T2-weighted sequences, and if inflamed, the cyst wall may be thickened [10]. We do not routinely utilise MRI, however would consider it selectively, particularly in complex or recurrent cases.

9.2.7 Management

Surgery is recommended for most branchial cleft cysts, to prevent infective complications. The aim of surgical excision is to resect both the cyst and ligate the tract as proximally as possible. If the cyst is not palpable, ultrasound may be useful to mark the location of the cyst.

9.2.7.1 Surgical Procedure

The procedure is performed under a general anaesthetic with the patient in a supine position and the neck in extension. A skin crease incision is made overlying the cyst, and subplatysmal flaps are raised. We perform a capsular dissection on the cyst wall, which can help to protect significant structures at risk including marginal mandibular branch of the facial nerve, the spinal accessory, vagus and hypoglossal nerves and the internal and external carotid arteries and internal jugular vein. Staying in a capsular plane also helps to identify and dissect the tract, and for a second branchial cleft cyst, it will pass between the internal and external carotid arteries and will be closely related to the internal jugular vein. We aim to isolate and ligate the tract as proximally as possible.

9.3 Ranula

A ranula is a mucocele of the floor of mouth, which progressively enlarges and extends into the surrounding soft tissue. It can be limited to the oral cavity or may extend to the neck as a 'plunging ranula' [15]. The plunging variant extends from the floor of mouth to the submandibular space by herniating through the mylohyoid, through a hiatus, which is estimated to be present in between 35 and 45% of the population and is often unilateral [15, 16].

This is commonly associated with the sublingual salivary gland and duct of Rivinus in the majority of cases, but may also be rarely associated with the submandibular gland, often due to trauma or obstruction of the duct [15]. The sublingual gland is located between the mucosa of the floor of mouth and mylohyoid and hyoglossus muscles and is closely related to the lingual nerve and submandibular duct. The duct of Rivinus drains the sublingual gland to the oral cavity, but rather than a single duct, there are often multiple ducts, which drain along the plica sublingualis [16]. Ranulas are extravasation pseudocysts, meaning that, following removal of the source of salivary secretion, the cavity will involute [17].

The pathophysiology of the ranula is thought to relate to the continuous secretion of mucous from the sublingual gland, and following rupture of the duct or acini, mucous is extravasated, leading to an inflammatory reaction, with the formation of granulation tissue. The sublingual gland is resistant to the subsequent surrounding fibrosis and continues to leak saliva, whereas both the submandibular and parotid glands are less resistant against the fibrosis, which can help to contain the extravasation [16].

9.3.1 Clinical Presentation

Patients often present with a unilateral, progressive, soft swelling in the floor of mouth and submandibular region. Most ranulas are greater than 2 cm at presentation, and as they increase in size, they typically have a blue appearance. They may be 'reduced' from the neck to cause an increase in swelling in the floor of mouth. Rarely, as they increase in size they may be associated with difficulties with speech and swallowing; however, the size may fluctuate over time [15].

9.3.2 Imaging

Imaging is not routinely required for diagnosis as often it is a clinical diagnosis based on history and examination. FNA with aspiration and testing of the fluid for amylase and cytology has been proposed as a routine part of the workup; however, this is only performed if there is diagnostic uncertainty in our practice [17].

9.3.2.1 Ultrasound

The ranula appears as a hypoechoic cystic mass and may contain internal echoes, and if extending to the submandibular space, the dehiscence in the mylohyoid muscle can often be seen, which is a diagnostic feature. US is also useful to assess the submandibular gland and identify any suspicious features related to the cyst, which may warrant further investigation.

9.3.2.2 Cross-Sectional Imaging

CT or MRI is not routinely used except in cases of diagnostic uncertainty or recurrent cases; however, MRI has been suggested to provide superior diagnostic accuracy of plunging ranulas compared with CT by demonstrating a 'tail sign' with extension of the submandibular cyst into the sublingual space [18]. Exclusion of other cystic differentials may still require FNA with fluid analysis to confirm salivary extravasation.

9.3.3 Management

Management of ranulas varies with a range of approaches and techniques described in the literature. As the vast majority of cases are related to the sublingual gland, treatment focuses on the removal of this gland often through an intraoral approach.

Variations of management include partial sublingual gland excision, incision and drainage, marsupialisation of the cyst and limited sublingual gland resection. Marsupialisation of the cyst is associated with higher recurrence rates; however, 'packing' the marsupialised cyst to block the salivary leak has been associated with lower recurrence rates [16]. Our preferred approach is to resect the sublingual gland through a transoral approach with either excision of the extravasation cyst or aspiration of the cyst. Manually reducing the cyst into the sublingual space can help with the excision of the cyst.

9.4 Metastatic Carcinoma Presenting as a Neck Cyst

Metastatic nodal deposits can also present as cystic masses and must be considered when assessing a neck mass in an adult. Cystic nodal metastasis is far more common than branchial cleft cyst in adults, despite the incidence of radiological reporting to the contrary. While the potential primary site can vary, common causes of cystic metastases of the neck include papillary thyroid carcinoma, HPV-associated oropharyngeal SCC and metastatic cutaneous SCC. When assessing patients with cystic neck masses, it is therefore important to have a high degree of suspicion about potential differentials and to perform a thorough history and examination including any history or evidence of skin malignancy, palpation and ultrasound of the thyroid and assessment of the oral cavity and pharynx (including tonsils and tongue base).

Point-of-care ultrasound and cross-sectional imaging may give a clue to the presence of an obvious or likely primary lesion and can exclude further nodal disease. If there is any concern, then an FNA of the cyst wall is prudent. Aspiration of fluid may be used as a cell block for cytology and can also be sent for biochemical analysis (e.g. thyroglobulin estimation to exclude differentiated thyroid carcinoma or calcitonin levels to exclude medullary thyroid carcinoma).

Take-Home Points

1. Always consider malignancy when assessing an adult with a cystic neck mass.
2. A detailed history and clinic examination can often provide an indication of the aetiology of the lesion.
3. Understanding the aetiology and underlying embryological basis for many neck cysts forms the basis of the surgical approach to minimise the risk of recurrence.
4. Ultrasound provides rapid, non-invasive and detailed information about the nature of the cyst, which should be considered as an adjunct to clinical examination.
5. If there is doubt regarding the aetiology or malignant risk of the cyst, FNA should be considered.

References

1. Kurt A, Ortug C, Aydar Y, Ortug G. An incidence study on thyroglossal duct cysts in adults. Saudi Med J. 2007;28(4):593–7.
2. Goldsztein H, Khan A, Pereira KD. Thyroglossal duct cyst excision-the Sistrunk procedure. Oper Tech Otolaryngol Head Neck Surg. 2009;20(4):256–9. https://doi.org/10.1016/j.otot.2009.09.001.
3. Enepekides DJ. Management of congenital anomalies of the neck. Facial Plast Surg Clin North Am. 2001;9(1):131–45.
4. Mondin V, Ferlito A, Muzzi E, et al. Thyroglossal duct cyst: personal experience and literature review. Auris Nasus Larynx. 2008;35(1):11–25. https://doi.org/10.1016/j.anl.2007.06.001.
5. Rohof D, Honings J, Theunisse HJ, et al. Recurrences after thyroglossal duct cyst surgery: results in 207 consecutive cases and review of the literature. Head Neck. 2015;37(12):1699–704.
6. Forest VI, Murali R, Clark JR. Thyroglossal duct cyst carcinoma: case series. J Otolaryngol Head Neck Surg. 2011;40(2):151–6. https://doi.org/10.2310/7070.2011.100153.
7. Simon LM, Magit AE. Impact of incision and drainage of infected thyroglossal duct cyst on recurrence after Sistrunk procedure. Arch Otolaryngol Head Neck Surg. 2012;138(1):20–4. https://doi.org/10.1001/archoto.2011.225.
8. Sistrunk WE. The surgical treatment of cysts of the thyroglossal tract. Ann Surg. 1920;71(2):121.
9. Wong J, Lee JC, Grodski S, Yeung M, Serpell J. Cancer in thyroglossal duct cysts. ANZ J Surg. 2022;92(3):443–7. https://doi.org/10.1111/ans.17369.
10. Valentino M, Quiligotti C, Carone L. Branchial cleft cyst. J Ultrasound. 2013;16(1):17–20. https://doi.org/10.1007/s40477-013-0004-2.
11. Chavan S, Deshmukh R, Karande P, Ingale Y. Branchial cleft cyst: a case report and review of literature. J Oral Maxillofac Pathol. 2014;18(1):150. https://doi.org/10.4103/0973-029X.131950.
12. Bagchi A, Hira P, Mittal K, Priyamvara A, Dey AK. Branchial cleft cysts: a pictorial review. Polish J Radiol. 2018;83:204–9. https://doi.org/10.5114/PJR.2018.76278.
13. Benson MT, Dalen K, Mancuso AA, Kerr HH, Cacciarelli AA, Mafee MF. Congenital anomalies of the branchial apparatus: embryology and pathologic anatomy. Radiographics. 1992;12(5):943–60. https://doi.org/10.1148/radiographics.12.5.1529135.
14. Meng F, Zhu Z, Ord RA, Zhang T. A unique location of branchial cleft cyst: case report and review of the literature. Int J Oral Maxillofac Surg. 2019;48(6):712–5. https://doi.org/10.1016/j.ijom.2018.11.014.
15. Kolomvos N, Kalfarentzos E, Papadogeorgakis N. Surgical treatment of plunging ranula: report of three cases and review of literature. Oral Maxillofac Surg Cases. 2019;5(1):100098. https://doi.org/10.1016/j.omsc.2019.100098.
16. Harrison JD. Modern management and pathophysiology of ranula: literature review. Head Neck. 2010;32(10):1310–20.
17. Lesperance MM. When do ranulas require a cervical approach? Laryngoscope. 2013;123(8):1826–7. https://doi.org/10.1002/lary.23937.
18. Kurabayashi T, Ida M, Yasumoto M, et al. MRI of ranulas. Neuroradiology. 2000;42(12):917–22. https://doi.org/10.1007/s002340000341.

Tracheal Surgery and Tracheostomy

10

Michael Zhang, Faruque Riffat, and Carsten Palme

10.1 Introduction

Tracheal neoplasms are inherently uncommon, with an estimated incidence of 2–3 in 1,000,000 people per year. Accounting for just over 0.2% of all respiratory tract malignancies and 0.02–0.04% of all recorded malignancies, malignancies of the larynx and bronchi 40 and 400 times more common respectively. In adults, tracheal malignancies may be either primary or secondary, with over 90% of all primary tracheal neoplasms being malignant. Squamous cell carcinoma (SCC) and adenoid cystic carcinoma (ACC) are the most common subtypes of primary tracheal malignancies [1]. Secondary tracheal tumours are more common than primary tracheal malignancy and predominantly arise from direct invasion of tumours of surrounding structures (such as the thyroid and oesophagus), with distant metastasis to the trachea is considerably rarer.

The rarity of tracheal tumours and their insidious, non-specific presentations (such as dyspnoea, cough and wheeze) greatly reduces the likelihood of early diagnosis. Optimal management of this spectrum of malignancies hinges upon the extent of disease (tumour location, size, locoregional spread and metastases) and the patient's own co-morbidities, with treatment regimens necessitating multidisciplinary input involving shared airway management, complex resection, reconstruction and potential adjuvant therapy in the form of radiotherapy and chemotherapy.

This chapter seeks to focus primarily on the workup and management of malignant diseases of the trachea (primary and secondary), relevant adjuvant therapy, surgically relevant anatomy and tracheostomy.

10.2 Anatomy of the Trachea

The trachea begins at the level of the C6 vertebrae and is a hollow tubular structure that provides a conduit between the larynx and the main bronchi of the lungs. Embryologically, it develops from an endodermal bud growing into the splanchnic mesoderm at approximately 4 weeks of gestation. It has a cervical component and a thoracic component, with a diameter of approximately 2 cm and a variable length of between 10–13 cm, dependent on inspiration. The trachea is comprised of 18–22 incomplete C-shaped hyaline cartilaginous 'rings' separated by annular or intercartilagenous ligaments derived from the mesoderm, creating its anterior and lateral walls. Posteriorly, a visceral, smooth muscle called 'trachealis' traverses the length of the trachea, connecting the two arms of

M. Zhang (✉) · F. Riffat · C. Palme
Department of Head and Neck Surgery, Chris O'Brien Lifehouse, Camperdown, NSW, Australia

The University of Sydney, Sydney, NSW, Australia
e-mail: Michael.Zhang4@health.nsw.gov.au; Carsten.Palme@lh.org.au

B. Ashford (ed.), *Head and Neck Surgery for General Surgeons*,
https://doi.org/10.1007/978-981-19-7900-2_10

the 'C.' The trachealis muscle and the hyaline cartilaginous C-shaped rings confers structural support during the negative intrathoracic pressure experienced during inspiration.

The luminal mucosa of the trachea, derived from endoderm, is lined with ciliated pseudostratified columnar epithelium (commonly known as respiratory epithelium), with mucous producing goblet cells. The mucous and cilia together form the 'mucociliary escalator' which synergistically traps and expels particulates that enter the airway. Chronic irritants may cause temporary and/or permanent damage to both the mucociliary escalator and the respiratory epithelium and can result in squamous metaplasia.

At its upper border, the cricotracheal ligament facilitates the trachea's superior attachment to the lower border of the cricoid. In adults, as the trachea passes inferiorly towards the thorax, it runs progressively deeper as it approaches the thoracic inlet; from a lateral viewpoint, it dives from anteriorly (subcutaneously) at the neck to posteriorly in the chest. It enters the thoracic inlet at midline, posterior to the manubrium, to bifurcate into the main bronchi at the carina, which is usually at the level of T4, right of midline and just below the lower border of the manubrium. From the carina, the right main bronchus continues more vertically, with the left main bronchus taking a more horizontal, acute angle with respect to the trachea.

There are several important organs and structures which surround the trachea. Anteriorly, the thyroid isthmus is adherent to the second and third cartilaginous tracheal rings, with the respective thyroid lobes situated anterior and lateral to the cervical trachea. Posteriorly, the cervical trachea lies upon the anterior cervical oesophagus, with the recurrent laryngeal nerves running in the tracheoesophageal groove.

10.2.1 Blood Supply

Understanding the vascular supply of the trachea is critical in minimising avascularisation of the trachea during surgical dissection, and thus minimising subsequent tracheal stenosis, necrosis or anastomotic failure. Fundamentally, the trachea is segmentally supplied by branches which create anastomotic networks and enter the trachea through lateral tissue pedicles. As these segmental arteries approach the trachea, they divide into superior and inferior branches in a longitudinal manner, forming anastomoses with the segmental branches above and below. Within the intercartilagenous or annular ligaments, the tracheal arteries again divide into anterior and posterior branches which travel circumferentially within the tracheal submucosa. These anastomose with the corresponding tracheal arteries from the contralateral side at the midline, creating submucosal capillary plexuses, which are the primary source of blood supply to the tracheal cartilage. Therefore, if this segmental blood supply is disrupted, it can potentiate tracheal ischaemia and its sequelae, reducing the potential extent of tracheal dissection [2, 3].

The upper half of the trachea (cervical trachea) is most commonly supplied by three tracheoesophageal branches of the inferior thyroid artery, from the thyrocervical trunk that branch off the subclavian artery on either side. The first tracheoesophageal branch supplies the lower cervical trachea, second supplies the middle cervical trachea and the third supplies the upper cervical trachea. Whilst the superior thyroid artery does not directly supply the trachea, it does anastomose and provide collateral to the inferior thyroid artery in supplying the thyroid isthmus and also the adjacent anterior trachea. The lower half of the of the trachea (thoracic trachea) and carina is generally supplied by three bronchial arteries – superior bronchial, middle bronchial and inferior bronchial arteries – which originate directly off the aorta itself [3]. The venous drainage of the entire length of the trachea is to the inferior thyroid venous plexus, which drains into the brachiocephalic veins.

10.2.2 Lymphatic Drainage

The primary lymphatic drainage of the cervical trachea is to the inferior group of deep cervical lymph nodes, whereas the thoracic trachea primarily drains to the pretracheal, paratracheal and subcarinal lymph nodes. Tumours of the trachea most commonly drain to the nearest lymphatic group, with skipped nodal metastases very uncommon.

10.3 Primary Tracheal Tumours

Tracheal tumours arise from the epithelial cells, mesenchymal structure or glands of the trachea. Most tracheal tumours, however, are secondary in nature and occur via direct invasion from nearby structures; however, of the primary tracheal tumours, over 90% are malignant.

10.3.1 Benign Tracheal Neoplasms

In adults, benign tracheal neoplasms are inherently uncommon, comprising only 10% of all adult primary tracheal tumours. In contrast, in children, over 70% tracheal neoplasms are benign. The most common benign tracheal tumours are squamous papillomas, which are caused by the human papilloma virus (HPV), usually by strains HPV-6 and HPV-11, and may be a manifestation of recurrent respiratory papillomatosis (RRP). These benign papillomatous lesions have a reported 3–7% risk of malignant transformation, especially in the presence of risk factors such as smoke or radiation exposure. These lesions are typically managed either medically with interferon, systemic antiviral, intralesional antiviral (cidofovir) therapy or surgically with excision via cold steel or a carbon dioxide laser. Further detailed discussion on the management of recurrent respiratory papillomatosis, or other benign tracheal pathology is outside the remit of this chapter.

10.3.2 Malignant Tracheal Neoplasms

In adults, over 90% of all primary tracheal neoplasms are malignant, with squamous cell carcinoma (SCC) and adenoid cystic carcinoma (ACC) being the most common subtypes.

10.3.2.1 Squamous Cell Carcinoma

Squamous cell carcinoma (SCC) is the most common histopathological type of malignant tracheal cancer, with a peak incidence in the seventh decade of life. Almost 90% of patients diagnosed report a history of smoking, and 15% having a history of prior respiratory tract malignancy. Males are 2–4× more likely to be affected than women. SCCs of the trachea are histologically identical to SCCs of the lung and can have an exophytic or ulcerative appearance. These tumours are very aggressive and have a predilection to local invasion and early metastasis. It is important to note that up to 30% of patients with primary tracheal SCC have synchronous or metachronous respiratory tract malignancies. Due to ulceration and mucosal irritation, haemoptysis is the most common presenting symptom, reported in over 60% of patients. As such, these tumours are generally diagnosed earlier, usually within 4–6 months of the onset of symptoms.

Prognosis amongst patients with SCC is generally quite poor, and heavily contingent on the surgical resectability of the tumour at time of presentation. The mean survival time was 38 months with resected SCC compared to 8.8 months with unresectable SCC. At 5 years, there was a 39.1% survival rate in patients with resected disease, compared with 7.3% in patients with unresectable disease. At 10 years, there was a survival rate of 18% in resected patients compared to 4.9% in unresectable patients. Patients who underwent complete resection (negative airway margins) had more favourable prognoses, with tumour size or extent of resection not significantly correlating with increased survival [4]. Unfavourable prognostic factors include extension into thyroid gland and lymphatic invasion [5].

10.3.2.2 Adenoid Cystic Carcinoma

Adenoid cystic carcinoma (ACC) is the second most common histopathological type of malignant tracheal cancer, and the most common glandular/salivary type tracheal cancer, with a peak incidence in the fifth decade of life. There are no known risk factors, with no gender predisposition, and no significant correlation with a history of smoking. Usually arising in the distal third of the trachea, ACCs of the trachea are histologically identical to those found in salivary glands. Insidious in its growth, the tumour tends to exert a mass effect on the trachea and nearby structures as opposed to direct invasion. Consequently, the most common presenting symptoms are dyspnoea and cough. Due to the non-specific nature of the presentation, adults are typically first misdiagnosed with airway disease such as adult-onset asthma or other forms of obstructive pulmonary disease, with a formal diagnosis usually coming a year after symptom onset.

Despite their slow growth, these tumours have a propensity for submucosal extension and perineural invasion but are less inclined to lymphatic spread to regional nodes. Despite this, patients are generally good operative candidates; however, there is often submucosal extension and perineural invasion at the time of operation, necessitating more extensive resection. ACCs are also prone to late locoregional and distal recurrences, in some cases up to 30 years after treatment.

Prognosis in patients with ACC is more favourable than that of SCC, with a mean survival time of 69 months in patients with resected ACC, and 41 months in patients with unresectable ACC. At 5 years, there was a 52.4% survival rate in patients with resected ACC compared to 33.3% for unresectable ACC. At 10 years, survival in patients with resected ACC was 29% compared to 10% in unresected patients. The greatest factors affecting prognosis in patients with ACCs are completeness of resection, perineural invasion and extramural extension [6]. Table 10.1 provides a comparison between the distinguishing features of the two most common histopathological subtypes of primary tracheal malignancies.

Table 10.1 Comparison between the two most common primary tracheal malignancies squamous cell carcinoma (SCC) and adenoid cystic carcinoma (ACC)

Squamous cell carcinoma (SCC)	Adenoid cystic carcinoma (ACC)
Most common primary tracheal malignancy (50–60%)	Second most common primary tracheal malignancy (10–15%)
Males 2–4× more likely to develop SCC	No gender predominance
Onset around 60–70 years	Onset around 40–50 years
Very strong association with smoking	No association with smoking, no clear risk factors
Can be ulcerative or exophytic, commonly presents with haemoptysis	Exerts a mass effect, commonly presents with dyspnoea
Rapid growing and usually diagnosed within 4–6 months of symptom onset	Slow growing and usually diagnosed >1 year after symptom onset
Prone to early metastases – Up to 30% may have synchronous or metachronous primaries	Likely to have submucosal and perineural invasion, and prone to late recurrences.
Prognostic factors: Resectability, thyroid invasion and lymph node extension	Prognostic factors: Resectability, perineural invasion and extramural extension

10.3.2.3 Other Malignant Tracheal Tumours

A variety of other epithelial, mesenchymal and glandular tumours have been reported and collectively represent the remaining 25–30% of all primary tracheal malignancy. Malignancy other than SCC or ACC of the trachea represent quite a heterogeneous group of tumours with carcinoids, mucoepidermoid tumours and sarcomas found to be most frequent, in that order. Table 10.2 provides a useful classification of tracheobronchial tumours. The rarity of these tumours makes accurate assessment of survival difficult, however similar to SCC and ACCs prognostication is contingent on tumour resectability. 5-year survival rates are reported to be 86% in patients with resected carcinoid tumours, 100% for resected mucoepidermoid tumours and 78% for sarcomas [7].

Table 10.2 Classification of primary tracheal neoplasms

	Benign	Malignant
Epithelial	• Fibroma/fibromatosis • Haemangioma • Paraganglioma • Glomus • Leiomyoma • Chrondroma • Schwannoma • Histiocytoma	• Chondrosarcoma • Rhabdomyocsacroma • Lymphoma • Malignant fibrous histiocytoma Melanoma
Mesenchymal	• Squamous papilloma	• Squamous cell carcinoma • Adenocarcinoma • Large cell undifferentiated carcinoma • Neuroendocrine tumours (NETs) – Typical carcinoid – Atypical carcinoid – Large cell neuroendocrine tumours • Small cell carcinoma
Glandular /salivary	• Pleomorphic adenoma • Oncocytoma • Mucous gland adenoma • Myoepithelioma	• Adenoid cystic carcinoma • Mucoepidermoid carcinoma • Carcinoma ex pleomorphic adenoma

10.4 Staging of Primary Tracheal Malignancies

Given the rarity of primary tracheal malignancy, there is currently no established, universally accepted staging system for primary tracheal malignancies. The most utilised system is a 'TNM' staging system proposed by Bhattacharyya, which is based on the Surveillance, Epidemiology, and End Results (SEER) 1973–2000 database and is shown in Table 10.3. Despite its adoption, there are inherent limitations due to the small number of cases, lack of differentiation between histological subtypes and their individual prognostic factors which impairs the comparison of the results of treatment and the ability of this system in predicting long-term survival.

Table 10.3 Proposed TNM staging system for primary tracheal malignancy Bhattacharyya et al. (2004) [11]

T-Staging	**Definition**
T_1	Primary tumour confined to the trachea; tumour size <2.0 cm
T_2	Primary tumour confined to the trachea; tumour size >2.0 cm
T_3	Spread outside trachea but not to adjacent structures or organs
T_4	Spread to adjacent structures or organs
T_x	Unknown; cannot be assessed
N—staging	**Definition**
N_0	No evidence of regional nodal disease
N_1	Presence of regional nodal disease
N_X	Unknown; cannot be assessed
M—staging	**Definition**
M_0	No evidence of distant metastases
M_1	Presence of distant metastases
M_X	Unknown; cannot be assessed
Overall staging	**Definition**
I	T_1 N_0 M_0
II	T_2 N_0 M_0
III	T_3 N_0 M_0
IV	T_4 N_0, any N_1 disease, or any M_1 disease

10.5 Secondary Tracheal Tumours

Secondary tracheal tumours are, by definition, malignant and can occur via direct invasion of the trachea from tumour or nodal metastases nearby or through systemic, haematogenous spread. These tumours almost universally have a very poor prognosis, with only secondary lesions from the thyroid and lung considered potentially curable. Secondary tracheal tumours from the direct invasion of oesophageal, head and neck, mediastinal malignancy or haematogenous distant metastases from breast cancer, colon cancer, melanoma (which may, extremely rarely, also be a primary tracheal tumour) and renal cell carcinoma are considered incurable and are managed with palliative intent.

Thyroid cancers are the most common source of secondary tracheal malignancy, with aerodigestive extension reported in over 6% of all cancers. Despite the aggressive reputation of anaplastic thyroid carcinoma, 76% of all laryngotracheal invasion by thyroid carcinoma was found to be histologically well-differentiated [8]. Shin et al. [9] proposed a 4-stage classification system to describe the depth of invasion of papillary thyroid cancer into the trachea. Stage 1 is where the carcinoma is limited to the glandular parenchyma. Stage 2 refers to the invasion of cartilage of tracheal rings, or intercartilagenous tissue. Stage 3 refers to the invasion of the lamina propria of the tracheal mucosa without any endotracheal change. Stage 4 refers to full thickness invasion with visible ulceration or neoplastic change in the lumen (see Table 10.4).

Table 10.4 Shin classification of tracheal invasion of papillary thyroid carcinoma [9]

Shin stage	Description
1	Thyroid carcinoma limited to the glandular parenchyma
2	Thyroid carcinoma invading tracheal rings or intercartilagenous tissue
3	Thyroid carcinoma invading the lamina propria of the tracheal mucosa, without endotracheal/luminal change
4	Full thickness invasion with visible ulceration/change within the lumen

Following evaluation of potential locoregional and distant metastases, where the thyroid tumour and its tracheal extension is considered surgically resectable, controversy exists as to whether a radical resection, window resection or shave excision of the trachea should be performed. Although no survival benefit was conferred in patients undergoing shave excision compared to radical resection if resection margins were clear of disease, generally a radical resection is preferred when tumour has invaded tracheal mucosa.

10.6 Clinical Presentation

Tracheal masses pose a diagnostic challenge, with their slow growth and vague symptomatology leading to a delayed presentation to a primary care clinician in the first instance, and secondarily a delayed diagnosis due to early symptoms being mild and attributed to common, benign pathology such as pneumonia, chronic obstructive pulmonary disease (COPD) and adult-onset asthma. As such, early diagnosis of tracheal malignancy requires an extremely high index of suspicion and a thorough elucidation of potential red flags on history and examination (see Table 10.5).

10.6.1 Common Features on History and Examination

The most common presenting complaints have been dyspnoea, cough and wheeze, with only the SCC subtype of tracheal cancer having a tendency

Table 10.5 Red flags for tracheal malignancy on history and examination

Red flags for tracheal malignancy on history	Red flags for tracheal malignancy on examination
Haemoptysis	Airway obstruction
Unexpected weight loss	Persistent stridor
History of smoking	Subtle long-term dysphonia
History of previous respiratory malignancy	Inspiratory dyspnoea exacerbated by lying flat
Dyspnoea unresponsive to medical therapy	Wheeze unresponsive to medical therapy

for presenting with haemoptysis. Patients typically do not experience significant breathlessness until the lumen of their airway is considerably narrowed, with exertional dyspnoea usually not evident until the airway narrowed by 50%, with dyspnoea at rest only apparent narrowing of greater than 70%. Patients reporting these early, non-specific symptoms of dyspnoea and cough frequently undergo a workup with a chest radiograph and pulmonary function testing. The chest x-ray is likely to miss an obstructive tracheal lesion in up to 75% of cases, with pulmonary function testing demonstrating a similar obstructive pattern and responsiveness to bronchodilators found in asthma. Patients are prescribed a regimen of bronchodilators and steroids; and it is only when this medical therapy begins to fail, do these patients undergo a CT which reveals the tracheal malignancy. A subset of patients will present with dysphonia as their primary complaint, as a result of direct invasion of the trachea from a thyroid primary malignancy. This is readily seen on nasoendoscopy, which should be a routine component of the workup of thyroid malignancy.

10.7 Investigations

10.7.1 Imaging

10.7.1.1 Chest X-Ray

Patients are often first investigated with chest x-rays given their universal accessibility and low cost. Chest radiographs are notoriously poor at diagnosing tracheal or bronchial malignancy, however, may be helpful in excluding other infective pathology. Only when tracheal malignancy is causing significant airway compression or narrowing where obstructive findings (e.g. hyperinflation) may be noted. As such the sensitivity of the chest radiograph is low, with less than one-third of all tracheal tumours are diagnosed with this modality.

10.7.1.2 Computed Tomography (CT)

CT is the mainstay of non-invasive investigation in the workup for potential tracheal lesions. Not only do they offer vital information about the primary tumour size, but its assessment of characteristics such as calcification, invasion of the tracheal wall, extension into the surrounding structures and locoregional lymphatic spread provides invaluable information into the extent of the disease itself and allows the surgeon to plan their operative approach and subsequent management.

In recent times, contrast-enhanced thin-slice multidetector CT (MDCT) scans are integral to the diagnosis and work-up of tracheal tumours. Modern MDCTs are readily available at most centres and are able to obtain high-quality images in a small amount of time. Multiplanar reformats are also possible, with two-dimensional axial, coronal, sagittal and oblique images centring on the tumours revealing the location, morphology, internal features and extramural invasion of tumours. Three-dimensional, virtual bronchoscopy reformats are also possible from the same scan, allowing clinicians to truly appreciate the complexity of the lesion itself within the lumen of the trachea. Imaging can also be performed on full inspiration and/or at full expiration to assess the dynamic states such as tracheomalacia, and the impact of the primary tumour on distal airways.

Differentiating between benign and malignant tracheal lesions on imaging alone can be quite difficult. Benign tracheal tumours typically are intraluminal with narrow bases or peduncles, show minimal spread along the tracheal wall and exhibit a well-circumscribed, homogenous appearance. They are generally less than 2 cm in size. The presence of calcium within the lesions is more consistent of lesions with a benign histology; however it very rarely may represent sarcoma. Lesions greater than 2 cm with irregular luminal stenoses, invasion of tracheal walls, heterogenous densities with associated mediastinal lymphadenopathy are quite suggestive of malignancy.

10.7.1.3 Magnetic Resonance Imaging (MRI)

Magnetic resonance imaging (MRI) has also been used in the workup of tracheal tumours. CT scans are less unreliable in assessing soft tissue and presence of perineurial disease, thus determining the presence and extent of submucosal spread of tumour, as well as additional prognostic features is challenging. Especially in adenoid cystic carcinomas and invasive thyroid malignancy, MRI has been shown to provide additional information regarding extent of invasion of the tracheal wall. Despite these advantages, MRI has not been specifically been shown to confer any significant additional diagnostic benefit.

10.7.1.4 Positron-Emission Tomography (PET)

Fluorine 18-fluorodeoxyglucose (FDG) positron-emission tomography (PET) and fused PET/CT images can be helpful in distinguishing between malignant and benign tumours. Benign tumours typically exhibit minimal or no standardised uptake values (SUV), whereas malignant lesions often demonstrate high SUVs. It can also be helpful in establishing whether disease has metastasised to regionally to lymph nodes, or to distant sites. This modality can also help assess response to adjuvant treatment and determine the presence of residual or recurrent disease, with follow-up PET scans typically performed at 8 weeks post adjuvant radiotherapy.

10.7.1.5 Ultrasonography

Whilst not utilised to diagnose tracheal malignancies, the use of ultrasonography and ultrasonographically guided biopsies of lymph nodes can be a useful adjunct in assessing progression of disease.

10.7.2 Pulmonary Function Testing

Pulmonary function testing (PFTs) has a limited role in the diagnosis of tracheal malignancies. They can suggest upper airway obstruction with flattening of the inspiratory and/or expiratory flow-volume loops. This can differentiate between both proximal and distal airway disease as well as intratracheal or extratracheal compression. The presence of these findings does not diagnose a tracheal tumour, and their absence does not preclude one; further investigation with imaging and endoscopy is required. Following treatment of tracheal malignancies, serial pulmonary function testing can be utilised to track progress, with peak flows easily self-administered to detect subtle early changes.

10.7.3 Endoscopic Evaluation and Biopsy

Bronchoscopy and biopsy is the gold-standard for diagnosing tracheal tumours and is a critical step in the workup of these masses. Initial flexible bronchoscopy can be performed to visualise the lesion. In patients with non-obstructing distal lesions, biopsies can be taken via the flexible bronchoscope. Despite both flexible and rigid bronchoscopy allowing for visualisation of the trachea down to the level of the carina and biopsy, the simplest way to evaluate tracheal lesions is via microlaryngoscopy and a rigid endoscope whilst the patient is either spontaneously breathing, or being oxygenated via jet ventilation or THRIVE. Any lesions can then be biopsied, and if necessary, the surgeon can debulk the tumour with laser or coblation and/or perform airway dilatations. Another advantage rigid bronchoscopy offers is the ability to apply pressure in the event of bleeding from the tumour or biopsy sites.

10.8 Management of Tracheal Malignancy

The management of tracheal malignancies is complex and necessitates multidisciplinary approach with detailed input from surgeons (ENT, Head and Neck, Thoracic), physicians (respiratory and intensivists) and anaesthetics for management of the shared airway, radiologists, pathologists, medical and radiation oncologists. Given the scarcity of these tumours, there are no randomised controlled trials to suggest the most effective treatment approach. Treatment regimens are based on basic oncologic principles and contingent on the surgical resectability of the tumour, with adjuvant therapy determined by histopathological subtype and other high-risk factors including positive margins, perineural invasion, lymphovascular invasion and extracaspsular spread.

10.8.1 Endoscopic Assessment and Management

If examination under anaesthesia via microlaryngoscopy and rigid endoscopy has not been performed previously, it should be done immediately prior to resection. This allows the surgeon to comprehensively assess the lesion and airway, plan the exact nature of the approach to the lesion and precise location of incisions. Depending on disease progression and patient suitability for surgery, tracheal lesions may be debulked to improve the airway with either coblation or laser, avoiding a long-term tracheostomy whilst enabling definitive, curative treatment via radiotherapy.

10.8.2 Surgical Resection

Surgical resection is the core treatment modality in tracheal malignancy, with tumour resectability a key factor in long-term survival.

The three governing surgical principles in tracheal surgery for malignancy are:

1. Ensuring all tumour is resected with adequate margins to optimise outcomes.
2. Limiting lymph node dissection and excessive tracheal mobilisation to preserve arterial supply, minimising risk of tracheal ischaemia, necrosis and stenosis.
3. Achieving a tension-free anastomosis.

10.8.3 Airway Management during Tracheal Surgery

The management of the airway during tracheal surgery requires clear communication between a surgical and anaesthetic team, with experience in managing these complex cases. The initial establishment of an airway, followed by maintenance of an airway after tracheal resection are the two main challenges. Ideally, the airway is stabilised prior to definitive surgical resection with debulking; however, it is not uncommon to have patients in respiratory distress. In these cases, slow induction with inhalational gases, avoidance of paralysis and the maintenance of spontaneous ventilation may be required. A tracheostomy is generally only utilised in patients with proximal tracheal lesions, as it may hinder subsequent tracheal anastomosis.

During resection, the nature of the lesion and type of resection will dictate the manner in which the airway is managed. For simple window resections, the endotracheal tube can often be left in situ (or advanced beyond), with care taken to avoid puncturing the cuff. Where segmental tracheal resection is required, ventilation via an on table endotracheal tube needs to be planned (so-called 'cross-field' ventilation). Generally, the distal incision is made first, with the distal tracheal stump intubated directly from the surgical bed. This is done under apnoea. A silk suture can be placed through Murphy's Eye of the original endotracheal tube to allow for easy retrieval at the end of the procedure. The on table tube is then secured and the orotracheal tube is left in the larynx and out of the way of the resection. Once the resection is complete, the posterior anastamotic sutures are placed. The existing endotracheal tube is then advanced beyond the transection, allowing for the anterior anastamotic sutures to be placed and the anastomosis to be completed. Typically, all sutures are interrupted with the knot placed on the external surface of the trachea.

Depending on the location of the tumour, other methods such as passing a small jet ventilation catheter into the distal airway, or for more distal lesions, intubating the right and left main bronchi directly are possible. Jet ventilation needs to be utilised with caution, as the constant insufflation of air can cause barotrauma due through progressive lung hyperinflation and increased ventilating pressures. Cardiopulmonary bypass remains an option; however, it comes with significant thrombotic risk and is rarely required.

10.8.4 Approach

Different incisions can be utilised to provide access to allow for resection and reconstruction, depending on the size and location of the primary tumour. Upper and mid-tracheal lesions can be accessed with a low cervical collar incision, with the option of a further vertical limb or partial/full median sternotomy providing access inferiorly. For more distal tracheal lesions, access may be gained through a right posterolateral thoracotomy through the fourth intercostal space. When using a cervical incision, the patient is positioned with the neck in a fully extended position with the assistance of a shoulder roll. In a similar fashion to a tracheostomy, the subplatysmal plane is developed and the trachea is exposed by separation of the strap muscles at the midline. Major mediastinal vasculature, especially the innominate artery, need to be identified and protected.

Mobilisation of the trachea depends on the extent of resection required and additional procedures such as thyroidectomy and or lymph node dissection. In general, the trachea should be mobilised only on its anterior surface to the level of the carina. At the point of resection, dissection should remain close to the trachea to protect the recurrent laryngeal nerves. Alternatively, these can be fully dissected and formally identified after removal of the thyroid gland and associated lymphatic tissue. Should resection of the cricoid cartilage be necessary, it is important to stay deep to its external perichondrium in order to avoid the recurrent laryngeal nerve at the level of Berry's Ligament and the criocothryoid joint, whilst preserving vascularity.

10.8.5 Extent of Resection

10.8.5.1 Tracheal Shave

This is the simplest method of tracheal excision, typically performed in patients with thyroid cancer. A margin is shaved off the surface of the trachea, with postoperative radioactive iodine relied upon to control and residual tumour should it be present. Despite this method perhaps being simpler and initially effective, the tumour is more predisposed to recur, especially if the trachea shave demonstrated disease involvement.

10.8.5.2 Simple Segmental Tracheal Resection

This is the most common type of tracheal resection, where a tracheal segment with disease/tumour involvement is resected. Important anatomical structures and landmarks such as the thyroid isthmus, cricoid, trachea and innominate artery are identified (Fig. 10.1a). The trachea is then mobilised on its anterior surface only to the level of the carina, ensuring dissection remains close to the trachea itself, and that superior mediastinal structures are avoided (Fig. 10.1b). Based on the extent of disease and accounting for margins, the superior and inferior limits of resection are then identified (Fig. 10.1c). The trachea is then mobilised circumferentially at the level of the resection, along the trachea-oesophageal groove; taking care to protect the recurrent laryngeal nerves bilaterally (Fig. 10.1d).

After the excised segment is mobilised, the inferior cut can be made. The endotracheal tube is withdrawn slightly if required, allowing the distal tracheal stump to be directly intubated via the surgical bed with a flexible, sterile endotracheal tube (Fig. 10.1e, f). When the airway has been established, the resection is completed with the superior cut and division of the trachealis muscle posteriorly.

Silk stay sutures are placed laterally around the superior and inferior tracheal rings and are brought together, allowing the surgeon to assess the level of tension of the anastomosis (Fig. 10.1h). Generally, a monofilament suture such as PDS is used, and the neck is placed in flexion to further reduce tension. The posterior sutures are placed first in a continuous manner, with the knot of the suture on the external surface of the trachea. The endotracheal tube may be intermittently inserted and removed, balancing the need for ventilation with repair of the posterior tracheal wall (Fig. 10.1i). The anastomosis is completed anteriorly with the placement of interrupted sutures around the adjacent anterior tracheal rings (Fig. 10.1j). Once the anastomosis is almost complete, the original endotracheal tube is pushed back down, distal to the anastomosis to facilitate normal ventilation. A 'reminder' or 'guardian' chin-to-chest suture is placed to prevent hyperextension (Fig. 10.1k). The patient should be extubated postoperatively.

10.8.5.3 Window Resection and Repair

This type of resection most encountered during thyroid surgery, where there is evidence of tumour adherence to the tracheal wall. A horizontal cervical incision is made to expose the thyroid isthmus, allowing the cricoid and trachea to be identified (Fig. 10.2a). The trachea is mobilised, and the window to be excised is delineated (Fig. 10.2b). Care must be taken to avoid inadvertent injury to the recurrent laryngeal nerves. The area is excised and the tracheal lumen is entered (Fig. 10.2c). Following resection, there are a number of methods by which the defect can be addressed. Should the defect be mainly anterior, a tracheostomy tube can be inserted, and the window can be allowed to heal via secondary intention after decannulation.

For small non-circumferential defects, a local flap is a simple option for immediate repair; with the sternocleidomastoid located nearby (Fig. 10.2d). The sternocleidomastoid can either be divided superior (Fig. 10.2e) and rotated medially to cover the defect (Fig. 10.2f) or mobilised inferior with the periosteum of the clavicle (Fig. 10.2g) and rotated medially to cover the defect (Fig. 10.2h). When suturing in the muscle, tension of the muscle is required to prevent collapse of the muscle into the trachea during inspiration.

10.8.5.4 Cricotracheal Resection and Thyrotracheal Anastomosis

This method involves resection of the cricoid, with subsequent thyrotracheal anastomosis achieved in either a sliding or step-wise fashion.

Slide

The area to be resected is exposed, including the thyroid isthmus, anterior arch of the cricoid cartilage and tracheal rings below (Fig. 10.3a). The thyroid isthmus is divided and the thyroid lobes are dissected off the lateral tracheal walls with care taken to avoid injury to the recurrent laryngeal nerves (Fig. 10.3b).

The anterior arch of the cricoid is mobilised from above and removed. The cricotracheal ligament laterally is also mobilised, staying deep/inside the external perichondrium, protecting the recurrent laryngeal nerves which run outside this layer. The internal cricoid perichondrium is mobilised posteriorly in continuity with the trachealis muscle, allowing detachment of the trachea from the remaining posterior cricoid lamina. The trachea can then be mobilised off the oesophagus (Fig. 10.3c).

The inferior cut is made, and the distal stump of the trachea is directly intubated through the surgical bed with a flexible sterile endotracheal tube. The oro-endotracheal tube is withdrawn to facilitate this, but not removed as it will be required after anastomosis (Fig. 10.3d). The excision is completed with the superior cut, with care taken to avoid inadvertent injury to the oesophagus posteriorly (Fig. 10.3e).

Stay sutures are placed laterally, bringing the segments together in a tension-free fashion. The trachea inferiorly will telescope into the cricoid and approximate the thyroid cartilage (Fig. 10.3f). The posterior wall is repaired first by placing sutures through the subglottic mucosa and part of the posterior cricoid lamina using a monofilament continuous suture (PDS).

The oro-endotracheal tube is retrieved back into the distal airway, and the anterior wall of the trachea is repaired with interrupted sutures placed around the thyroid cartilage superiorly and tracheal ring inferiorly. Soft drains are placed, the wound is closed in layers and a chin-to-chest reminder suture preventing hyperextension is placed. Extubation is preferred; however, a small tracheostomy tube can be placed if there are airway concerns (Fig. 10.3g).

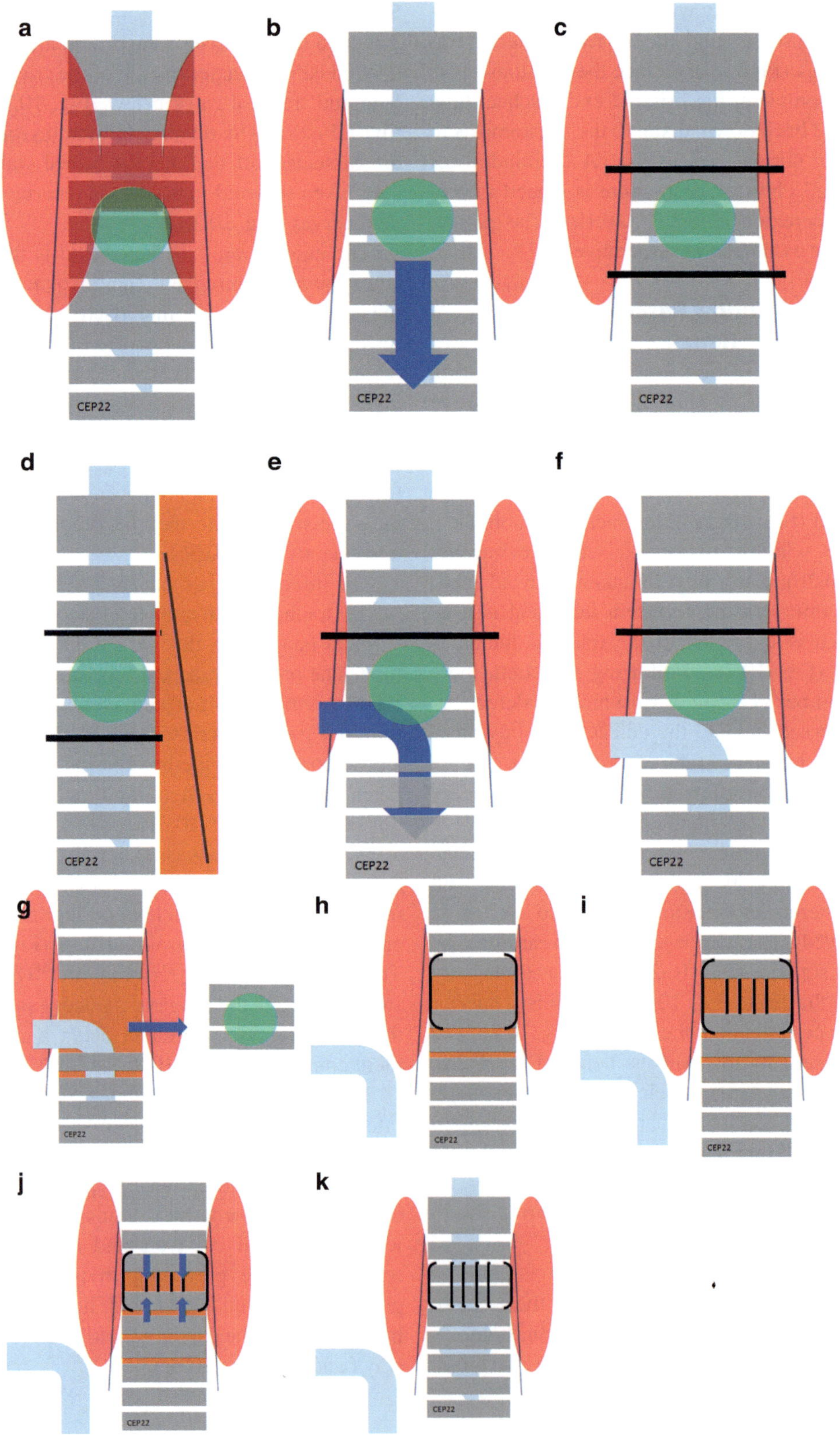
a
b
c
CEP22
CEP22
CEP22
d
e
f
CEP22
CEP22
CEP22
g
h
i
j
k

Fig. 10.1 (**a**) The thyroid isthmus is exposed, with important anatomical landmarks (cricoid, trachea and innominate artery inferiorly) identified. (Key: *red* thyroid, *green* tumour, *light blue* endotracheal tube, *grey* trachea, *thin black lines* recurrent laryngeal nerves). (**b**) The trachea is mobilised bluntly on its anterior surface only to the level of the carina, taking care to avoid injury to superior mediastinal vascular contents. (Key: *red* thyroid, *green* tumour, *light blue* endotracheal tube, *grey* trachea, *thin black lines* recurrent laryngeal nerves). (**c**) The superior and inferior extent of resection are identified. (Key: *red* thyroid, *green* tumour, *light blue* endotracheal tube, *grey* trachea, *thin black lines* recurrent laryngeal nerves, *thick black line* superior and inferior margins of resection). (**d**) Circumferentially mobilise the trachea at the level of resection, avoiding injury to the oesophagus by separating the trachea-oesophageal groove region. (Key: *red* trachea-*oesophageal groove*, *green* tumour, *light blue* endotracheal tube, *grey* trachea, *thin black lines* recurrent laryngeal nerves, *thick black line* superior and inferior margins of resection*)*. (**e**) The trachea is entered via the inferior cut, the endotracheal tube is withdrawn and the distal stump is intubated via a separate endotracheal tube, through the operative field. *(*Key: *red* thyroid, *green* tumour, *light blue* endotracheal tube, *dark blue* intubation of distal tracheal stump, *grey* trachea, *thin black lines* recurrent laryngeal nerves, *thick black line* superior and inferior margins of resection). (**f**) The trachea is entered via the inferior cut, the endotracheal tube is withdrawn, and the distal stump is intubated via a separate endotracheal tube, through the operative field. *(*Key: *red* thyroid, *green* tumour, *light blue* new endotracheal tube, *grey* trachea, *thin black lines* recurrent laryngeal nerves, *thick black line* superior and inferior margins of resection). (**g**) The resection is completed by making the superior cut and dividing the trachealis posteriorly. *(*Key: *red* thyroid, *green* tumour, *light blue* endotracheal tube, *grey* trachea, *thin black lines* recurrent laryngeal nerves, *orange* defect*)*. (**h**) Silk stay sutures are placed laterally around the superior and inferior tracheal rings and test bringing the segments together in a tension-free manner. You may need to remove the shoulder roll and place the neck in slight flexion to reduce tension. *(*Key: *red* thyroid, *green* tumour, *light blue* endotracheal tube, *grey* trachea, *thin black lines* recurrent laryngeal nerves, *thick black line* stay silk sutures, *orange* defect*)*. (**i**) Commence your repair by placing sutures posteriorly first. You might use a monofilament (PDS) in a continuous manner. Utilise the stay sutures to bring the posterior wall together to facilitate a tension-free repair. Endotracheal tube may be intermittently inserted and removed intermittently to facilitate oxygenation, or to expose the posterior wall fully. *(*Key: *red* thyroid, *green* tumour, *light blue* endotracheal tube, *grey* trachea, *thin black lines* recurrent laryngeal nerves, *thick black line* sutures, *orange* defect). (**j**) The anastomosis is completed anteriorly by placing sutures around the adjacent tracheal rings using interrupted sutures (PDS). *(*Key: *red* thyroid, *green* tumour, *light blue* endotracheal tube, *grey* trachea, *thin black lines* recurrent laryngeal nerves, *thick black line* sutures, *orange* defect). (**k**) Once the repair is nearly complete, push the endotracheal tube back down to facilitate normal ventilation. Insert soft drains to prevent subcutaneous emphysema and close the wound in layers. Place a 'reminder stitch' between the mentum and the sternum to prevent inadvertent hyperextension. Aim to extubate the patient at the end of the procedure. *(*Key: *red* thyroid, *light blue* endotracheal tube, *grey* trachea, *thin black lines* recurrent laryngeal nerves, *thick black line* sutures, *orange* defect)

Step-Wise

This technique is ideally suited to tumours located at the level of the cricotracheal groove and Berry's Ligament, with sacrifice of the recurrent laryngeal nerve potentially necessary. The trachea is first mobilised on its anterior surface to the level of the carina (Fig. 10.4a). The tumour is then excised with sections of the cricoid cartilage and adjacent tracheal rings. If possible, dissection should stay inside or deep to the external perichondrium of the cricoid, protecting the recurrent laryngeal nerves. (Fig. 10.4b). A step-wise cut is fashioned in the distal trachea, with the corresponding segment removed (Fig. 10.4c). The distal segment is advanced into the superior resection margin, with stay sutures helpful in bringing the segments together (Fig. 10.4d). The posterior wall is repaired first, and then the anterior walls are brought together with interrupted monofilament sutures (PDS). The repair can be completed while the endotracheal tube remains in situ taking care to avoid injury to the cuff (Fig. 10.4e).

10.8.6 Principles of Anastomosis

Following resection, the patient's neck is restored to a flexed position to allow for anastomosis. Depending on the segment excised, anastomoses can be performed in an end-to-end, end-to-side or sliding fashion utilising continuous sutures inter-

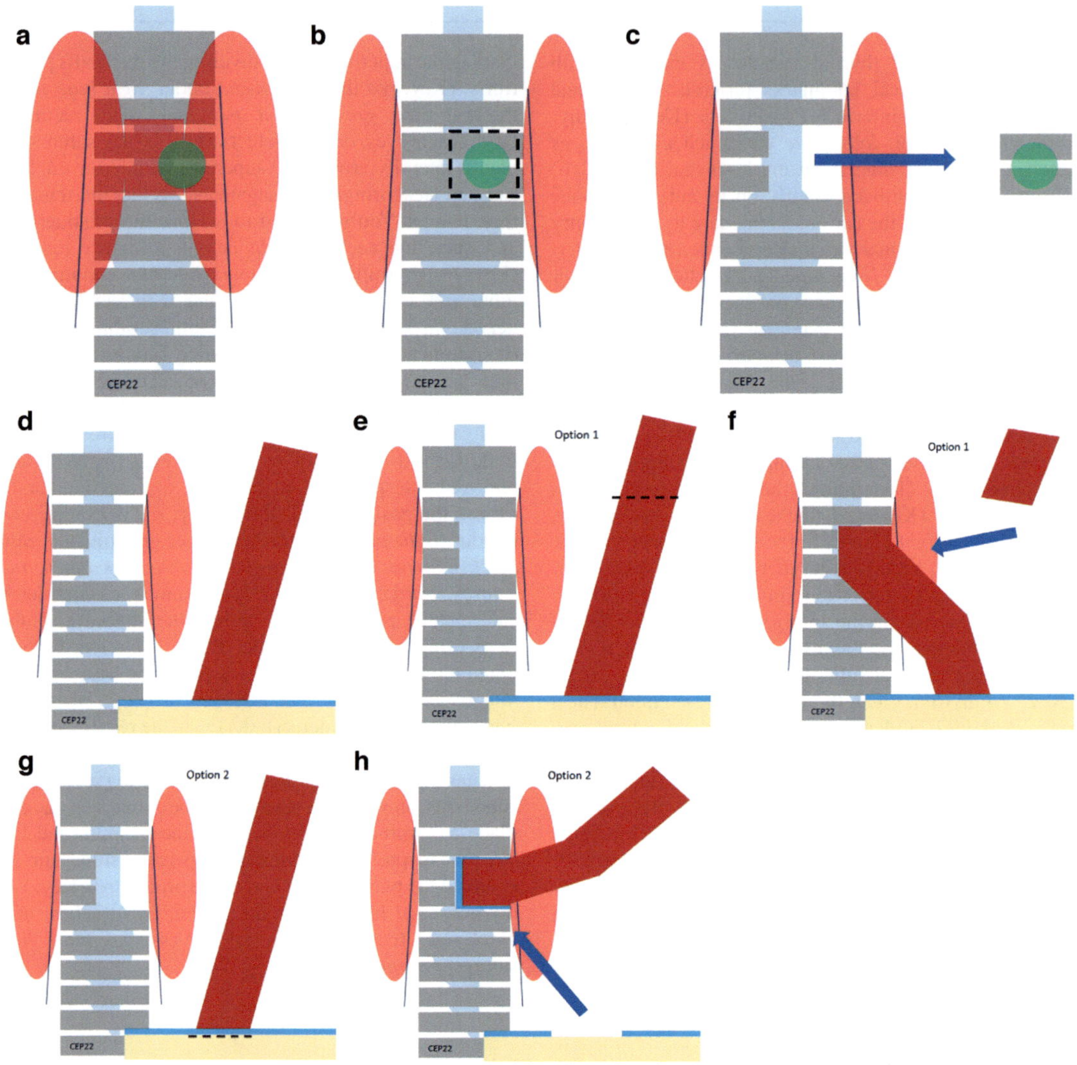

Fig. 10.2 (**a**) Expose trachea via a horizontal cervical incision. Identify cricoid above and trachea below the thyroid isthmus. (Key: *red* thyroid, *green* tumour, *light blue* endotracheal tube, *grey* trachea, *thin black lines* recurrent laryngeal nerves). (**b**) The trachea is carefully mobilised, with the window to be excised delineated. Care is taken to avoid injury to the recurrent laryngeal nerve. (Key: *red* thyroid, *green* tumour, *light blue* endotracheal tube, *grey* trachea, *thin black lines* recurrent laryngeal nerves, *thick black lines* window resection). (**c**) The area is excised, the tracheal lumen is entered and tumour removed. (Key: *red* thyroid, *green* tumour, *light blue* endotracheal tube, *grey* trachea, *thin black lines* recurrent laryngeal nerves). (**d**) The adjacent sternocleidomastoid muscle is ideally located. (Key: *light red* thyroid, *dark red* sternocleidomastoid, *green* tumour, *light blue* endotracheal tube, *grey* trachea, *thin black lines* recurrent laryngeal nerves, *yellow* clavicle, *blue* periosteum of clavicle). (**e**) Option 1—The sternocleidomastoid muscle is partially divided superiorly, taking care to avoid injury to the accessory nerve and underlying carotid sheath. (Key: *light red* thyroid, *dark red* sternocleidomastoid, *green* tumour, *light blue* endotracheal tube, *grey* trachea, *thin black lines* recurrent laryngeal nerves, *yellow* clavicle, *blue* periosteum of clavicle). (**f**) Option 1—The superior portion of the sternocleidomastoid is rotated into the defect medially. This is sutured into the edge of the defect ensuring adequate tension to avoid collapse into the tracheal lumen during respiration. (Key: *light red* thyroid, *dark red* sternocleidomastoid, *green* tumour, *light blue* endotracheal tube, *grey* trachea, *thin black lines* recurrent laryngeal nerves, *yellow* clavicle, *blue* periosteum of clavicle). (**g**) Option 2—The sternocleidomastoid muscle can be mobilised inferiorly together with periosteum of the clavicle below. (Key: *light red* thyroid, *dark red* sternocleidomastoid, *green* tumour, *light blue* endotracheal tube, *grey* trachea, *thin black lines* recurrent laryngeal nerves, *yellow* clavicle, *blue* periosteum of clavicle). (**h**) Option 2—The inferior mobilised muscle is rotated medially and sutured to the edges of the tracheal defect, ensuring some degree of tension in order to avoid collapse into the tracheal lumen. (Key: *light red* thyroid, *dark red* sternocleidomastoid, *green* tumour, *light blue* endotracheal tube, *grey* trachea, *thin black lines* recurrent laryngeal nerves, *yellow* clavicle, *blue* periosteum of clavicle)

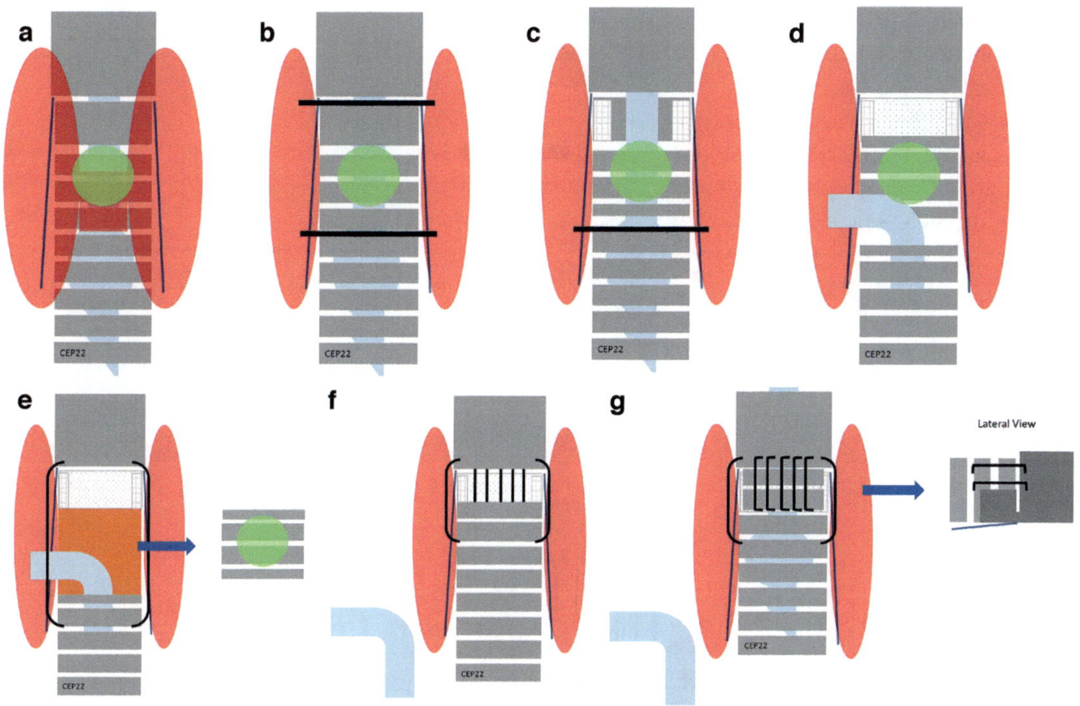

Fig. 10.3 (**a**) Expose the area to resected which includes the anterior arch of the cricoid cartilage and the tracheal rings below. (Key: *light red* thyroid, *green* tumour, *light blue* endotracheal tube, *grey* trachea, *thin black lines* recurrent laryngeal nerves). (**b**) The thyroid isthmus is divided, and the thyroid lobes are mobilised off the lateral tracheal walls, taking care to avoid injury to the recurrent laryngeal nerves. (Key: *light red* thyroid, *green* tumour, *light blue* endotracheal tube, *grey* trachea, *thin black lines* recurrent laryngeal nerves, *thick black lines* superior and inferior limit of resection). (**c**) The anterior arch of the cricoid is mobilised from above and removed. The cricotracheal ligament laterally is also mobilised, staying deep/inside the external perichondrium, protecting the recurrent laryngeal nerves which run outside this layer. The internal cricoid perichondrium is mobilised posteriorly in continuity with the trachealis muscle, allowing detachment of the trachea from the remaining posterior cricoid lamina. The trachea can then be mobilised off the oesophagus. (Key: *light red* thyroid, *green* tumour, *light blue* endotracheal tube, *grey* trachea, *thin black lines* recurrent laryngeal nerves, *thick black lines* superior and inferior limit of resection). (**d**) The inferior cut is made, and the distal stump of the trachea is directly intubated through the surgical bed. The oro-endotracheal tube is withdrawn to facilitate this, but not removed as it will be required after anastomosis. A silk suture may be placed through Murphy's Eye in order to allow retrieval after anastomosis. (Key: *light red* thyroid, *green* tumour, *light blue* endotracheal tube, *grey* trachea, *thin black lines* recurrent laryngeal nerves, *thick black lines* superior and inferior limit of resection). (**e**) The resection is completed following the superior excision, taking care to avoid injury to the oesophagus posteriorly. (Key: *light red* thyroid, *green* tumour, *light blue* endotracheal tube, *grey* trachea, *thin black lines* recurrent laryngeal nerves, *orange* defect). (**f**) Stay sutures are placed laterally, bringing the segments together in a tension-free fashion. The trachea inferiorly will telescope into the cricoid and approximate the thyroid cartilage. The posterior wall is repaired first by placing sutures through the subglottic mucosa and part of the posterior cricoid lamina using a monofilament continuous suture (PDS). (Key: *light red* thyroid, *green* tumour, *light blue* endotracheal tube, *grey* trachea, *thin black lines* recurrent laryngeal nerves, *thick black lines* sutures, *orange* defect). (**g**) The orotracheal tube is brought back into the distal airway and the repair of the anterior wall is completed using interrupted sutures placed around the thyroid cartilage superiorly and the tracheal ring inferiorly. Soft drains are placed and the wound is closed in layers. A 'reminder stitch' preventing neck hyperextension is placed. Extubation is preferable, but placement of a small tracheostomy tube is appropriate where there are airway concerns. (Key: *light red* thyroid, *light blue* endotracheal tube, *grey* trachea, *thin black lines* recurrent laryngeal nerves, *thick black lines* sutures, *orange* defect)

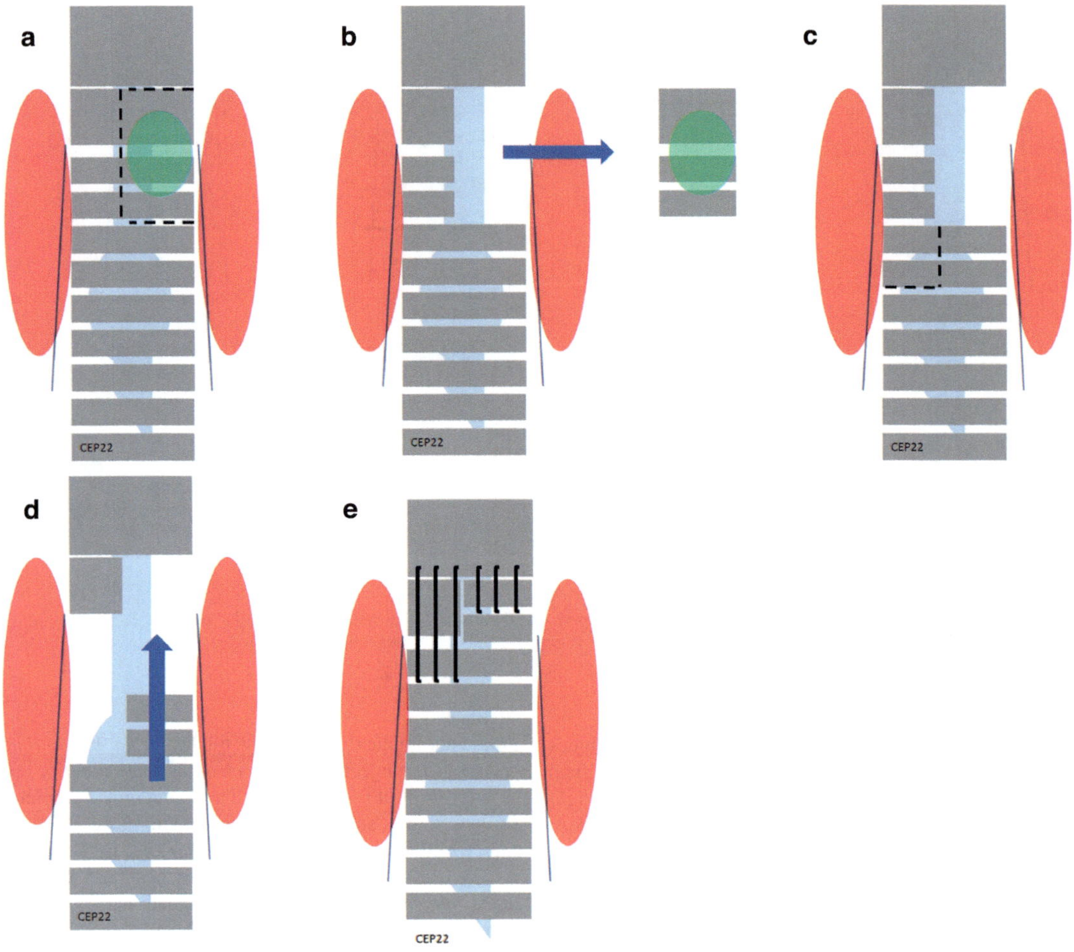

Fig. 10.4 (**a**) Mobilise the trachea on its anterior surface only to the level of the carina. (Key: *red* thyroid, *green* tumour, *light blue* endotracheal tube, *grey* trachea, *thin black lines* recurrent laryngeal nerves, *dotted thick black line* limit of resection). (**b**) The tumour is excised with sections of the cricoid cartilage and adjacent tracheal rings. If possible, dissection should stay within the external perichondrium of the cricoid cartilage to protect the recurrent laryngeal nerves. Avoid injury to the oesophagus posteriorly. (Key: *red* thyroid, *green* tumour, *light blue* endotracheal tube, *grey* trachea, *thin black lines* recurrent laryngeal nerves). (**c**) A step-wise cut is created and the corresponding segment of the trachea is removed. (Key: *red* thyroid, *light blue* endotracheal tube, *grey* trachea, *thin black lines* recurrent laryngeal nerves, *dotted thick black line* step-wise tracheal cut). (**d**) The distal segment is mobilised into the superior resection margin. Stay sutures laterally are helpful and bringing the segments together. (Key: *red* thyroid, *light blue* endotracheal tube, *grey* trachea, *thin black lines* recurrent laryngeal nerves). (**e**) The posterior wall is repaired first, and then the anterior walls are brought together with interrupted monofilament sutures (PDS). The repair can be completed while the endotracheal tube remains in situ taking care to avoid injury to the cuff. (Key: *red* thyroid, *light blue* endotracheal tube, *grey* trachea, *thin black lines* recurrent laryngeal nerves, *thick black lines* sutures)

rupted or a combination of both, with the goal of creating a tension-free join. If following the required resection, there is still an unacceptable tension on the potential anastomosis, release manoeuvres can be performed to further mobilise the trachea. Supra-laryngeal release procedures allow further mobilisation of the tracheal inferiorly, with the suprahyoid and/or infrahyoid release potentially generating an additional 1–2 cm of movement inferiorly each. Infra-laryngeal release procedures such as hilar release, pretracheal dissection and incision of the annular ligaments provide an additional 1–2 cm of movement superiorly each. These manoeuvres are not without their own challenges and complications – with supra-laryngeal release manoeuvres placing the patient at a high risk of significant dysphagia, and infra-laryngeal release procedures requiring input from thoracic surgeons.

Following anastomosis, a local, regional, or free flap can be utilised to 'cover' the anastomotic site, especially if there has been previous irradiation. In the neck, the strap musculature or a pedicled sternocleidomastoid muscle may be used, whereas in the chest pericardial fat, pedicled chest wall muscle, or omental flaps may be used. A soft drain (such as an open penrose drain) is placed at the anastomotic site to reduce subcutaneous emphysema and a chin-to-chest 'guardian' or 'reminder' suture (otherwise, eponomyously known as the Grillo suture) is often placed from the submental skin to the sternal skin to hold the neck in flexion for 7 days, preventing neck extension and rupture of the anastomosis.

Following resection and anastomosis, it is imperative that mechanical ventilation is avoided, secretions are controlled, and prophylactic antibiotics are administered to prevent wound breakdown. If the patient requires re-intubation, a small endotracheal tube should be placed under rigid endoscopic vision ideally distal to the anastomotic junction. High ventilation pressures should be avoided where possible.

10.8.7 Risks and Complications

Tracheal surgery is complex, and as such it has significant intraoperative risk and postoperative complications, which can be life-threatening in nature through imminent loss of the airway. Intraoperative risks include bleeding, damage to surrounding vasculature, damage to nearby structures and injury to the recurrent laryngeal nerves.

Early complications can include airway obstruction from postoperative oedema and bleeding, aspiration and anastomotic dehiscence or rupture. With larger and recurrent resections, or patients who are immunocompromised or have previously received radiotherapy to the area, there is an increased risk of anastomotic complication. Pulmonary complications such as retained secretions, aspiration (especially after suprahyoid release manoeuvres or recurrent laryngeal nerve injury) is also common and may require management with antibiotics and swallow rehabilitation.

Later complications can include stenosis of the anastomotic junction requiring bronchoscopy and dilatation, development of granulation tissue, dysphagia, dehiscence of the anastomosis and fistula to surrounding viscera or vessels. See Table 10.6 for a breakdown of early and late complications from tracheal surgery.

Table 10.6 Comparison of early and late complications following tracheal surgery

Early complications	Late complications
Airway obstruction (from oedema)	Tracheal stenosis
Bleeding	Development of granulation tissue
Infection	Tracheomalacia
Anastomotic leak, dehiscence or rupture	Fistula (tracheoesophageal, tracheo-inominate, tracheopulmonary)
Subcutaneous emphysema	Dehiscence of anastomosis.
Dysphonia (laryngeal oedema/ RLN injury)	Dysphagia

10.9 Non-Surgical and Adjuvant Management

10.9.1 Radiotherapy

Radiotherapy can be utilised with curative intent as an adjuvant following surgical resection in patients with histopathologically aggressive disease. The presence of positive or close surgical margins, perineural or lymphovascular invasion indicates the use of adjuvant radiotherapy and has been shown to increase median survival times and 5-year survival rates. Palliative radiotherapy for unresectable tumours or patients who are medically unfit for a general anaesthetic can also be given for disease suppression and symptom control [10].

10.9.2 Chemotherapy

The use of chemotherapy in tracheal surgery remains unclear given the paucity of literature on tracheal tumours and its management. Currently, there is perhaps a role for chemotherapy in radiosensitisation, management of distant disease, or for palliation. Further research is required into its use, particularly in different subtypes of tracheal cancer.

10.9.3 Immunotherapy

In more recent times, immunotherapy has come into the fore with regards to cancer management. Depending on the pathology, differing targeted therapies such as Lenvatinib and Pembrolizumab may be able to be offered. Research is continuing with regards to the future role of immunotherapy in tracheal cancer.

10.9.4 Palliative Therapy

In patients with advanced, unresectable disease, palliation or best supportive care may be the most appropriate management option. In these patients, tracheal stents may be inserted to provide symptomatic relief to patients. Palliative radiotherapy may also be considered in these patients for symptomatic relief and disease suppression.

10.10 Tracheostomy and Tracheotomy

A tracheotomy is an incision in the trachea, whereas a tracheostomy is the removal of a small portion of the anterior tracheal wall, with the difference between the two often disregarded. A tracheostomy may be short-term or long-term in nature and is performed for the bypass of a current or anticipated upper airway obstruction, facilitate prolonged and more efficient ventilation (through reduction of dead space), protect the airway against chronic aspiration and/or to enable a pulmonary toilet.

10.10.1 Procedure

The procedure itself may be performed percutaneously or surgically, under general or local anaesthesia. The patient is positioned supine with a shoulder roll with or without a head ring facilitating neck extension, bringing the trachea to the surface of the neck. Relevant surgical landmarks including the thyroid eminence, cricoid, sternal notch, anterior borders of the sternocleidomastoid and the anticipated incision line are marked.

A transverse skin incision is usually made at least 2 cm (or 2 finger breadths) above the sternal notch (Fig. 10.5a), or a vertical skin incision is made along the midline. Transverse skin incisions are preferred as they confer more desirable cosmetic outcomes; however, vertical skin incisions provide more expedient access in the event of an emergency where cosmesis takes a lower priority. The subplatysmal plane is developed, noting that the platysma may be dehiscent in the midline, with the anterior jugular veins retracted aside or ligated. The next layer encountered is the infrahyoid strap muscles and their midline raphe, which is incised. The strap muscles are retracted laterally to expose the isthmus of the thyroid and the anterior tracheal wall. The isthmus of the thyroid may be retracted superiorly/inferiorly, or divided between clamps or with a vessel sealing device (Fig. 10.5b). The innominate artery must always remain in the back of the surgeon's mind, as these may be high riding in some patients. Continual, repeated digital palpation through the wound is imperative to ensure the surgeon remains midline, inadvertent dissection lateral to the trachea is avoided, and critical structures such as the innominate artery remains away from the site of tracheostomy.

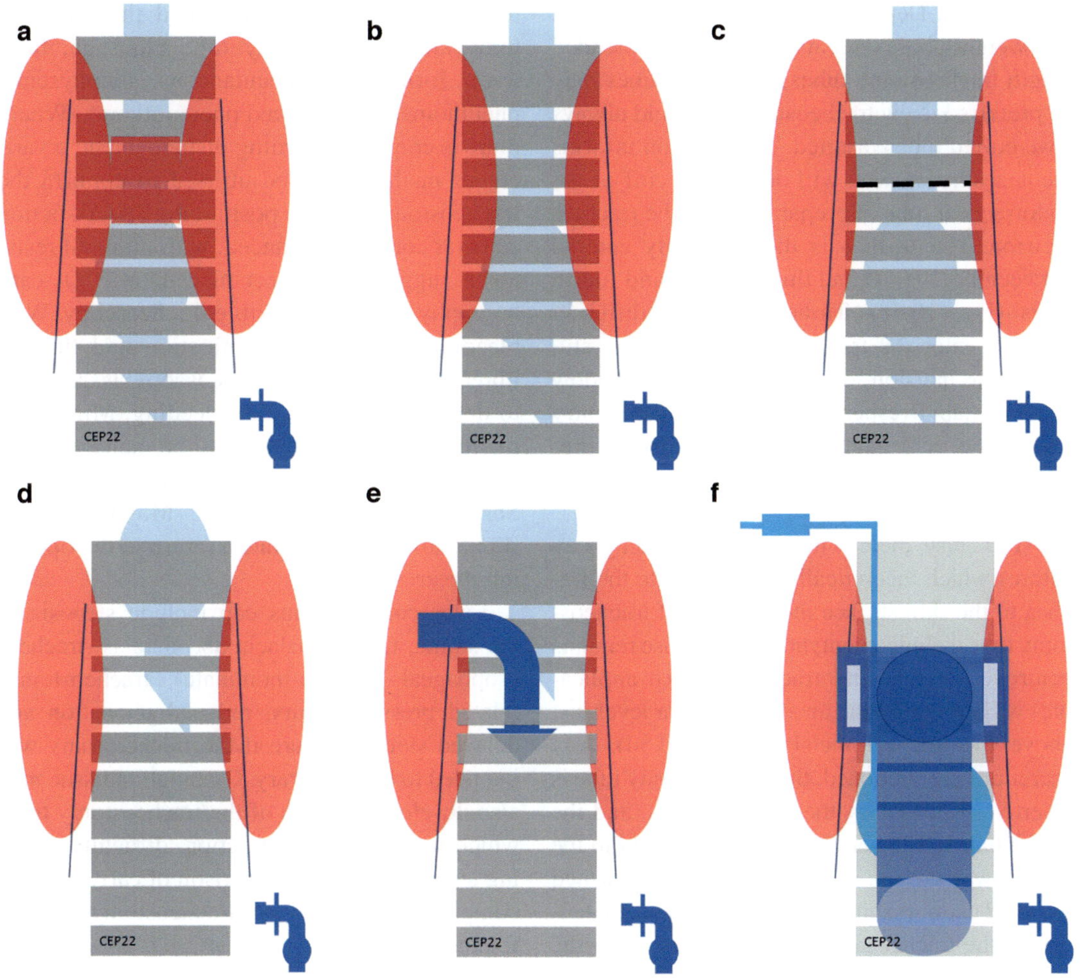

Fig. 10.5 (**a**) A skin crease incision is made above sternal notch. The midline raphe is entered, strap muscles are retracted, and the cricoid cartilage, thyroid isthmus and trachea are identified. (Key: *red* thyroid, *light blue* endotracheal tube, *dark blue* tracheostomy tube, *grey* trachea, *thin black lines* recurrent laryngeal nerves). (**b**) The thyroid isthmus is divided to expose the tracheal rings. (Key: *red* thyroid, *light blue* endotracheal tube, *dark blue* tracheostomy tube, *grey* trachea, *thin black lines* recurrent laryngeal nerves). (**c**) A tracheotomy between the second and third, or third and fourth tracheal rings is made. (Key: *red* thyroid, *light blue* endotracheal tube, *dark blue* tracheostomy tube, *grey* trachea, *thin black lines* recurrent laryngeal nerves, *thick black lines* tracheotomy). (**d**) The endotracheal tube is withdrawn under direct vision by the anaesthetist and secretions are suctioned. (Key: *red* thyroid, *light blue* endotracheal tube, *dark blue* tracheostomy tube, *grey* trachea, *thin black lines* recurrent laryngeal nerves). (**e**) The tracheostomy tube cuff is inserted in a gentle twisting motion under direct vision into trachea. Communicate with anaesthetist and ensure ease of ventilation and evidence of CO_2 return. (Key: *red* thyroid, *light blue* endotracheal tube, *dark blue* tracheostomy tube, *grey* trachea, *thin black lines* recurrent laryngeal nerves). (**f**) The tracheostomy tube is secured to skin via sutures or tapes, the cuff is inflated and the distal airway is suctioned. Insert the inner cannula. (Key: *red* thyroid, *light blue* endotracheal tube, dark blue *tracheostomy tube*, *grey* trachea, *thin black lines* recurrent laryngeal nerves)

Prior to entering the trachea, the appropriately sized tracheostomy tube (as well as the size below) needs to be readily available, with the cuff tested for leaks, the introducers inserted and lubricated. Tracheostomy tube selection is closely dependent on patient factors, with a variety of cuffed and cuffless, fenestrated and non-fenestrated, extended length and adjustable length tubes. Depending on patient factors (e.g. overweight/obese patients may require extended length tracheostomy tubes), different tubes may be preferred. New tracheostomies should always have cuffed tubes inserted. The surgeon informs the anaesthetist, who will deflate the cuff of the endotracheal tube in preparation for the tracheal incision. The trachea is then typically entered between the second and third or third and fourth rings (Fig. 10.5c). There are many differing ways to enter the trachea – via a midline slit, transverse incision, creation of a small window or Bjork flap. Irrespective of this, cold steel entry via scalpel and Metzembaum scissors is preferred over energy devices to nullify the risk of an airway fire.

After entry, there is the option of placing stay sutures which theoretically helps elevate the trachea to the skin surface in the event of tracheostomy tube dislodgement; however, its use remains controversial. The endotracheal tube (if applicable) withdrawn by the anaesthetist to a level just above the tracheal incision (Fig. 10.5d). Any secretions are suctioned, the tracheostomy tube is inserted, followed by the inner cannula, and the cuff inflated. The ventilator is reconnected to the new airway circuit, and positioning is confirmed via CO2 capnography (Fig. 10.5e, f). The phalanges of the tracheostomy tube are secured to the skin bilaterally via silk sutures and/or via tracheostomy ties. Note, in patients who have undergone free flap reconstruction, ties around the neck are generally avoided due to the pressure they may apply onto the vascular pedicle and anastomoses. In these patients, the phalanges of the tracheostomy tube may intentionally be cut to prevent any ties (and thus pressure to the anastomosis) being applied.

10.10.2 Complications of Tracheostomy

The complications following tracheostomy can be classified into early and late. In the immediate aftermath of the procedure, early complications can include dislodgement of tracheostomy tube, bleeding, infection around the tracheostomy site, tracheostomy tube blockage, false tract formation, subcutaneous emphysema, pneumomediastinum and pneumothorax. Where there is concern regarding dislodgement, a variety of methods can be utilised to confirm the tracheostomy tube's positioning. A Y-suction catheter could be advanced, with minimal resistance suggesting correct placement, CO_2 capnography or formal flexible tracheoscopy. With bleeding, a detailed examination and flexible fibreoptic endoscopy/tracheoscopy is required to delineate the source of bleeding. Minor stomal bleeding is likely able to be managed with intravenous tranexamic acid and placement of Surgicel around the wound. Major bleeding should always necessitate a return to the operating theatre.

Later complications can include stenosis of the stoma, tracheomalacia and fistulas (tracheoesophageal, trachea-inominate), tracheostomy-related pressure injury, reduced phonation and delayed stomal closure if the tracheostomy was intended to be temporary. Granulation tissue may also develop at the tip of the tracheostomy tube, which may lead to obstruction, difficulty toileting and bleeding. A comparison of early and late complications following tracheostomy can be found in Table 10.7.

Table 10.7 Comparison of early and late complications following tracheostomy

Early complications	Late complications
Bleeding from stomal site	Tracheal stenosis and tracheomalacia
Obstruction of tube	Development of granulation tissue, which may cause obstruction and bleeding
Dislodgement of tube (immature tract)	Fistulas (tracheoesophageal, trachea-inominate)
False tract formation	Tracheostomy-related pressure injury
Pneumothorax, pneumomediastinum, subcutaneous emphysema	Delayed tracheostomy closure

10.10.3 Decannulation

Before decannulation can be considered, the patient's original pathology requiring tracheostomy should have resolved, their respiratory function and intrinsic airway protection (via coughing to clear secretions) must be optimised, and a fibreoptic examination of their upper airway should be performed to ensure patency. Only then, is a sequential approach is used to assess the patient's suitability in successfully tolerating decannulation, or smaller uncuffed tracheostomy tubes or a continuous period of having their tracheostomy capped.

Following decannulation, the tracheostomy site is dressed, with patients encouraged to apply pressure to their stoma site during phonation to promote airflow through their native airway rather than out the stoma site, to encourage expedient closure and healing.

10.11 Conclusion

Despite being exceedingly rare, the majority of tracheal tumours are malignant; most of which are metastatic lesions. Of primary tracheal malignancy, the two most common histological subtypes are squamous cell carcinoma and adenoid cystic carcinoma. They are often difficult to diagnose early as their symptomatology is quite non-specific. Investigation is primarily with CT and PET, with diagnostic biopsies obtained through bronchoscopy. Secondary tracheal malignancy is more prevalent than primary tracheal malignancy, with the most common form being invasion from adjacent structures (most commonly thyroid). Surgical management and adjuvant radiotherapy remains the mainstay of management with the resectability of the tumour being the primary determinant of long-term survival. Care must be taken to ensure surgical dissection preserves blood supply and subsequent anastomoses are tension free to minimise complication. Patients will require extensive follow-up, with the best long-term survival seen in patients with resectable ACCs.

Top Five Takeaways

1. 90% of tracheal lesions are malignant, most of which is secondary in nature. The two most common primary tracheal malignancy are SCCs and ACCs whereas secondary tracheal neoplasms occur from direct invasion from surrounding structures such as the thyroid and oesophagus.
2. A high index of suspicion is required to diagnose tracheal malignancy early, owing to its rarity and non-specific constellation of presenting symptoms. Fine-slice contrast enhanced CT with 3D tracheal reconstructions is the imaging modality of choice, with bronchoscopy the gold-standard for biopsy and diagnosis.
3. The management of tracheal cancer is multimodal, typically incorporating surgical resection and adjuvant radiotherapy. During surgical resection, the three governing principles are to resect the tumour with clear margins, maintain the blood supply to the trachea and ensure a tension-free anastomosis. Adjuvant radiation is critical in preventing disease recurrence.
4. Prognosis is more favourable in the ACC histological subtype and are largely dependent whether the tumour has been completely resected.
5. Patients will require close, long-term follow-up with repeated imaging and investigation to exclude recurrence.

References

1. Honings J, van Dijck JAAM, Verhagen AFTM, van der Heijden HFM, Marres HAM. Incidence and treatment of tracheal cancer: a Nationwide study in The Netherlands. Ann Surg Oncol. 2007;14(2):968–76.
2. Grillo HC. Surgery of the trachea and bronchi. Ontario, Canada: BC Decker Inc.; 2004. p. 890.
3. Furlow PW, Mathisen DJ. Surgical anatomy of the trachea. Ann Cardiothorac Surg. 2018;7(2):255–60.
4. Gaissert HA, Grillo HC, Shadmehr MB, Wright CD, Gokhale M, Wain JC, et al. Long-term survival after resection of primary adenoid cystic and squamous cell carcinoma of the trachea and carina. Ann Thorac Surg. 2004;78(6):1889–96. discussion 96-7.

5. Honings J, Gaissert HA, Ruangchira-Urai R, Wain JC, Wright CD, Mathisen DJ, et al. Pathologic characteristics of resected squamous cell carcinoma of the trachea: prognostic factors based on an analysis of 59 cases. Virchows Arch. 2009;455(5):423.
6. Honings J, Gaissert HA, Weinberg AC, Mark EJ, Wright CD, Wain JC, et al. Prognostic value of pathologic characteristics and resection margins in tracheal adenoid cystic carcinoma. Eur J Cardiothorac Surg. 2010;37(6):1438–44.
7. Gaissert HA, Grillo HC, Shadmehr MB, Wright CD, Gokhale M, Wain JC, et al. Uncommon primary tracheal tumors. Ann Thorac Surg. 2006;82(1):268–72; discussion 72–3
8. Gaissert HA, Honings J, Grillo HC, Donahue DM, Wain JC, Wright CD, et al. Segmental laryngotracheal and tracheal resection for invasive thyroid carcinoma. Ann Thorac Surg. 2007;83(6):1952–9.
9. Shin D-H, Mark EJ, Suen HC, Grillo HC. Pathologic staging of papillary carcinoma of the thyroid with airway invasion based on the anatomic manner of extension to the trachea: a clinicopathologic study based on 22 patients who underwent thyroidectomy and airway resection. Hum Pathol. 1993;24(8):866–70.
10. Zeng R, Wang H, Cai X, Guo X, Ping Y, Yang Q. Radiotherapy for primary tracheal carcinoma: experience at a single institution. Technol Cancer Res Treat. 2021;20:15330338211034273.
11. Bhattacharyya N. Contemporary staging and prognosis for primary tracheal malignancies: a population-based analysis. Otolaryngol Head Neck Surg. 2004;131(5):639–42.

Carotid Body Tumours and Paragangliomas

11

Timothy Eviston and Kevin Higgins

11.1 Introduction

Paragangliomas in the head and neck are vascular-associated tumours of neural crest origin and are a type of extra-adrenal neuroendocrine tumour. They are sometimes called glomus tumours and can be classified according to their location and whether they are secretory or not. These are uncommon tumours typically occurring in mid-life (4th–6th decade). The first priority for the clinician seeing a suspected paraganglioma is to rule out primary or metastatic malignancy of head and neck sites including mucosal (oral cavity, oropharynx, nasopharynx, larynx and hypopharynx), skin and salivary gland (submandibular, parotid, minor salivary gland).

As a general approach, three attributes ("SLS") will help diagnose and classify head and neck paragangliomas:

1. Symptoms: this can be local mass effect, nerve deficit or secondary to secretory catecholamines.
2. Location: this will give insight into the nerve of origin and structures at risk if it grows and focus your examination and differential diagnosis.
3. Syndromes: whether the paraganglioma of the neck is just the tip of the iceberg for the patient with regards to other tumours, surveillance, genetic testing and/or distant disease.

Unlike adrenal neuroendocrine tumours which tend to be predominantly secretory, head and neck paragangliomas tend to be predominantly non-secretory. This is due to their parasympathetic origin and so usually present as an asymptomatic finding on cross-sectional imaging. They may also exert mass effect or with a nerve deficit from the nerve of origin or adjacent nerves. Secretory head and neck paragangliomas do also occur and this is still important to test for as this will become one of the considerations in deciding management. Symptoms can include labile hypertension, tachycardia, headache, palpitations and/or tremor.

A small minority of paragangliomas are malignant (approximately 3–5%) or bilateral (5–10%), occurring predominantly in familial cancer syndromes or with genetic mutations (e.g., *SDH* mutations). Malignancy is defined by the hallmark presence of regional lymph node metastases. Histologically, benign and malignant paragangliomas are otherwise indistinct with the same features of chief cells surrounded by sustantecular. This means a pathologist is unable to determine malignancy based on a biopsy, and distant sites of disease could be representative of

T. Eviston (✉)
Department of Surgery, Mater Private Hospital, Brisbane, Australia
e-mail: Tim.Eviston@mater.org.au

K. Higgins
University of Toronto, Toronto, ON, Canada
e-mail: kevin.higgins@sunnybrook.ca

B. Ashford (ed.), *Head and Neck Surgery for General Surgeons*,
https://doi.org/10.1007/978-981-19-7900-2_11

multifocality, unless the sine qua non of regional metastatic disease is evident. When they occur, typical sites of metastases may also include haematogenous spread to lung and liver like other neuroendocrine tumours.

The spectrum of head and neck paragangliomas includes carotid body tumours (neural crest cells of the carotid body), glomus vagale (vagus nerve) and glomus jugulare (tumour located at the skull base). These tumours can be confused with schwannomas which are neurogenic tumours arising from Schwann cells and which tend to occur on the vagus nerve or along the sympathetic chain, typically the superior or middle ganglia. Despite their distinct clinical nature, both paragangliomas and neurogenic tumours present in a similar clinical picture: The patient is usually in their 4th–sixth decade with a soft tissue density lesion found on cross sectional imaging or as a slowly enlarging mass felt in the neck. More rarely, these tumours may present with cranial nerve deficits (e.g., X, XI, XII). These tumours can present challenges from a management perspective due to their relationship to important clinical structures and the need to balance the risk of removal against the risk of progression and/or malignant transformation. In the case of paragangliomas, they can also have pulsatile tinnitus, symptoms relatable to catecholamine secretion (up to 5%), metastatic disease or as part of a familial cancer syndrome (e.g., SDH, MEN2B, tuberous sclerosis, NF1, VHL). The most common genetic association is with SDH mutations and broadly anyone with a paraganglioma diagnosis should consider genetic testing [1].

11.2 Key Elements of History

The goal of the work up of these patients is to:

1. Exclude the mass being metastatic malignancy from a mucosal, skin or salivary primary.
2. Established functional deficit (e.g., Vocal cord palsy or impaired swallowing from vagal nerve dysfunction, Horner's syndrome as a result of carotid encasement for sympathetic chain origin, any functional or secretory symptoms).
3. Establish rate of growth to educate treatment decisions.
4. Establish whether solitary or multiple and could it be part of a broader familial or genetic cancer syndrome.

With these tumours, particular history relating to other cancers and a family history of cancers is particularly important due to their common associations with genetic mutations (*SDH*) or syndromes (MEN2, NF1, Tuberous sclerosis, Von Hippel Lindau).

11.3 Clinical Examination Pearls

Typical presentation of paragangliomas include:

1. A firm neck mass in level II (below the angle of the mandible, under the SCM, behind the submandibular gland).
2. A parapharyngeal extension of the mass: look for signs of palate deviation, and an oropharyngeal bulge and retromandibular fullness.
3. Cranial nerve or sympathetic nerve deficits: examine for voice and swallow function (X), shoulder shrug against resistance and trapezius wasting (XI), tongue wasting and movement (XII), and signs of Horner's syndrome (ipsilateral ptosis, anhidrosis (decreased sweating), meiosis (pupillary constriction)).

The first part of assessing a patient with a neck mass includes thorough clinical history and examination with the goal of ensuring the mass does not represent metastatic disease from a mucosal, skin or salivary site. Paragangliomas are firm soft tissue density masses which on clinical examination cannot be easily distinguished from metastatic nodal disease, particularly in the case of carotid body tumours. Careful observation and documentation of cranial nerve function is critical as this will inform management with particular attention paid to the lower cranial nerves (X, XI, XII). The age of the patient may influence the decision tree with a bias towards surgery for earlier tumours in younger patients with a greater chance of lifetime progression.

General assessment of the patient including blood pressure, heart rate may give insight into whether the mass is secretory and stigmata of familial cancer syndromes, e.g., Thyroidectomy scar or thyroid masses for MENII, subungal fibromas for tuberous sclerosis, neurofibromas for NF1, abdominal examination for concomitant adrenal or liver masses should be examined for.

The location of the tumour may give good insight into its likely nerve of origin and a broader assessment of the patient may give you an understanding of the likelihood of this being a localized tumour or part of a broader issue. Carotid body tumours are often pulsatile and classically exhibit Fontaine's sign as they are often mobile laterally in the horizontal plane but not vertically.

11.4 Investigations and Their Limitations

As a starting point, all patients with a suspected paraganglioma should have their blood pressure and heart rate assessed and documented, followed by a flexible nasal endoscopy, cross-sectional imaging (either MRI with gadolinium or contrast enhanced CT)) and biochemical assays for plasma and 24 h urinary catecholamines. For carotid body tumours, the diagnosis is made on imaging findings and a biopsy should not be performed if the imaging findings are wholly consistent. This is different for atypical non-carotid body glomus tumours or schwannomas where there may be a suspicion for other potentially sinister pathology, however, be prepared for the biopsy to be non-diagnostic if it is a glomus tumour or schwannoma. The relevant immunohistochemical staining of paraganglioma is presented in Fig. 11.1.

Once a diagnosis of a paraganglioma is established, cross-sectional imaging of the adrenal glands should be performed to look for concomitant adrenal tumours along with genetic testing (*SDH* mutations, NF1, *RET*, and VHL at a minimum). If a genetic mutation is established, testing of first degree relatives (and potentially second degree relatives in some mutations) should then occur under the guidance of a genetic counsellor. Other SDH-associated tumours to be mindful of include GIST, renal cell carcinomas and pituitary adenomas.

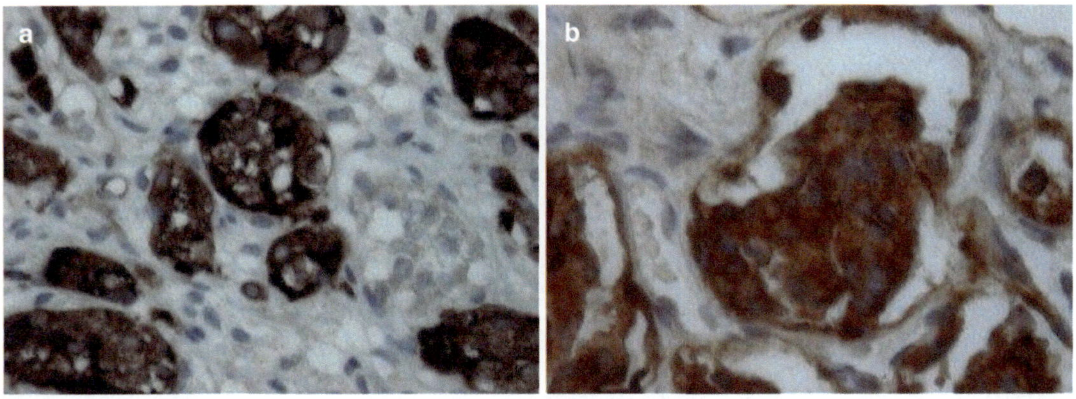

Fig. 11.1 Immunohistochemistry of a cervical paraganglioma staining with chromogranin (**panel a**) and synaptophysin (**panel b**). The cellular architecture is arranged with chief cells surrounded by sustentacular cells in collagen stroma. Chief cells act as chemoreceptors for oxygen (PaO_2), carbon dioxide ($PaCO_2$) and pH. They contain neurotransmitter granules and transmit afferent signal via Hering's nerve (a branch of the glossopharyngeal nerve (IX))

11.5 Imaging

Cross-sectional imaging is critical in the diagnosis of paragangliomas and examining their relationship to the great vessels (Fig. 11.2). Vagal lesions separate the IJV and common carotid and often pushed the carotid artery anteromedially. Sympathetic chain lesions push the carotid sheath anterolaterally within the parapharyngeal space. Carotid body tumours lie at the carotid bifurcation and have the classic "salt and pepper" pattern on post gadolinium MRI and splay the internal and external carotid vessels (Lyre sign). Schwannomas have a classic hypointense signal on T1 and hyperintense signal on T2 and have a fusiform or tapered appearance on sagittal and coronal imaging. In determining the location and extent, interrogation in at least two planes (coronal and axial) is critical for forming a diagnosis and guiding treatment decisions. It is also of note

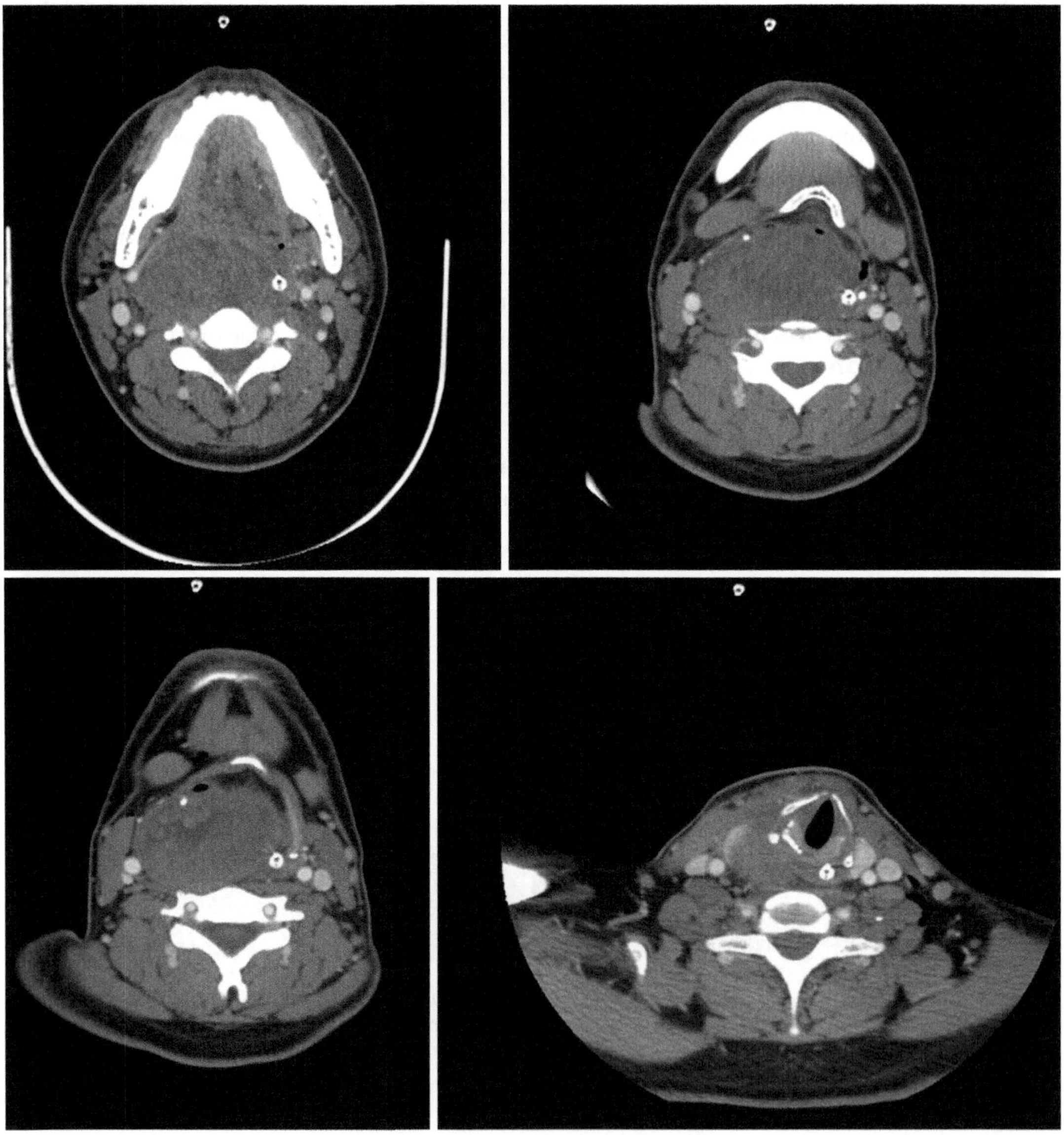

Fig. 11.2 A large sympathetic chain schwannoma presenting as a submucosal mass centred in the oropharyngeal/hypopharangeal region. Symptoms at presentation included sleep apnoea, voice change ("hot potato" voice) and weight loss

that schwannomas may have a cystic appearance and be confused for other cystic lesions such as branchial cleft cysts; however, it is rare for them to be completely cystic. Positron emission tomography (PET) or MIBG is the best test for assessing for malignant paragangliomas where metastatic disease and/or other paragangliomas will be evident based on their metabolic activity.

Carotid body tumour	Vagal tumour	Sympathetic chain tumour
Internal and external carotid splayed (lyre sign). Mass located at carotid bifurcation.	Carotid and internal jugular vein separated by lesion with carotid pushed anteromedially	Carotid vessels displaced anterolaterally

11.5.1 CT

On CT, paragangliomas are soft tissue density, they will fill with contrast due to their vascularity and they are usually well demarcated from surrounding tissue (Fig. 11.2). Their anatomical location and the relationship to the great vessels as described above will give insight into the nerve of origin.

The extent of arterial encasement on CT will assist in determining their grading (Fig. 11.3: Shamblin 1 < 180 ° carotid encasement; Shamblin 2180–270 ° carotid encasement; Shamblin 3 > 270 ° of internal carotid encasement). Glomus vagale and vagal schwannoma tumours will separate the jugular vein and carotid vessels with the arteries displaced anteromedially. Sympathetic chain schwannoma will displace the carotid sheath anterolaterally.

11.5.2 MRI

Paragangliomas have a classical feature of 'salt and pepper' appearance on T1 weighted MRI with gadolinium enhancement where high signal foci represent blood from extravasation and the low signal represent flow voids from tumour vessels. It is important to review the superior extent of the tumour as vagal tumours can commonly extend into the jugular foramen and occasionally intracranially. Although schwannomas may be difficult to distinguish from paragangliomas, findings of hypointense signal on T1 and hyperintense signal with T2 sequencing is helpful in making the distinction. Schwannomas are usually homogenously enhancing, fusiform or tapered in coronal or sagittal plane and may show extension to neural foramina. They will also occasionally demonstrate cystic change. If the mass extends to the jugular foramen, schwannomas will remodel/expand the foramen while paragangliomas will demonstrate permeative erosion of the foramen.

11.5.3 Interventional Radiology

As carotid body tumours are intensely vascular and sacrifice of the great vessels may be required for resection (particularly in Shamblin II or III tumours), selective angiography (Fig. 11.4) and balloon occlusion testing have an important role in determining potential operability. Preoperative super-selective embolization (approx. 70% reduction in vascularity) has an adjunctive role but cannot be definitive due to the risks of cranial nerve toxicity/ischaemia. Stroke, intimal dissection and bleeding are also potential complications. Microparticles and/or bleomycin are commonly used; however, there is a dose constraint with bleomycin due to lung and bladder toxicity.

11.6 Surgical Approaches

Some special issues need to be considered with regard to head and neck paragangliomas due to their delicate location and the potential for permanent disabling cranial nerve injury due to surgical misadventure or required nerve resection in the course of tumour extirpation. Broadly, the decision to operate on paragangliomas of the head and neck should be well justified and ideally involve multidisciplinary input and a long-term view of what is likely to result in the best outcome for the patient. The anatomic location of the tumour and its relationship to the great ves-

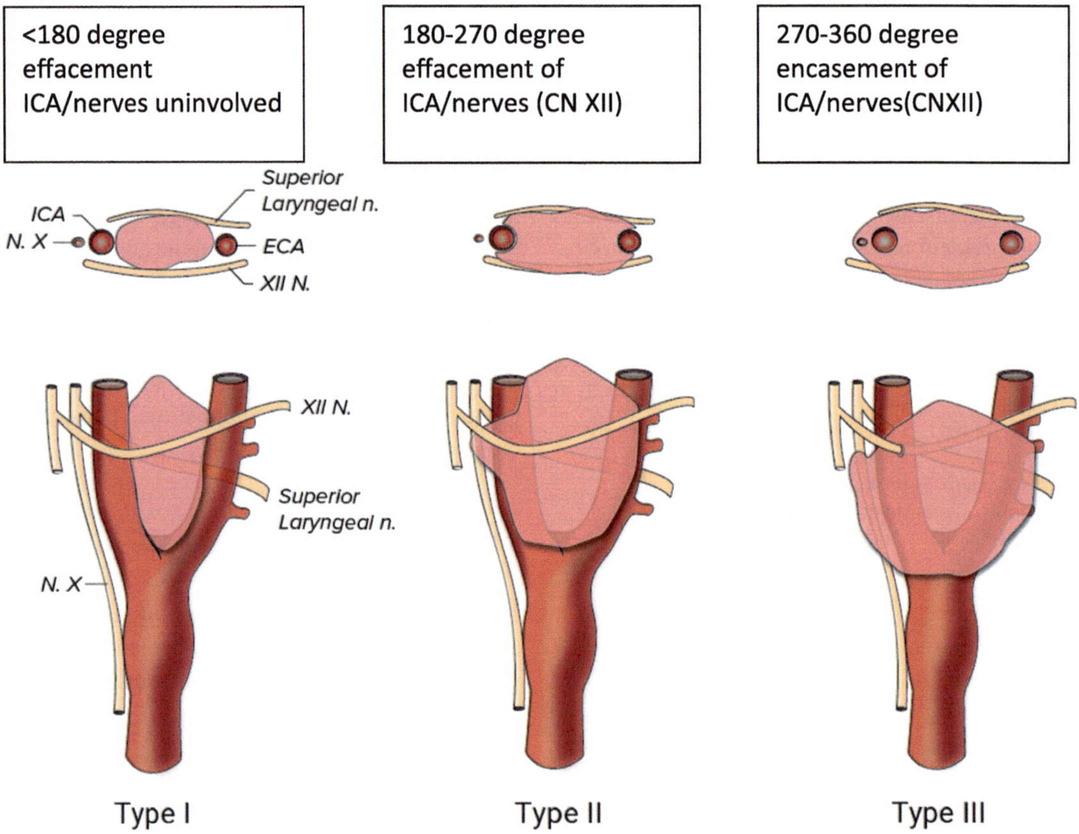

Fig. 11.3 The Shamblin classification of carotid body tumours. Type I tumours are localized and resectable. Type II includes tumours adherent or partially surrounding vessels. Type III tumours intimately surround or encase the vessels. Reproduced from Hallett et al. [2]. *ICA* internal carotid artery, *ECA* external carotid artery, *N* nerve, *sup. laryn. n.* superior laryngeal nerve. Take away: Even with a Shamblin 1, the external carotid artery could be completely encased and require sacrifice for extirpation. *(Artwork courtesy of Alex Eviston Design)*

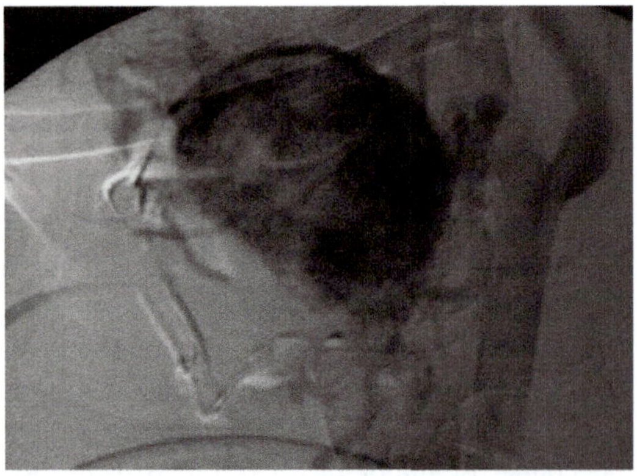

Fig. 11.4 Selective angiography demonstrating intense vascular "blush" of a glomus laryngeal tumour

sels and skull base will inform the likely nerve of origin and what nerve deficit(s) are likely from observation. Observation, radiation and in some cases, medical management for symptomatic secretory paraganglionic tumour may be used in these tumours to preserve cranial nerve function and in patients with advanced age and/or poor performance status.

Typical scenarios where surgery should be considered include younger patients (<55 years of age), with malignant tumours or functional secretory tumours.

11.6.1 Carotid Body Tumours

The surgery to resect a carotid body tumour is one of anatomical dissection and critical structure preservation. Wide exposure and proximal and distal control of vessels are essential (Fig. 11.5). Close collaboration with anaesthesia, interventional radiology and vascular surgery colleagues is advised should shunting or resection/replacement be required as part of the procedure.

Preoperatively a concomitant phaeochromocytoma should be excluded by both biochemical catecholamine measurement and by abdominal imaging (given the pheochromocytoma/paraganglioma familial syndrome is the most common genetic syndrome). If the tumour is secretory, an endocrine consultation for blood pressure/alpha antagonist control will be undertaken to avoid any malignant hypertensive crisis. Preoperative consultation by the anaesthetic team is also essential. The extent of the tumour is assessed and graded according to its Shamblin classification and vascular surgery is involved as needed. As these tumours are highly vascular, preoperative embolization will be considered to reduce the intraoperative vascular burden. This intervention has to be carefully timed ideally with within 24 h of embolization to avoid the risk of collateralization and fibrosis that can affect ease of dissection, especially cranial nerve dissection. Risks of the embolization procedure include the risk relating to groin hematoma, pseudoaneurysm formation, dissection, stroke, cranial neuropathy, facial pain, skin necrosis, etc. This should generally be considered for the larger tumours where one may also be considering balloon test occlusion at the same time. Careful assessment of the imaging in the coronal plane will give insight into the cephalad extent and the access required to achieve superior control of the vessels. The patient will be placed supine position with a head ring and a shoulder role and the head will be rotated to the contralateral side. If the tumour extends under the mandible, a nasal intubation is advised to allow the dentition to occlude giving an extra couple of centimetres of parapharyngeal

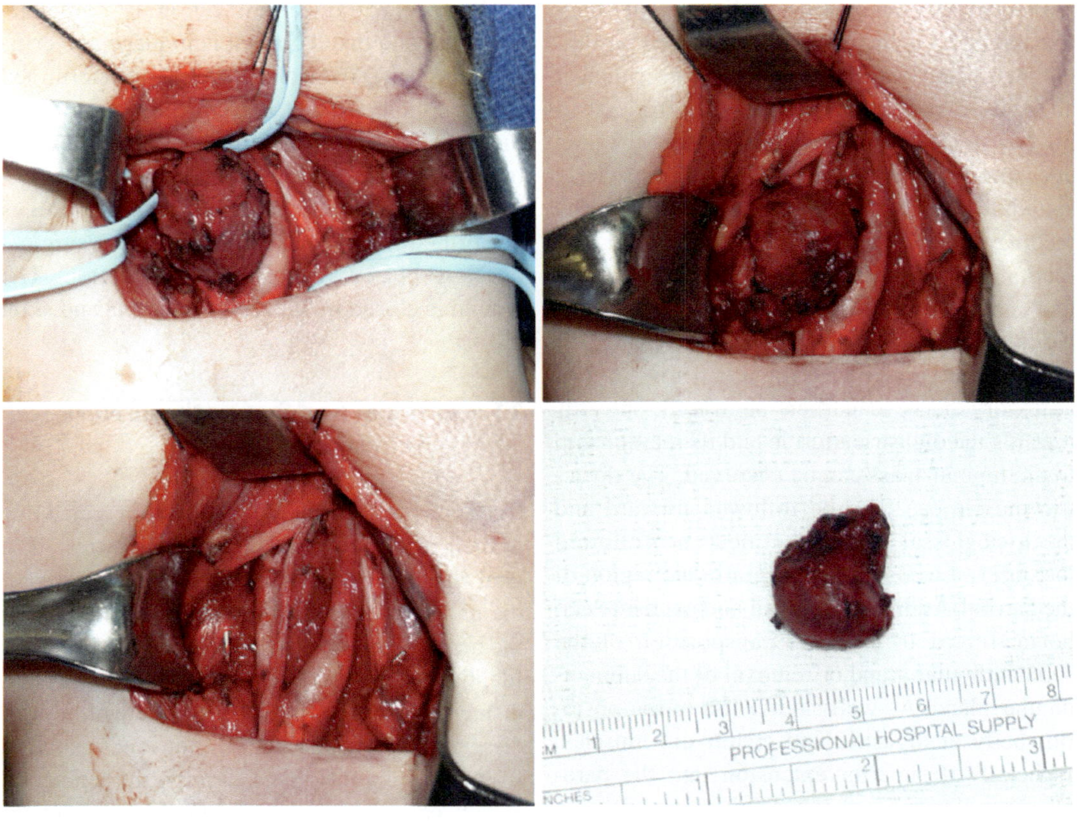

Fig. 11.5 Intraoperative images from a carotid body tumour resection. Courtesy: A/Prof Kevin Higgins, Sunnybrook Health Sciences Centre, Toronto ON

access from below. Additional manoeuvres can include use of the temporal bone Fisch retractor to sublux the jaw anteriorly, the use of a premoulded orthognathic appliance to achieve temporary type III occlusion, or even by employing a vertical subsigmoid mandibular osteotomy with anterior and superior rotation of the posterior fragment.

A cervical crease incision will be placed in the mid neck with elevation subplatysmal flaps to allow full exposure. Care will be taken not to injure the marginal mandibular nerve when raising the subplatysmal flaps, this lies beneath a layer of fascia over the submandibular gland 1-2 cm below the mandible. The fascia of the anterior border of the SCM is incised and the SCM is retracted posteriorly to expose the jugular vein. The carotid artery will sit just anterior and deep to the jugular vein in the carotid sheath. The next step of the operation is to identify and preserve critical structures, in particular the accessory nerve, the hypoglossal nerve and the vagus nerve including the important superior laryngeal branches penetrating the thyrohyoid membrane. Careful haemostasis is critical at all times to ensure adequate vision for identifying key structures, with judicious use of the jeweller microbipolar forceps which are especially suited to deal with the numerous adventitial feeding vessels. Superiorly, in the field of dissection, the accessory nerve (XI) will be identified entering the SCM under a perforator vascular leash typically entering the SCM just anterior and sometimes slightly below it. The accessory nerve can then be traced upwards towards the digastric muscle and its relationship to the tumour mass can be observed. The digastric muscle can then be followed forward and the hypoglossal nerve identified and followed just inferior to its lower margin in the region of the carotid. Additional control and exposure can be facilitated by anterior transposition of the submandibular gland or removal of the submandibular gland. As well as division of the posterior belly of digastric and stylohyoid muscles, especially if superior extension into the parapharyngeal space is noted. The authors prefer to place vessel loop around the hypoglossal nerve anterior to the tumour mass to assist in its rapid reidentification and retraction/dissection. Neurolysis of the hypoglossal nerve will allow it to be dissected free of the tumour mass. The lymphatic/fatty tissue overlying the vessels in level 2 between the SCM, digastric and submandibular gland will usually be removed to allow clear visualization of the vascular structures. The digastric muscle will usually need to be divided over a haemostat to allow access to the carotid bifurcation and to get above the tumour. The jugular vein will need to be retracted and the facial vein divided to expose the length of the carotid. Vessel loops will be placed around the common carotid, the internal carotid, the external carotid and the internal carotid taking care to ensure the vagus nerve which lies at the posterior border of the carotid is not included in the dissection and vessel loop. Passing the vessel loops around twice loosely will allow the vessels to be rapidly controlled if there is any vascular injury during the course of resection. Once the anatomical dissection is complete, proximal and distal control is in place and critical nerves and the extent of tumour determined the tumour is dissected from the adventitia of the carotid vessels ensuring careful haemostasis of feeding vessels during the course of dissection. Following tumour removal, a Valsalva is performed to assess haemostasis and a surgical drain is placed to the site of resection. The wound is closed in 2 layers—platysma and skin.

11.6.2 Vagal and Sympathetic Nerve Schwannomas

Occasionally these tumours may be resected due to their mass effect and cosmetic deformity. The goal of the procedure in this case is to preserve the underlying nerve if possible while debulking the benign tumour growth surrounding the nerve. Identification of the nerve of origin proximal and distal to the tumour is a useful guide with careful dissection along the nerve allowing separation from the tumour mass. Rarely the epineural sheath can be split longitudinally to allow for tumour enucleation and preservation of at least some axonal fibres to maintain at least bulk and tone beyond the motor endplate.

11.7 Non-surgical Management

For many patients, observation is a justifiable treatment approach. The work by James Netterville and colleagues [3] was important in this respect. In a cohort of 43 patients with 47 tumours (28 carotid body tumours; 19 vagal tumours) followed for a median of 5 years (1–17 years), 42% (19 tumours) remained stable in size over the monitoring period and 20% (9 tumours) regressed in size. Of the 38% (19 tumours) which increased in size during the observation period, the average rate of growth was 0.2 cm/year. Given this exceptionally slow rate of growth for these tumours and the high likelihood of severe morbidity with difficult to excise tumours or those involving critical cranial nerves, observation is highly valid in many circumstances.

For those patients where observation is not suitable, single modality treatment with radiation (external beam or stereotactic) has an important role where operative risks are high due to patient factors or where the nerve of origin is critical for quality of life. As these tumours are rare, there is a paucity of high-level long-term data; however, retrospective series from large centres does provide important insight. In a seminal work by Rich et al. [4], 84 patients over a 22 year period treated with single modality radiation demonstrated a 10-year tumour control rate of 89% based on radiographic stability. The cohort comprised predominantly of glomus jugulare (61.9%), carotid body (16.7%) and glomus vagale (14.3%) tumours treated with between 26–51 Gy (mean 36.8) over 13–25 fractions (mean 16).

Top Five Takeaways

1. Getting the diagnosis correct and not missing an occult malignancy is the first critical step.
2. Paragangliomas need to be assessed in the context of symptoms, location and whether they are secretory, as well as age of the patient performance status and the timeframe for symptom evolution.
3. Broader thought as to whether consideration should be given to they are part of a broader genetic or familial syndrome and testing for SDH allele mutation undertaken.
4. Surgery is not necessary for all paragangliomas and carries significant risk of permanent disability, especially for Shamblin 3 tumours and glomus jugulare with lower cranial nerve palsy and glomus vagale with high vagal palsy. When surgery is required, it is best addressed in expert centres. For many patients, observation or radiation and/or medical therapy will be sufficient and offer the best functional outcome in the long term.
5. The anatomic relationship of the great vessels to the mass on CT will give insight into the likely pathology, carotid body tumours splay the ICA and ECA (lyre sign), vagal schwannomas and glomus vagale tumours push the ICA and ECA anteromedially and the separate them from the jugular vein. Sympathetic chain schwannomas push all the vessels forwards and anterolaterally.

References

1. Muth A, Crona J, Gimm O, Elmgren A, Filipsson K, Stenmark Askmalm M, Sandstedt J, Tengvar M, Tham E. Genetic testing and surveillance guidelines in hereditary pheochromocytoma and paraganglioma. J Intern Med. 2019;285(2):187–204. https://doi.org/10.1111/joim.12869. Epub 2019 Jan 15
2. Hallett JW Jr, Nora JD, Hollier LH, Cherry KJ Jr, Pairolero PC. Trends in neurovascular complications of surgical management for carotid body and cervical paragangliomas: a fifty-year experience with 153 tumors. J Vasc Surg. 1988;7:284–91.
3. Langerman A, Athavale SM, Rangarajan SV, Sinard RJ, Netterville JL. Natural history of cervical paragangliomas: outcomes of observation of 43 patients. Arch Otolaryngol Head Neck Surg. 2012;138(4):341–5. https://doi.org/10.1001/archoto.2012.37.
4. Rich JT, Kristen OJ, Franklin JH, Goldstein DP, Yu E, Bartlett E, Cummings BJ, Gullane PJ n.d.. Radiotherapy as single-modality treatment for head and neck paragangliomas: twenty-two year results from a single center Presented July 23, 2012 at the 8th international conference on head and neck cancer, Toronto Canada.

12 Mucosal Malignancy: Management of the Oral Cavity and Facial Skeleton

Szymon Mikulski and N. Gopalakrishna Iyer

12.1 Oral Cavity Anatomy and Function

The relatively small yet complex oral cavity plays an integral role in various sophisticated processes vital to the patient's quality of life. Its normal functioning relies on the three-dimensional anatomical juxtaposition and functional interplay of rigid and soft tissues, which are subject to disruption by pathology and disease. In endeavoring to address oral mucosal malignancy, the surgeon must appreciate the complex anatomy and function of the oral cavity, so as to carefully consider the potential morbidity resulting from surgical treatment, especially major oncologic resection, as well as the possible avenues for structural reconstruction and functional restoration.

Anatomically, the oral cavity begins anteriorly at the mucocutaneous junction between the skin of the face and the vermillion border of the upper and lower lip. Posteriorly, it is separated from the oropharynx by the junction between the hard and soft palate superiorly, anterior tonsillar pillars (or palatoglossal arches) laterally, and the chevron of circumvallate papillae inferiorly, which divide the tongue into anterior two-thirds (oral portion) and posterior one-third (pharyngeal portion). See Fig. 12.1.

The anterior external opening of the oral cavity is the oral fissure and the posterior communication with the pharynx is the oropharyngeal isthmus. The superior and inferior dental arches divide the oral cavity into the anterior oral vestibule, and the oral cavity proper, which is situated behind the teeth. The oral cavity is divided from the adjacent nasal cavity by the hard and soft palate.

With the teeth in occlusion, the oral cavity proper is mostly filled by the tongue, which rests against the posterior aspect of the incisors and up against the palate. The tip and anterior two-thirds of the oral tongue are freely movable, while the immobile posterior one-third of the tongue lies in the oropharynx.

The bony framework of the oral cavity is contributed primarily by the paired immobile maxillae and the unpaired mobile mandible (with minor contributions from the palatine, temporal, sphenoid, and hyoid bones).

Functionally, the oral cavity constitutes the uppermost part of the digestive tract and contributes to the vocal tract, as well as to the upper respiratory tract by providing an alternate breathing pathway in case of increased respiratory demand or nasal blockage.

S. Mikulski (✉) · N. G. Iyer
Department of Head and Neck Surgery, Singapore General Hospital and National Cancer Centre Singapore, Duke-NUS Medical School, Singapore, Singapore
e-mail: szymon.mikulski@singhealth.com.sg; gopaliyer@singhealth.com.sg

B. Ashford (ed.), *Head and Neck Surgery for General Surgeons*,
https://doi.org/10.1007/978-981-19-7900-2_12

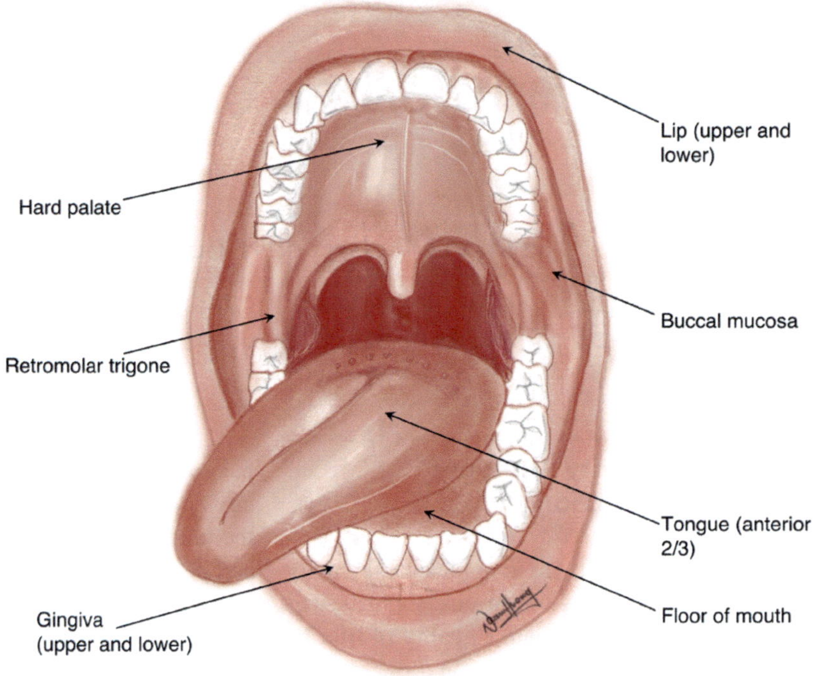

Fig. 12.1 Anatomy and subsites of the oral cavity

The oral cavity is the site of food and liquid ingestion, perception of taste, mastication, and the oral phase of deglutition (swallowing). Chemical digestion also begins in the oral cavity, with the enzyme salivary amylase excreted into the oral cavity in saliva, via ducts from nearby major salivary glands and directly from minor salivary glands embedded throughout the oropharyngeal submucosa.

Speech articulation is mediated by varying the size and shape of the oral cavity through adjusting the relative position of the lips, tongue, teeth, and palate.

Finally, as a gateway to the aerodigestive tract, the oral cavity mucosa forms an immune barrier, which defends the internal systems from continuous exposure to external environment and foreign material.

The various physiologic, metabolic, and immune functions of the oral cavity are mediated by the large and diverse microbial community, which colonizes its surfaces. The rich oral microbiome is key to the maintenance of oral homeostasis and thus integral to oral health and disease processes.

The entire oral cavity is lined by oral mucosa covered in stratified squamous epithelium with varied degrees of keratinization depending on the specific location, function, and mechanical requirements. The immobile tightly bound masticatory mucosa lining surfaces exposed to masticatory loads is keratinized and covers the hard palate, gingiva, and alveolar ridges. In contrast, the mobile mucosa overlying the lips, vestibular sulcus, buccal surfaces, retromolar trigone, and ventral tongue is non-keratinized. Finally, the dorsum of the tongue is lined by specialized keratinized gustatory mucosa, which contains taste receptors. Like the rest of the upper aerodigestive tract epithelium, the oral submucosa is also host to countless minor salivary glands.

12.2 Epidemiology

The overwhelming majority (90%) of oral cavity malignancies are squamous cell carcinomas arising from the oral mucosa, with the remaining 10% originating from minor salivary glands, bone, melanocytes, as well as from lymphoid, bone, dental, connective, or neurovascular tissue, or as distant metastasis [1].

Upward of 370,000 people were diagnosed with squamous cell carcinoma of the lip and oral cavity and almost 180,000 died from it globally in 2020 (oropharynx excluded), rendering lip and oral cavity cancer the 16th most common worldwide in terms of incidence, prevalence, and mortality alike. However, the geographic distribution of lip and oral cancer is not uniform, with South-Central and South-East Asia being overrepresented, and the former accounting for 45% of all cases globally. While lip and oral carcinoma represented merely 2% of all new cancer diagnoses worldwide in 2020, it was the second most-commonly diagnosed malignancy in India, Pakistan, Sri Lanka, and Papua New Guinea. In India, lip and oral cancer was the leading cause of cancer-related mortality among males and the sixth among females, together accounting for 75,000 deaths. Moreover, the burden from lip and oral cancer is projected to rise, the increase disproportionately affecting countries with lower human development index (HDI), where the annual incidence and mortality are expected to double by the year 2040. Of the subsites of the oral cavity, tongue is the most common site of cancer in populations among whom tobacco or betel nut chewing is not endemic. In the latter, buccal carcinoma predominates [2].

The highest rates of oral cancer are seen in older males (in their sixth or seventh decade of life), who are affected twice as frequently as females. However, global epidemiological data suggests a relative increase in the incidence of oral cancer among younger patients and among women [3].

12.3 Risk Factors

Although the etiology of all malignancies is multifactorial and mirrors ethnic and genetic variability, tobacco consumption has been demonstrated to be the major modifiable risk factor for development of oral cancer, with a combination of heavy smoking and heavy alcohol drinking conveying a multiplicative deleterious effect. The carcinogenic effect on the oral mucosa is conferred by both smoked and smokeless (i.e. chewed) tobacco, as well as by prolonged exposure to secondary smoke. However, the disproportionately high incidence of oral cancer in certain geographic regions is likely attributable to chewing of betel (Areca catechu) nut, which is widely practiced among some populations of South, South-East Asia, and the Pacific. Although betel nut chewing is an independent factor predisposing to the development of oral mucosal malignancy, the effect is synergistic with those of tobacco and alcohol consumption. There is insufficient evidence to link poor oral hygiene, sharp teeth, badly fitting dentures, or regular use of mouthwash to oral carcinogenesis. However, using alcohol-containing mouthwash more than once daily or for more than 35 years has been associated with an increased oral cancer risk. In contrast to oropharyngeal cancer, human papilloma virus (HPV) infection is not an established cause of oral cancer. Finally, other risk factors common to head and neck malignancies include prior exposure to ionizing radiation and immunosuppression.

12.4 Key Elements of Presentation and History

Patients with oral cancer will typically present following a referral to a head and neck surgeon from a general practitioner or dentist, after a suspicious lesion had been detected incidentally or in response to the patient's symptoms. The following complaints should alert the clinician to a likelihood of an underlying oral malignancy: mouth or tongue ulceration or sore persisting beyond 3 weeks in duration; mouth, tongue, or jaw lump or swelling; bleeding; loose teeth; uncomfortable or poorly fitting dentures; pain on eating or swallowing; difficulty with swallowing or with speech articulation. Occasionally, patients may present with referred otalgia (earache of non-otologic etiology), which may even be the first symptom of head and neck carcinoma. Finally, patients may seek specialist medical attention for neck lumps suggestive of cervical lymphadenopathy or for constitutional symptoms indicative of advanced metastatic disease.

A thorough history must be elicited, and the details of the patient's symptoms, including their onset, duration, and progression clearly documented. Note should be made of any of the above attendant risk factors, and the use of any carcinogenic substances should be quantified. The patient's past medical history should be obtained, with significant comorbidities, which may increase the risk of surgical intervention or general anesthesia identified and potentially optimized. Medication history including drug allergies should be recorded and antiplatelet agents or anticoagulants may need to be suspended in anticipation of tissue biopsy. The patient's premorbid and current functional status (e.g. ECOG) should be documented, and an effort should be made to obtain ample social history, elements of which will prove pertinent in preparation for major surgical resection and/or adjuvant treatment, as well as a potentially prolonged recovery and rehabilitation. It is paramount that the surgeon gathers the history personally, so as to be neither biased nor limited by the information contained within the referral letter.

12.4.1 Allied Health

Once the diagnosis of oral cancer is strongly suspected or confirmed, assistance of allied health professionals should be sought in order to establish a functional baseline, and optimally prepare the patient for the upcoming treatment. Ideally, the allied health team should have a special interest in and be familiar with the principles and challenges of head and neck oncology. In our institution, each patient is routinely referred to a dietitian, physiotherapist, speech therapist, medical social worker, and psychologist, all of whom specialize in the care of cancer patients, and attend to them at a dedicated one-stop allied-health clinic as soon as an individualized treatment plan is laid out. Doing so at the outset of the patient's journey, and especially prior to any ablative surgery is important in helping to align the patient's expectations and enables continuity of care in the post-operative phase.

Special consideration should be given to nutritional assessment and perioperative supplementation, which occasionally may necessitate the insertion of a feeding tube. A nasogastric catheter is adequate if nutritional supplementation is expected to be short term, whereas a gastrostomy should be considered if the patient's swallowing is expected to remain significantly compromised following treatment.

12.5 Clinical Examination Pearls

A proper physical examination should preferably be conducted in a dental chair and, if available, a head lamp should be used to ensure optimal lighting. The patient is instructed to remove any dental prosthesis (dentures) and the oral cavity is inspected completely by dividing it into seven following anatomical subsites: lips, gingiva (vestibular and lingual aspects), bilateral buccal surfaces, bilateral retromolar trigones, the floor of mouth, the tongue, and the hard palate (Fig. 12.1). The mucosa of each subsite is then carefully visualized with the aid of a tongue depressor and cheek retractors. The patient should be instructed to protrude his tongue, point it upward, and to either side, to enable full exposure of its dorsal, ventral and both lateral surfaces. The tongue may be grasped with a gauze and pulled anteriorly to examine its posterior portion. Special care must also be taken to visualize the anterior hard palate, as it can be easily overlooked unless the surgeon bends down to direct his gaze upward behind the patient's incisors. Inspection is followed by careful palpation of all subsites with a gloved finger, and bimanual examination of the cheeks and the floor of mouth. The soft palate including the uvula, tonsillar pillars, and fossae, as well as the posterior tongue and posterior pharyngeal wall, although parts of the oropharynx rather than the oral cavity, should be examined for completeness. Finally, the neck is systematically palpated for cervical lymphadenopathy across the six nodal levels.

The surgeon must scrutinize the oral mucosa, deliberately looking out for features of malignancy or premalignant change. Oral squamous cell carcinoma (SCC) may present as an ulcer, induration or mass, whereas common potentially precancerous lesions include erythroplakia (fiery-red sharply demarcated patches), leukoplakia (white patches that unlike thrush from *Candida albicans* cannot be wiped away), lichenification (reticular pattern of white lines, papules or patches), and oral submucous fibrosis. The latter is a progressive condition affecting all of oral submucosa occurring exclusively in individuals who chew betel (areca) nuts. A high index of suspicion must be held, keeping in mind that the presence of one pathology does not exclude another, and several may present in combination (Fig. 12.2). Although SCC may arise from normal-appearing mucosa, most malignancies occur on the background of premalignant change. Finally, besides identification of the aforementioned suspicious lesions, the clinician should be able to recognize normal mucosal variants including physiologic pigmentation frequently encountered on the oral mucosa of darker-skinned individuals, or the staining/tattooing of mucosa from dental amalgam.

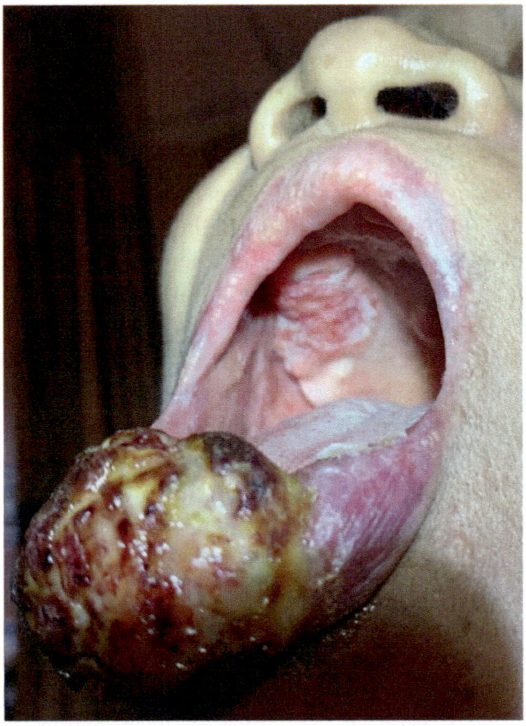

Fig. 12.2 Synchronous lip and maxillary alveolar SCC

The purpose of the clinical examination is to identify and characterize any suspicious findings, and to begin surgical planning. Once a lesion suspicious for malignancy is found, the surgeon should characterize and document the following features: tumor subsite/location, laterality/crossing of midline, size, presence of ulceration and whether it appears exophytic/fungating or infiltrative. Note should be made of any affected/loose dentition, apparent bony or skin involvement, as well as of any functional deficit due to deep tissue invasion, including limitation of the range of motion of the tongue, dysarthria, or trismus, which suggest advanced disease. The clinical examination is completed by performing flexible nasoendoscopy to assess the mucosa of nasopharynx, oropharynx, hypopharynx, and larynx for irregularities, and to ascertain the symmetry and mobility of the vocal cords. Although, in some cases, the location and characteristics of the tumor may be immediately apparent, it is critical that the surgeon does not truncate the clinical examination and that the entirety of the upper aerodigestive mucosa is thoroughly examined for every patient. This is to avoid missing a second malignancy (Fig. 12.2) within the oral cavity or at another subsite, which may occur both synchronously and metachronously secondary to field cancerization of large segments of mucosa affected by exposure to carcinogens. In instances of late presentation with advanced disease, whereby mouth opening is significantly restricted by trismus, or assessment is otherwise limited by pain, an examination under anesthesia (EUA) should be arranged. Likewise, prompt dental evaluation should be arranged for treatment and clearance prior to surgery or radiotherapy, as well as to obtain dental impressions. Finally, if resection followed by reconstruction is anticipated, a reconstructive surgery consultation should be scheduled. All pertinent positive and negative clinical examination findings should be clearly documented, ideally with the aid of digital photographs (Table 12.1).

Table 12.1 Pertinent findings on physical examination: identification of premalignant changes, detailed description of suspicious lesion

Premalignant changes	Notable features of suspicious lesion
Erythroplakia	Location/subsite/laterality/crossing of midline
Fiery-red demarcated patches	Size
Leukoplakia	Induration/ulceration
White patches that cannot be wiped away	Whether exophytic/fungating/infiltrative
Lichenification	Loose dentition
Reticular pattern of lines/papules/patches	Bone/skin involvement
Submucous fibrosis	Tongue range of motion
Submucosal hardening (exclusive to betel nut chewers)	Dysarthria/trismus

12.6 Investigations and their Limitations

12.6.1 Biopsy

At the cornerstone of initial evaluation of suspected oral cavity cancer is the diagnostic tissue biopsy, which must be invariably obtained prior to definitive treatment. Provided that the primary tumor is safely accessible, this can be performed in the clinic after administration of local anesthetic. Conversely, in advanced disease presenting with trismus, biopsy should be performed during EUA. An adequate sample at the periphery of the lesion should be taken, such that adjacent segments of normal and abnormal mucosa are available for assessment of invasion by the pathologist. The biopsy must also be of sufficient depth, such that the tumor depth-of-invasion (DOI, Fig. 12.3) can be measured and the indication for prophylactic neck dissection determined. In patients who are not candidates for definitive surgical resection (due to advanced disease or prohibitive performance status), the pathologist should be instructed to evaluate the biopsy sample for epidermal growth factor receptor (EGFR) as well as programmed death ligand 1 (PDL-1) expression (combined positive score/tumor proportion score) to predict potential benefit from targeted- and immunotherapy.

There is usually no need to perform a biopsy of cervical lymph nodes at initial presentation, because clinically apparent lymphadenopathy warrants a formal surgical neck dissection. A cervical nodal biopsy may be useful however, when the site of primary tumor cannot be determined, when synchronous malignancies are diagnosed (e.g. lung carcinoma) and the origin of the metastatic lymphadenopathy is in question, or when cancer recurrence is suspected. An open biopsy, core biopsy, or fine-needle aspiration cytology (FNAC) may be performed depending on the clinical context. Percutaneous techniques are best deployed under ultrasonographic guidance, and the assistance of the interventional radiologist may be sought to minimize the chance of a false-negative result.

12.6.2 Imaging

The purpose of imaging in evaluation of all newly diagnosed cancer patients is to assess for local invasion, involvement of regional lymph nodes, distant metastasis (i.e. local, regional, and systemic staging), or for the presence of a second aerodigestive tract malignancy. Cross-sectional imaging is preferred, with limited yield from plain radiography and the role of preoperative ultrasonography limited to interrogation of cervical lymph nodes.

A fine-cut computed tomograph (CT) with intravenous contrast should be initially obtained of the neck to evaluate the primary tumor size, extent, and invasion into surrounding structures. Specifically for cancers of the oral cavity, a "puffed cheek" view is advantageous, and oblique cuts may be taken to minimize metallic artifact from dental work. A CT of the chest is added to exclude metastatic disease. Alternatively, especially in patients with advanced disease, multiple palpable cervical lymph nodes or synchronous second primary on physical examination, a whole-body fluorodeoxglucose positron emis-

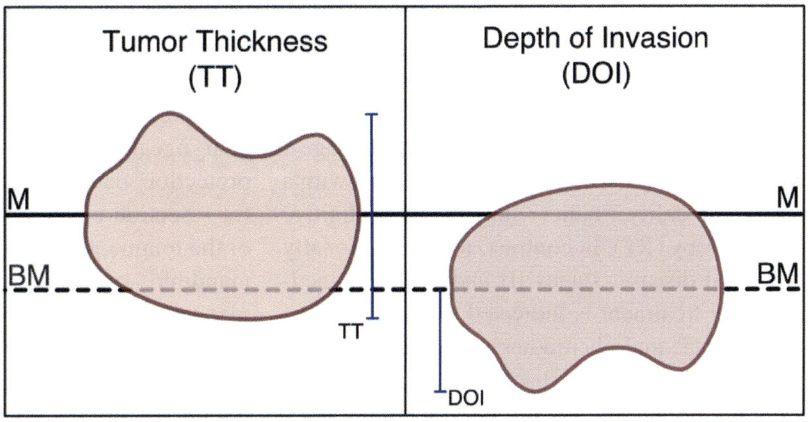

Fig. 12.3 Tumor thickness vs. depth of invasion (DOI); *M* mucosa, *BM* basement membrane

sion tomography (FDG-PET) co-registered with CT (FGD-PET/CT) may be preferred to CT of the thorax alone as means of regional and distant staging. FDG-PET/CT is superior to both CT and MRI in detection of regional nodal metastases, distant metastases, and synchronous second primary malignancies. In doing so, it serves as a replacement for panendoscopy (direct laryngoscopy, nasopharyngoscopy, and esophagoscopy).

Magnetic resonance (MRI) offers superior soft tissue imaging in comparison with CT, with T1- and T2-weighted sequences with fat suppression commonly used. MRI is advantageous for superficial mucosal tumors, tumors of the tongue, and for detection of bone marrow or cartilage invasion, perineural spread, skull base, or intracranial involvement. In contrast, CT remains superior to MRI in detection of bony cortical erosion and of cervical nodal metastases. The quicker CT may also be preferrable to MRI in elderly patients who often find staying supine and still for prolonged image acquisition uncomfortable, or in those who may find the MRI scanner claustrophobic.

A fine-cut CT or MRI should be ordered, and both axial and coronal views routinely reconstructed. Sagittal views may be obtained when indicated. A contrasted CT or MRI angiogram should be specifically requested, when delineation of vascular anatomy is required.

An orthopantomogram (OPG) is a single specialized panoramic radiograph of the maxilla, mandible, and teeth. An OPG is usually performed during initial workup as a means of convenient preliminary assessment of potential bony destruction, mandible height, and of dental anatomy and pathology.

All imaging should be obtained prior to biopsy so as to minimize tissue distortion and inflammation from invasive procedures, which may mimic radiologic neoplastic features and either falsely upstage the disease or mask neoplastic metabolic activity.

If the patient is planned for major bony resection followed by reconstruction, additional dedicated imaging of donor skeleton and vasculature (e.g. CT/MRI angiogram) may be indicated, though this is best arranged following the consultation with and by the reconstructive surgeon.

Finally, in addition to initial evaluation, serial re-assessment with cross-sectional imaging, either CT, MRI, or FDG-PET/CT (or sometimes a combination thereof) is used to monitor treatment response and as surveillance for potential locoregional or distant recurrence. The initial post-treatment scan may be scheduled at 3–4 four months, but the interval and subsequent frequency must be adjusted based on the degree of clinical concern.

12.7 Surgical Management Including Risks

The overwhelming majority of cancers of the oral cavity are squamous cell carcinomas arising from the oral epithelium. Clinical staging is performed based on preoperative imaging in accordance with the latest eighth edition of the Tumor, Node, Metastases (TNM) staging system of the American Joint Committee on Cancer (AJCC) and the Union for International Cancer Control (UICC) updated in 2017 [4]. Generally, stage I and II are considered early, and are treated with a single modality: either surgery or definitive radiotherapy (RT). In contrast, for locoregionally advanced disease (stages III and IV) combined-modality treatment is indicated, with the role of surgery, RT, and chemotherapy decided following multidisciplinary discussion (Table 12.2). Notably, primary surgical resection followed by adjuvant therapy (as opposed to concurrent chemoradiotherapy) remains the mainstay of treatment even in advanced oral cavity cancer wherever feasible [6]. The surgical component of management is discussed below. For comprehensive clinical practice guidelines, the reader may refer to the latest publication from the National Comprehensive Cancer Network [5] or other expert groups.

Other than for very small and superficial lesions, major oral cavity surgery is performed under general anesthesia, with the patient in a supine position. Unless a tracheostomy is performed as the initial step of the surgery, endotracheal intubation should be trans-nasal and the nasotracheal tube oriented north. Once the patient is under anesthesia, a nasogastric feeding tube is placed and secured to the membranous nasal septum with a silk stitch or with a nylon tape looped around the choana (assuming a gastrostomy tube is not already in place). A shoulder roll is usually placed, and the head is draped across the labial philtrum, leaving the mouth exposed. A temporary prophylactic tracheostomy should be considered in patients planned for major oral resection to secure the airway in the post-operative period from obstruction due to tongue or laryngeal swelling and from aspiration due to copious oropharyngeal secretions or hemorrhage. Airway protection via tracheostomy is especially prudent for resection of locoregionally advanced tumors of the tongue, floor of mouth, those involving the mandible or when major reconstruction is planned. In contrast, prophylactic tracheostomy is not usually necessary with straightforward maxillectomy, or with relatively minor soft tissue resections limited to the oral cavity. In our practice, tracheostomy is performed first, after which the patient is re-cleaned and re-draped. Resection then begins with cervical lymphadenectomy (if indicated), followed by primary tumor resection. This sequence allows surgery to progress from a clean to a contaminated surgical field. However, other surgeons prefer the inverse, i.e. resection of the primary tumor followed by neck dissection. This sequence aims to minimize manipulation of the malignant cells and thus theoretically reduces the risk of tumor seeding or spread. In the absence of strong evidence supporting either approach, the decision to order primary resection and cervical lymphadenectomy thus depends on the surgeon's preference.

The main objective of oncologic surgery is complete extirpation of primary tumor with adequate margins of healthy tissue so as to minimize the risk of local recurrence and to optimize prognosis. Proper preoperative assessment and surgical planning are key to avoid incomplete excision, reoperation, and/or post-operative radiotherapy, where it might not be otherwise indicated by stage or other high-risk features. For close or

Table 12.2 Simplified overview of treatment of oral cavity cancer (adapted from NCCN Clinical Practice Guidelines in Oncology [5] (RT – radiotherapy; systemic therapy may consist of cytotoxic chemo-, targeted-, and immunotherapy)

Disease	Modality	Surgical		Non-surgical
Early (T1–2, N0)	Single	Surgery (preferred) Primary ± neck	or	Definitive RT
Advanced (T3–4 or N+)	Multi	Surgery Primary and neck	and	RT ± systemic therapy
Recurrent	Multi	Salvage surgery If resectable	and	Systemic therapy ± RT
Metastatic	Multi	Palliative surgery	and/or	Systemic therapy ± RT

positive surgical margins, re-resection rather post-operative radiotherapy is strongly recommended whenever feasible.

For cancers of the oral cavity, a minimum in vivo circumferential gross tissue margin of 1 cm is recommended to achieve a final pathologic margin of at least 5 mm following tissue shrinkage during specimen preparation. The surgeon should orient each resected specimen with sutures and photographs should be taken before the specimen is dispatched for histopathologic examination.

Because of the complex three-dimensional anatomy and close proximity of structures in the oral cavity and head and neck in general, achieving appropriate surgical margins may be difficult and/or lead to added functional morbidity. The surgeon must make a habit of regularly inspecting and palpating the tumor during resection to ensure the desired margin is taken. Where available, intraoperative frozen sections of resection margins should be performed and no effort should be spared to ensure negative margins are achieved, unless deliberately deemed unresectable due to prohibitive resultant morbidity. Otherwise, the surgeon should never compromise a negative surgical margin and leave its clearance up to post-operative radiotherapy. Likewise, the adequacy of oncologic resection should never be compromised by reconstructive considerations.

12.7.1 Oral Tongue

The majority of oral tongue SCC arise from the lateral surfaces of the middle third, near the border between the dorsal keratinized and non-keratinized epithelium contiguous with that of the floor of mouth. Tumors of the oral tongue should be worked up with an MRI to determine suspected invasion of extrinsic muscles. Imaging combined with intraoperative clinical findings confirm whether or not the tumor crosses the midline and informs the laterality of neck dissection. Intraoperatively, some may employ ultrasonography as an adjunct to palpation to assess tumor extent, ensure and confirm that adequate margins are taken, and to estimate tumor depth of invasion.

A partial glossectomy refers to a resection of less than one-third of the tongue, a hemiglossectomy involves resection of one-third to a half, a subtotal glossectomy involves resection of half to three-quarters, whereas a total glossectomy removes three-quarters of the tongue or more. Full thickness of the tongue is excised whenever possible. While early disease is treated with glossectomy alone, to achieve 1-cm circumferential gross margins, locally advanced disease of the oral tongue may require en-bloc resection of the posterior/pharyngeal portion of the tongue, the floor of mouth, or the mandible.

Occasionally, a mandibulotomy or lingual release may be necessary for posterior resections, in event of trismus, or when local involvement dictates that glossectomy is performed en-bloc with neck dissection. Otherwise, silk stay sutures placed broadly through the tip of the tongue, or tongue-holding forceps, may be used to retract the tongue anteriorly to aid with exposure during resection and closure. Circumferential and deep margins should be sent for intraoperative assessment with frozen section so that negative resection margins can be confirmed.

Smaller defects up to one-third of the tongue may be closed primarily or with the use of split thickness skin graft or absorbable mesh and/or fibrin sealant. Defects larger than one-third, or those involving the floor of the mouth usually require reconstruction. Suturing of the tongue to the floor of mouth and tethering of the mobile tongue tip should be avoided, as it impairs functional recovery (the tip of the tongue is required for proprioceptive awareness of tongue orientation). The final effect on speech and swallowing is determined by the extent of resection, presence and type of reconstruction, and the use of adjuvant radiotherapy.

12.7.2 Buccal Mucosa

The buccal mucosa is the most common subsite of oral cavity SCC among consumers of smokeless tobacco as well as betel nut chewers, in whom it may arise on the background of submucous fibrosis. Buccal cancers tend to present as advanced disease due to delayed diagnosis and the ease of spread to adjacent buccal structures including the external skin of the cheek (which implies T4a disease). Surgical resection with 1-cm three-dimensional margins will usually include the buccinator and may require a partial maxillectomy, marginal mandibulectomy, or cheek skin resection. As with all oral cancer resections, frozen section confirmation of negative margins is strongly recommended. Care should be taken to identify and preserve the opening and course of the parotid (Stensen's) duct if oncologically permitted. Otherwise, the duct should be repositioned or deliberately ligated to prevent sialoma formation.

Small excisions may permit primary closure or split thickness skin grafting, whereas larger resections necessitate a local flap such as the buccal fat pad, regional pedicled flap such as the pectoralis major myocutaneous flap, or microvascular free flap reconstruction, commonly utilizing a free radial forearm flap or anterolateral thigh flap. The flap may need to be folded into a bi-paddled configuration and the fold de-epithelialized if reconstruction of a full-thickness cheek defect is required. Leaving the buccal mucosal defect to heal by secondary intention predisposes to severe trismus. However, regardless of the closure method, post-operative mouth-opening jaw exercises are critical to prevent significant trismus and microstomia, especially in the setting of adjuvant radiotherapy.

12.7.3 Floor of Mouth

Squamous cell carcinoma is thought to affect the floor of mouth due to pooling of carcinogens dissolved in saliva over its non-keratinized epithelium. Because of the relatively small size of this subsite, SCC of the floor of mouth tends to spread to cervical lymph nodes early and invade adjacent sites including the tongue, the mandible, and even the submandibular glands. Hence, resection with 1-cm circumferential margins frequently involves a partial glossectomy and/or segmental mandibulectomy and may be performed en-bloc with upper cervical lymphadenectomy via a combined transoral and transcervical approach. In early-stage disease, the surgeon should take care to avoid the lingual nerve as it courses superficially in the floor of mouth. An attempt should also be made to preserve or reimplant the submandibular (Wharton's) ducts if neck dissection and submandibular gland excision is not done. Frozen section analysis of resection margins should be performed to ensure surgical clearance.

Closure of small defects may be achieved primarily, by secondary intention or with a skin graft. Larger defects may require a free tissue transfer or a composite flap if mandibulectomy is performed.

12.7.4 Retromolar Trigone

The retromolar trigone (RMT) is an area behind the third lower molar, below the maxillary tuberosity, medial to posterior buccal mucosa, and lateral to the anterior tonsillar pillar. Its mucosa overlies the ascending ramus of the mandible. Although SCC of retromolar trigone is statistically rare, it tends to present with advanced disease, often with trismus and invasion into adjacent structures including the buccal mucosa, mandible, maxilla, masticator space and the oropharynx. Hence, resection with 1-cm three-dimensional margins must extend to the affected subsites and may include a posterior inferior maxillectomy, marginal or segmental mandibulectomy, and oropharyngeal resection. Except for early disease which maybe resected trans-orally, retromolar trigone resection usually necessitates mandibulotomy, or a cervicofacial route for access. If ramus mandibulectomy is performed, the posterior extent of resection should include the pterygoid muscles. As with any resection, circumferential and deep margins should be analyzed by intraoperative frozen section to confirm negativity.

The resultant defects are likely to require a free flap reconstruction in order to reduce post-operative trismus and for optimal functional outcome, with local flaps and skin grafts reserved for relatively minor resections. Pedicled flaps such as the pectoralis major myocutaneous flap or the latissimus dorsi flap tend not to offer adequate reach to reconstruct the retromolar trigone and may result in posterior dehiscence, but may nevertheless prove a useful last resort in a salvage setting.

12.7.5 Hard Palate, Upper Alveolus, and Maxilla

Physical examination is adequate for assessment of the intraoral extent of palatal tumors. In contrast, involvement of the maxillary bone, maxillary sinus, and beyond is best assessed on CT or MRI coronal sections. Invasion into masticator space, pterygoid plates, the skull base, or encasement of the internal carotid artery signifies very advanced disease and may imply unresectability. Otherwise, maxillary resection is indicated in the event of suspected bony invasion or to achieve clear 1-cm surgical margins. Bony work may range from transoral wide excision of the upper alveolus or hard palate, to formal maxillectomy. Inferior maxillectomy is usually sufficient for oral cavity tumors and is achieved through a sublabial incision or midfacial degloving approach. A Weber-Ferguson incision with a cheek flap with or without subciliary extension is preferred for a total maxillectomy. Because bony work on the maxilla may result in significant blood loss, the steps of maxillectomy should be well sequenced. Specifically, all mucosal cuts should be completed, soft tissue elevated away in the subperiosteal plane, and bony cortex exposed before any osteotomies are made with a saw and the maxilla is down-fractured. As the last step, the posterior maxilla is disarticulated from the pterygoid plates with a curved osteotome and the intervening soft tissue is divided using heavy curved scissors. This enables prompt visualization of the pterygoid venous plexus so that pressure and judicious diathermy can be applied and hemostasis achieved. Unless oncologically indicated, the soft palate should be preserved to prevent velopharyngeal insufficiency.

Small maxillary defects may be closed with local flaps such as the buccal fat pad or facial artery musculo-mucosal (FAMM) flap. Larger defects must be reconstructed with microvascular free-tissue transfer or with a custom surgical obturator to separate the oral from the nasal cavity.

12.7.6 Lower Alveolus and Mandible

Locally advanced oral cavity tumors with suspected involvement of the mandible require mandibular resection. Lower alveolus-, tongue-, floor of mouth-, buccal-, and retromolar trigone-based tumors may all involve the mandible. The location and extent of mandibulectomy is dictated by cancer location and the need to achieve clear circumferential margins. Despite advanced imaging techniques, preoperative assessment of mandible invasion remains difficult. Hence, a deep bony margin deeper than the greatest tumor depth of invasion and a lateral bony margin in line with a 1-cm soft tissue margin is recommended. Frozen section analysis of bony margins is generally unreliable, hence it is not conducted. However, mucosal margins should be sent for intraoperative frozen section analysis routinely. If the remnant height of the mandible is sufficient (at least 1 cm), marginal (rim) mandibulectomy may be performed. Otherwise, or if the mandible had been previously irradiated (which confers an increased risk of osteoradionecrosis), segmental mandibulectomy is appropriate. For anterior or lateral tumors, mandibulotomies are best performed through sockets of extracted teeth, which prevents dental root damage and exposure, thus reducing the risk of later osteonecrosis. For tumors involving the retromolar trigone, mandibular resection may be performed through the sigmoid notch, involve the coronoid process, but preserve the temporomandibular joint.

Mandibular defects arising from marginal (rim) resection are amenable to primary closure, unless the extent of mucosal defect necessitates reconstruction, which may range from a skin graft, through a local pedicled flap (e.g. buccal fat pad, FAMM flap), to a free soft tissue transfer (e.g. free radial forearm or anterolateral thigh flap). In contrast, segmental mandibular defects are best reconstructed with a composite flap from the fibula, iliac crest, or the scapula.

12.7.7 Mandibulotomy for Access

The majority of early-stage oral cavity tumors can be resected via the transoral route, without the need for a separate neck incision unless required for cervical lymphadenectomy. On the other hand, more extensive resections of the tongue, floor of mouth, or those involving the mandible may require a combined transoral and transcervical approach. Occasionally, locoregionally advanced tumors, or those located posteriorly, or associated with significant trismus may benefit from a mandibulotomy with or without a lip split (mandibular swing) for adequate access, even though mandibular resection is not indicated. In those instances, the mandible should either be pre-plated, or upfront arch bars should be considered to ensure correct bony union and dental occlusion during subsequent healing. The mandibular osteotomy should be placed in a paramedian location anterior to the mental foramen to preserve the inferior alveolar nerve and thus the sensation to the lip (via the mental nerve).

12.7.8 Surgical Management of the Neck

For cancers of the oral cavity, decision making with regard to neck dissection depends on the anatomical subsite, presence of clinically detectable cervical lymphadenopathy, as well as on the size and extent of the primary tumor, i.e. the T and N stage. For all tumors of the lower alveolus and retromolar trigone, as well as for upper alveolus and hard palate tumors with T2 disease or greater, and for most buccal mucosal tumors, elective neck dissection is recommended even in node-negative necks (cN0 disease) based on a high risk of subclinical nodal involvement (occult metastases). For node-negative tumors of the oral tongue and of the floor of mouth, decision to perform a prophylactic neck dissection depends on the primary tumor's depth of invasion (DOI), as DOI has become an established predictor of occult nodal metastases, recurrence, and survival [7]. Although there is no consensus on the cut-off value of DOI for performing an elective neck dissection, the author applies a 3-mm DOI as an indication for prophylactic lymphadenectomy. It is hereby important to note the distinction between DOI, which represents the vertical extent of tumor growth deep to the basement membrane, and tumor thickness, which indicates the greatest vertical size of the tumor (Fig. 12.3). This approach highlights the importance of obtaining an adequate diagnostic biopsy to enable an accurate determination of DOI. Alternatively, DOI can be measured on intraoperative frozen section following primary resection, or approximated clinically. Occasionally, the surgeon may elect to await the final histologic evaluation of the resected primary tumor specimen and perform the neck dissection if indicated in a separate setting. In T1–2, cN0 disease limited to the oral tongue the decision to perform an elective neck dissection may also be guided by a sentinel lymph node biopsy.

The extent of prophylactic neck dissection also depends on the subsite of the primary tumor and is usually performed in a supraomohyoid fashion (taking lymph node levels I-III or I-IV, possibly sparing level Iib), with at least 18 nodes harvested for proper pathologic staging. In contrast, for all node-positive tumors and for T3–4 tumors regardless of cervical nodal status, a comprehensive neck dissection is usually indicated. In all neck dissections, care must be taken to preserve the spinal accessory nerve, internal jugular vein, and the sternocleidomastoid muscle unless gross invasion by metastatic nodal disease is identified thereof. A bilateral neck dissection should be performed if the primary tumor crosses or approaches the midline, or in the presence of bilateral cervical lymphadenopathy (cN2c). Although bilateral neck dissection is associated with an increased risk of edema due to lymph stasis, sparing of the jugular veins reduces the overall risk of edema through maintained venous return. Moreover, the surgeon must take care to preserve uninvolved vessels during neck dissection to facilitate microvascular anastomoses in event of free flap reconstruction.

(Please refer to Chap. 8 for a detailed discussion on neck dissection)

12.7.9 Reconstruction

Long-term deleterious effects of major oncologic resection on the complex anatomy and multiple functions of the oral cavity can be mitigated by appropriate reconstruction and post-operative rehabilitation. The choice of reconstructive strategy depends on the type and extent of resection, on the patient's medical fitness to undergo reconstructive surgery and prolonged anesthesia, on the availability of suitable donor tissue, as well as on the surgeon's reconstructive surgical expertise. Although minor resection defects may be amenable to primary closure, skin grafting, or to healing by secondary intention, better functional outcomes are generally achieved with the use of local flaps such as the buccal fat pad or the facial artery musculo-mucosal flap, especially for oral cavity subsites where post-operative trismus is likely (i.e. buccal mucosa, retromolar trigone). Larger defects, which result from major oral cavity resections generally benefit from microvascular free tissue transfer. These offer a more flexible reconstructive option than regional pedicled flaps and are usually performed by a dedicated reconstructive specialist surgical team.

Free fasciocutaneous flaps frequently used in oral cavity soft tissue reconstruction include the radial forearm flap and the anterolateral thigh flap. The former is preferred when thin pliable tissue is required, as in the reconstruction of the buccal mucosa or the floor of mouth, whereas the latter provides more bulk useful in a functional reconstruction of the tongue. Segmental defects of the mandible should be reconstructed with a composite free flap whenever feasible. Among other features, the osteofasciocutaneous free fibula flap based off the peroneal artery is often selected for its ample pedicle, consistent linear shape and adequate length, which permit segmentation via several osteotomies and the creation of a construct customized to match the original mandibular projection and facial contour. A digital reconstruction planning process (computer-aided design and manufacturing, CAD-CAM) is increasingly employed for optimal outcomes. Alternatives to the free fibula flap include vascularized scapula or iliac crest flaps. The choice of maxilla reconstruction depends on the defect size and ranges from local flaps to soft or composite free tissue transfer. Alternatively, satisfactory maxillary reconstruction can be achieved via a custom surgical obturator.

The success of the microvascular free tissue transfer depends on robust arterial and venous anastomoses to vessels in the neck. If adequate recipient vessels are not available, due to tumor involvement, anatomical variants, or prior surgery, or if the patient is otherwise not a good candidate for free-flap reconstruction, pedicled regional flaps (such as the pectoralis major, latissimus dorsi, or deltopectoral flap) may be used in select oral cavity reconstructions. Notably, pedicled flap utility is constrained by the length of the vascular pedicle, which limits the reach toward more posterior or superior defects such as those of the retromolar trigone. Despite this and other limitations however, the surgeon must never compromise the extent of oncologic resection based on reconstructive considerations. A two-team approach to resection and reconstruction allows each team to focus on only one of these seemingly conflicting priorities, while concurrent resection and flap harvest shortens the overall duration of the surgery.

(For an in-depth discussion of head and neck reconstruction, please refer to Chaps. 7, 18 and 19)

12.7.10 Recurrent Disease

Recurrent cancer of the oral cavity portends a poor prognosis and treatment options are limited by previous surgical and radiation therapy. However, surgical salvage is recommended in a select group of patients with recurrence limited to the primary site and/or isolated cervical lymph nodes, in the absence of distant metastases. Careful patient selection is paramount based on performance status and to ensure resectability. In order to reduce the risk of therapeutic failure in the recurrent setting, a radical surgical approach with wide margins and resection of adjacent structures (e.g. neck vessels, overlying skin, and bony skeleton), or the resection of entire anatomical compartment may be indicated. Salvage surgery is technically challenging and associated with an increased post-operative morbidity due to radicality of resection and the status of previously operated and/or irradiated tissues. These "hostile" surgical conditions also limit the reconstructive options, with pedicled flap reconstruction (e.g. pectoralis major) often preferred to eliminate the risk of microvascular anastomotic failure while ensuring adequate coverage. The complexities of management of recurrent head and neck cancer are best addressed by multidisciplinary teams in high volume centers, so that optimal multi-modality therapy can be tailored to each patient's specific condition.

12.7.11 Post-Operative Complications

General surgical complications, which are not unique to oral cavity resection, include post-operative bleeding, surgical site and deep space infection, wound breakdown or dehiscence, and fistula formation. Acute post-operative edema, while common to many surgeries, is potentially life threatening following oropharyngeal resection due to laryngeal airway obstruction, unless accompanied by a tracheostomy. Moreover, through alteration of normal anatomy, ablative surgical treatment to the oral cavity interferes with vital upper aerodigestive tract functions, which has the potential to significantly affect the patient's quality of life. Specifically, oral resection frequently results in deficits in speech articulation and swallowing, predisposing to aspiration and impairing nutrition. Finally, head and neck surgery in general carries potential deleterious psychosocial consequences imparted by any post-operative cosmetic deformity. Cervical lymph node dissection, especially when bilateral and involving internal jugular vein resection further contributes to head and neck (lymph-) edema. Specific to a left-sided level IV cervical nodal dissection is a risk of thoracic duct injury and resultant chyle leak, whereas level II and level V dissection risks injury to the spinal accessory, which may cause shoulder weakness. Although successful surgical reconstruction goes a long way to restore the affected anatomy and improve long-term function and quality of life, the reconstructive process predisposes the patient to risk of post-operative flap failure, donor site complications, and reoperation.

Surgical complications are exacerbated by those of adjuvant radiotherapy, which contributes to aerodigestive mucositis, dysphagia, trismus, xerostomia, dysgeusia, skin and soft tissue fibrosis, lymphoedema, and osteoradionecrosis. Perhaps the most feared long-term complication of combined-modality treatment for advanced oral cavity cancer is the acute carotid blowout syndrome, a surgical emergency whereby a sudden catastrophic hemorrhage from a weakened carotid artery or its major branches rapidly predisposes to airway compromise, hemodynamic instability, hypoxic-ischemic cerebral injury, and demise.

12.8 Relevant Non-Surgical Management

Occasionally, management of oral cavity malignancy may be approached non-surgically in technically unresectable disease, in situations where functional organ preservation is paramount, or in patients who are medically unfit or otherwise refuse surgical intervention. Moreover, non-surgical modalities of treatment may be employed in resectable yet advanced disease as a part of multi-modality therapy.

12.8.1 Radiation Therapy

For early (stage I and II) oral cavity cancer, single modality treatment with surgical resection is recommended whenever feasible. However, in patients for whom the surgical risk is prohibitive or where resection would result in unacceptable morbidity or functional deficit, definitive radiation therapy (RT) to the primary tumor serves as an alternative. RT may also be applied as a treatment modality to cervical lymph nodes in lieu of an elective neck dissection in node-negative (N0) early-stage disease.

In contrast, locoregionally advanced (stage III and IV) oral cavity cancer implies aggressive disease with a high risk of recurrence following either surgery or RT alone. Hence, a combined-modality management with a combination of surgery, RT to the primary tumor and neck and systemic treatment is indicated. Surgical resection remains the preferred first step whenever feasible, with RT, with or without concurrent chemotherapy, given in an adjuvant setting. Palliative RT (in combination with systemic therapy) is reserved for unresectable tumors or patients who are not surgical candidates.

For patients with high-risk features on final post-operative histopathology, adjuvant RT in combination with systemic chemotherapy is indicated. These include: more than one positive cervical node (N2 or N3 disease), nodal positivity in cervical levels IV or V, extranodal extension, resection margin positivity, perineural or vascular invasion.

Modern RT employs ionizing radiation administered via an intensity-modulated external beam (IMRT). The radiation oncologist carefully devises an individualized treatment plan, which aims to optimize the dose, field and schedule of treatment, such that the cumulative treatment dose is fractionated into smaller daily doses delivered over multiple sessions. The objective of radiation therapy is to administer the maximum prescribed dose of radiation to the tumor while sparing the surrounding normal tissues from radiation toxicities.

Acute toxicities of RT to the oral cavity include mucositis, xerostomia, loss of taste, and skin reactions, while later complications include trismus, skin or soft tissue atrophy, fibrosis, and osteoradionecrosis of the mandible. Moreover, irradiation of the oral cavity mucosa predisposes to the development of second (radiation-induced) oral malignancies in the future.

12.8.2 Proton Beam

Proton therapy is an emerging alternative to conventional IMRT with purported benefits of reduced collateral toxicity owing to the controllable sharp drop-off in energy of the radioactive particles as they penetrate irradiated tissue. Although clinical data demonstrating therapeutic advantage of proton beam over IMRT is currently lacking, the potential benefits for oral cavity and head and neck malignancies in general are noteworthy.

12.8.3 Cytotoxic Chemotherapy

Platinum-based concurrent chemoradiation therapy (CCRT) is indicated for non-surgical management of locoregionally advanced oral cavity squamous cell carcinoma (SCC) or as adjuvant treatment of patients in whom final histopathologic examination reveals features suggestive of high risk of recurrence [8]. Among other complications, the use of cytotoxic platinum-based systemic therapy is associated with risk of severe immunosuppression and infection, peripheral neuropathy, oto- and nephrotoxicity. Therefore, for older patients (70 years of age or more) or those with poor performance status, the risk of adding chemotherapy to RT may outweigh its benefits.

12.8.4 Targeted Therapy

Epidermal growth factor receptor (EGFR) overexpression in head and neck SCC is associated with poor prognosis. The human-murine chimeric monoclonal antibody cetuximab, which inhibits EGFR has been shown to improve overall survival when administered concurrently with RT compared to RT alone in patients with advanced head and neck SCC [9]. Hence, cetuximab is administered with RT in patients requiring systemic therapy but deemed not fit to undergo concurrent platinum-based chemoradiation.

12.8.5 Immunotherapy

One of the mechanisms by which cancer proliferates is via evasion of T-cell-mediated destruction by the immune system through expression of the inhibitory programmed cell death ligand (PDL-1) on the surface of tumor cells. As PDL-1 binds to the programmed cell death (PD-1) checkpoint protein on the surface of a T-cell, it inhibits apoptosis of the tumor cell, promotes peripheral exhaustion of T cells, and in turn enables the tumor cell to evade immune response.

If immunohistochemical staining of the histopathologic specimen (either resected SCC or biopsy) reveals heavy expression of PDL-1, checkpoint inhibitor drugs (e.g. pembrolizumab) can be used to re-sensitize the immune system and promote immune-mediated cellular cancer destruction. Such immunotherapy may be used for recurrent oral cavity SCC irrespective of previous treatment with platinum-based chemotherapy [10]. Use of immunotherapy in non-recurrent disease is currently investigational, pending KESTREL trial results.

12.8.6 Multidisciplinary Approach

The choice between surgical and non-surgical treatment options for oral cavity malignancy is complex and best performed at a large-volume center, under the care of multiple head and neck specialists with interest and experience in managing the condition. A multidisciplinary approach involving surgical, medical, and radiation oncologists, as well as radiologists, pathologists, dental, and reconstructive surgeons is key. At our institution, a head and neck multidisciplinary team meeting is convened weekly to ensure that an evidence-based individualized treatment plan is carefully devised for each patient, and that the clinical decision making reflects not just an individual but an institutional opinion, in line with accepted clinical practice guidelines.

In addition, because oral cavity cancer and its treatment can have a profound effect on the patient's quality of life, all complex oral cavity cancer patients are followed-up by speech therapists, dietitians, physiotherapists, and psychologists, and the patient's quality-of-life issues are discussed in a dedicated weekly meeting held between the clinical and allied health teams.

Top Five Takeaways

1. While obtaining a detailed history is essential, the clinician must take note that majority of oral cavity cancers are mucosal squamous cell carcinomas, which more commonly affect males with well-established risk factors of alcohol, tobacco, or betel nut consumption, and present with non-healing mouth lesions.
2. A thorough examination of the oral cavity with its seven anatomical subsites (lips, gingiva, buccal surfaces, retromolar trigones, hard palate, oral tongue, and floor of mouth) and of the remainder of the upper aerodigestive tract is critical during initial evaluation of suspected malignancy to identify potential synchronous lesions.
3. Workup of oral cavity malignancy centers on a diagnostic tissue biopsy adequately demonstrating tumor depth of invasion, followed by cross-sectional imaging for purposes of locoregional staging of the primary tumor and cervical lymph node status, determination of resectability and for surgical planning.
4. Principles of oncologic surgical resection include en-bloc extirpation of the oral cavity tumor with negative circumferential margins (inclusive of bony facial skeleton if involved) combined with either prophylactic or therapeutic neck dissection depending on the clinical cervical nodal status and primary tumor depth of invasion. Major resection defects benefit from immediate surgical reconstruction.
5. In general, early-stage oral cavity cancers are treated with a single modality: either surgery or radiation therapy, whereas advanced-stage disease is treated with multi-modality approach consisting of a combination of sur-

gery, radiation therapy, cytotoxic chemotherapy, targeted systemic therapy, and immunotherapy. Management of complex oral cavity cancers benefits from multidisciplinary team approach inclusive of allied health professionals.

References

1. Montero PH, Patel SG. Cancer of the oral cavity. Surg Oncol Clin N Am. 2015;24(3):491–508. https://doi.org/10.1016/j.soc.2015.03.006. Epub 2015 Apr 15. PMID: 25979396; PMCID: PMC5018209
2. Sung H, Ferlay J, Siegel RL, Laversanne M, Soerjomataram I, Jemal A, Bray F. Global cancer statistics 2020: GLOBOCAN estimates of incidence and mortality worldwide for 36 cancers in 185 countries. CA Cancer J Clin. 2021;71(3):209–49. https://doi.org/10.3322/caac.21660. Epub 2021 Feb 4
3. Ng JH, Iyer NG, Tan MH, Edgren G. Changing epidemiology of oral squamous cell carcinoma of the tongue: a global study. Head Neck. 2017;39(2):297–304. https://doi.org/10.1002/hed.24589. Epub 2016 Oct 3
4. Amin MB, Greene FL, Edge SB, Compton CC, Gershenwald JE, Brookland RK, Meyer L, Gress DM, Byrd DR, Winchester DP. The eighth edition AJCC cancer staging manual: continuing to build a bridge from a population-based to a more "personalized" approach to cancer staging. CA Cancer J Clin. 2017;67(2):93–9. https://doi.org/10.3322/caac.21388. Epub 2017 Jan 17
5. Pfister DG, Spencer S, Adelstein D, Adkins D, Anzai Y, Brizel DM, Bruce JY, Busse PM, Caudell JJ, Cmelak AJ, Colevas AD, Eisele DW, Fenton M, Foote RL, Galloway T, Gillison ML, Haddad RI, Hicks WL, Hitchcock YJ, Jimeno A, Leizman D, Maghami E, Mell LK, Mittal BB, Pinto HA, Ridge JA, Rocco JW, Rodriguez CP, Shah JP, Weber RS, Weinstein G, Witek M, Worden F, Yom SS, Zhen W, Burns JL, Darlow SD. Head and neck cancers, version 2.2020, NCCN clinical practice guidelines in oncology. J Natl Compr Canc Netw. 2020;18(7):873–98. https://doi.org/10.6004/jnccn.2020.0031.
6. Iyer NG, Tan DS, Tan VK, Wang W, Hwang J, Tan NC, Sivanandan R, Tan HK, Lim WT, Ang MK, Wee J, Soo KC, Tan EH. Randomized trial comparing surgery and adjuvant radiotherapy versus concurrent chemoradiotherapy in patients with advanced, non-metastatic squamous cell carcinoma of the head and neck: 10-year update and subset analysis. Cancer. 2015;121(10):1599–607. https://doi.org/10.1002/cncr.29251. Epub 2015 Jan 29. Erratum in: Cancer. 2015;121(19):3560
7. Tam S, Amit M, Zafereo M, Bell D, Weber RS. Depth of invasion as a predictor of nodal disease and survival in patients with oral tongue squamous cell carcinoma. Head Neck. 2019;41(1):177–84. https://doi.org/10.1002/hed.25506. Epub 2018 Dec 7
8. Cooper JS, Pajak TF, Forastiere AA, Jacobs J, Campbell BH, Saxman SB, Kish JA, Kim HE, Cmelak AJ, Rotman M, Machtay M, Ensley JF, Chao KS, Schultz CJ, Lee N, Fu KK, Radiation Therapy Oncology Group 9501/Intergroup. Postoperative concurrent radiotherapy and chemotherapy for high-risk squamous-cell carcinoma of the head and neck. N Engl J Med. 2004;350(19):1937–44. https://doi.org/10.1056/NEJMoa032646.
9. Bonner JA, Harari PM, Giralt J, Azarnia N, Shin DM, Cohen RB, Jones CU, Sur R, Raben D, Jassem J, Ove R, Kies MS, Baselga J, Youssoufian H, Amellal N, Rowinsky EK, Ang KK. Radiotherapy plus cetuximab for squamous-cell carcinoma of the head and neck. N Engl J Med. 2006;354(6):567–78. https://doi.org/10.1056/NEJMoa053422.
10. Burtness B, Harrington KJ, Greil R, Soulières D, Tahara M, de Castro G Jr, Psyrri A, Basté N, Neupane P, Bratland Å, Fuereder T, Hughes BGM, Mesía R, Ngamphaiboon N, Rordorf T, Wan Ishak WZ, Hong RL, González Mendoza R, Roy A, Zhang Y, Gumuscu B, Cheng JD, Jin F, Rischin D, KEYNOTE-048 Investigators. Pembrolizumab alone or with chemotherapy versus cetuximab with chemotherapy for recurrent or metastatic squamous cell carcinoma of the head and neck (KEYNOTE-048): a randomised, open-label, phase 3 study. Lancet. 2019;394(10212):1915–28. https://doi.org/10.1016/S0140-6736(19)32591-7. Epub 2019 Nov 1. Erratum in: Lancet. 2020;395(10220):272. Erratum in: Lancet. 2020 Feb 22;395(10224):564. Erratum in: Lancet. 2021;397(10291):2252

13 Mucosal Malignancy: Cancers of the Oropharynx

Joel C. Davies, Susannah C. Orzell, and Danny J. Enepekides

13.1 Background: Scope of the Problem

Our understanding of the complexities of cancer of the oropharynx has changed dramatically over time. Prior to the 1980s, the majority of patients presenting with oropharynx cancer had risk factors which were common to other sites of the head and neck, primarily exposure to tobacco and alcohol consumption [1, 2]. However, over the last two to three decades, there has been a rapid shift away from tumors that are driven by traditional risk factors such as alcohol and tobacco [2]. These patients presenting tended to be younger (40–59) and male [1]. It was discovered that in these patients, cancer of the oropharynx was driven by a viral-mediated mechanism through exposure to high-risk subtypes of the Human Papillomavirus (HPV) [3]. The rise of HPV-positive oropharyngeal cancer over the past few decades is significant and, since 2009, has surpassed that of cervical cancer [4]. Approximately 14,000 new cases of oropharynx were diagnosed in the USA in 2013 and account for 10–12% of all upper aerodigestive tract malignancies [2]. Although based on histology, the majority (>90%) of cancers in the oropharynx are squamous cell carcinomas (SCCs), at a cellular level 70% are now HPV-positive SCCs with the remainder being HPV-negative or indeterminate [1]. The most common subtypes of HPV associated with oropharyngeal cancer include HPV 16,18, 31, 33, and 35, with type 16 comprising close to 90% of HPV-positive OPSCC [5]. While tobacco and alcohol consumptions are the major risk factors for development of HPV-negative OPSCC, number of sexual partners and oral infection with HPV are the risk factors most associated with HPV-positive OPSCC [3, 6]. Given these known risk factors, physicians should be aware of the importance of recommending HPV vaccination in younger cohorts of boys and girls. Currently, the CDC recommends vaccination for boys and girls up to age 26 with a target of these patients receiving vaccination prior to their first sexual contact [5].

The prognosis of oropharynx cancer is highly dependent on HPV status and, to a lesser degree, the location of the primary tumor. Generally, those patients with HPV-positive malignancies tend to have a more favourable prognosis and this has been reflected in the most recent editions of the AJCC staging guidelines. For example, a

J. C. Davies
Department of Otolaryngology-Head and Neck Surgery, Sinai Health System, University of Toronto, Toronto, ON, Canada
e-mail: Joel.Davies@sinaihealth.ca

S. C. Orzell · D. J. Enepekides (✉)
Department of Otolaryngology-Head and Neck Surgery, Sunnybrook Health Sciences Centre, University of Toronto, Toronto, ON, Canada
e-mail: susannah.orzell@uhn.ca; danny.enepekides@sunnybrook.ca

B. Ashford (ed.), *Head and Neck Surgery for General Surgeons*,
https://doi.org/10.1007/978-981-19-7900-2_13

3 cm HPV-positive tumor of the tonsil with three ipsilateral-positive lymph nodes measuring 2 cm each without distant metastatic disease would be staged as cT2N1M0 (overall stage I) with a 5-year overall survival of 85% [7]. However, a tumor with the same dimensions and clinical profile that is HPV-negative would be staged as cT2N2bM0 (overall stage 4a) with a 5-year overall survival of 45% [7]. As a clinician evaluating a patient presenting with a tumor of the oropharynx, understanding the etiologic, clinical, and treatment-related differences between the two distinct entities is of utmost importance and will be the primary focus of this chapter.

13.2 Anatomy of the Oropharynx

The oropharynx is sub-divided into anatomic subsites including the tonsil, soft palate, base of tongue, and posterior pharyngeal wall (Fig. 13.1). It is bordered superiorly by the soft palate and inferiorly by the valleculae and hyoid bone. The circumvallate papillae form the anterior extent and the posterior pharyngeal wall the posterior extent. The lateral oropharynx is bounded by the palatine tonsils.

The soft palate originates at the posterior extent of the hard palate and is mainly comprised of skeletal muscle capable of tensing and elevating the palate. The primary function of the soft palate is to close off and separate the oropharynx from the oral cavity and nasopharynx. The palatine tonsils are comprised of lymphoid tissue and are located between the anterior and posterior tonsillar pillars which are formed by the palatoglossus and palatopharyngeal muscles, respectively. The base of tongue extends posteriorly from the circumvallate papillae back to the valleculae. The superficial base of tongue is predominantly lymphoid tissue, while the deep tongue is skeletal muscle. The posterior pharyngeal wall is formed by the superior constrictors and the mucosa overlying these constrictors. It extends superiorly from the soft palate and inferiorly down to the attachment of the epiglottis to the thyroid cartilage.

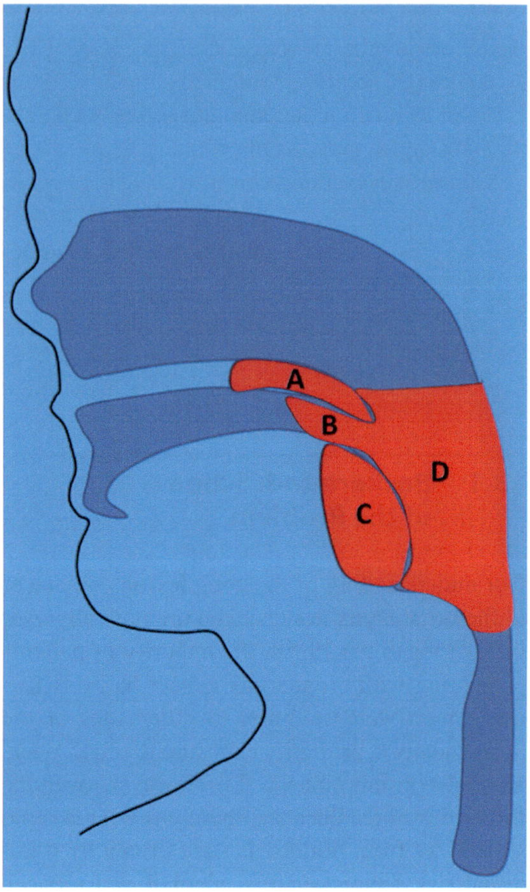

Fig. 13.1 Diagram of the upper aerodigestive tract (dark blue) demonstrating the oropharynx (red), including subsites: (**a**) soft palate, (**b**) palatine tonsils, (**c**) base of tongue, and (**d**) posterior pharyngeal wall

13.3 Key Elements of History

13.3.1 Signs and Symptoms of Oropharynx Cancer

While patients with oropharyngeal cancer may be referred with an obvious tumor of the tonsil or soft palate, these tumors may begin very small within tonsillar crypts or deep in the base of tongue. As a result, these tumors may go unnoticed for months or years before presenting for evaluation. Therefore, clinicians must be judicious in evaluation patients presenting with subtle signs and symptoms of oropharyngeal cancer.

Common presenting symptoms of oropharynx cancer:

- Dysphagia.
- Odynophagia.
- Otalgia.
- Pain.
- Globus sensation.

Common presenting signs of oropharynx cancer:

- Neck mass.
- Oral bleeding.
- Palpable mass in subsite of oropharynx.

Tumors of the oropharynx most commonly present within the tonsil. These patients will frequently complain of dysphagia, otalgia muffled voice, and/or trismus. The second most common subsite affected by oropharyngeal cancer is the base of tongue. Given that these tumors may be deep and, therefore difficult to detect, they more often present at an advanced stage. Common symptoms include dysphagia, ipsilateral referred otalgia, oral bleeding, and/or globus sensation. Oropharyngeal tumors of the soft palate are the third most common. These tumors, like tonsillar tumors, are more easily detected and therefore present at an earlier stage. Signs and symptoms are similar to tonsillar cancers. Lastly, tumors of the posterior pharyngeal wall are among the rarest of oropharynx cancers. Symptoms at presentation include dysphagia, odynophagia, and bleeding. Of note, all tumors of the oropharynx, with the exception of the tonsil, have bilateral lymphatic drainage to the neck and most commonly within levels II-IV. Therefore, a patient presenting with a neck mass within any combination of unilateral, contralateral, or bilateral levels II-IV must be examined for an oropharyngeal primary cancer.

13.3.2 Social and Sexual History

Although pathologic diagnosis is required to confirm HPV status, clinical suspicion may be heightened by obtaining a careful history. Specifically, social history can reveal important clues such as common risk factors for HPV-negative-driven cancers including exposure to tobacco and alcohol. A discussion regarding sexual history including number of sexual partners and age of first encounter with oral/vaginal intercourse is important as these factors have been found to be associated with HPV-positive OPSCC. For example, D'Souza et al. (2007) observed that high lifetime number of vaginal-sex (≥26) and oral-sex (≥6) partners was associated with HPV-positive OPSCC [6]. Lastly, there is some literature to suggest that marijuana users may be at an elevated risk for developing HPV-positive oropharyngeal cancer [8]. However, it is difficult to assess whether it is marijuana use itself or characteristics of the population using marijuana that increase their risk.

13.3.3 Special Consideration of Cancer of Unknown Primary

Although many patients may present with symptoms and signs of oropharynx cancer and have their primary tumors found during physical examination, a certain subset of these patients will present with a cervical lymph node that is positive for malignancy without an obvious primary tumor. Although a discussion regarding the workup of cancer of unknown primary (CUP) of the neck may be covered elsewhere in this book, it is important that clinicians be aware of the high likelihood that these CUPs are oropharyngeal tumors that are often too small to detect clinically. Close to 90% of all CUPs of the neck are metastases from oropharyngeal tumors and are approximately equally divided between the tonsil and base of tongue [5]. These patients tend to present with lymph nodes in levels II-IV that are cystic in nature and, despite small occult primaries, the nodes can be large. Although there are many benign etiologies with a similar presentation, one must always consider an oropharyngeal primary tumor in evaluating a patient presenting with a cystic lymph node of the neck.

13.4 Clinical Examination Pearls

As with other sites, evaluation of the oropharynx begins with a thorough inspection of the various subsites including the palatine tonsils, soft palate, base of tongue, and posterior pharyngeal wall. However, unlike the oral cavity, small tumors may be hidden from plain sight deep within crypts of the base of tongue or tonsil. Therefore, it is critical that the next stage of evaluation includes palpation of these areas. The examination continues with endoscopy (flexible or rigid) to further evaluate the base of tongue, posterior pharyngeal wall, and posterior palatine tonsils. It is important to provide the patient with topical anaesthetic/decongestant prior to evaluation to improve comfort and facilitate an accurate examination. During the examination, having a patient protrude their tongue can assist in identifying small base of tongue tumors. As an adjunct to an endoscopic examination, narrow band imaging may be performed to detect pre-malignant and early malignant tumors which otherwise may not be clinically apparent. Narrow band imaging has been demonstrated to provide a more accurate diagnostic assessment of malignancy than white light imaging [5]. If a tumor is identified during the examination, biopsies can be obtained through using a transnasal approach via side channels of a transnasal endoscope or transorally while simultaneously performing endoscopy. Lastly, bimanual palpation of the neck is required to identify and characterize lymph nodes of the neck to assess for possible regional metastases.

Although included within the next section on investigations, panendoscopy should also be considered an important part of the clinical examination as a more thorough assessment of the subsites can be performed with the patient under general anaesthesia.

13.5 Investigations and Limitations

13.5.1 Biopsy of the Primary Site

Prior to the commencement of treatment planning, a biopsy with histopathologic evaluation and immunohistochemistry is required. Many primary tumors of the oropharynx are amenable to transoral biopsy and are frequently performed safely in the office setting under local anesthetic. If there is concern about the vascularity of the tumor, such as when a neurofibroma or hemangioma is suspected, a transoral biopsy in the office setting may not be appropriate. Visible tumors of the oropharynx not accessible transorally may still be amenable to an in-office biopsy with a transnasal endoscope.

13.5.2 Biopsy of a Lymph Node

The initial presenting symptom for many oropharyngeal squamous cell carcinomas is a neck mass related to a metastatic disease within a lymph node, most often in the upper jugulodigastric lymphatic basin. HPV-associated tumors in particular are associated with early metastases to cervical lymph nodes, even with small or nonexistent primary tumors in the oropharynx. When a patient presents with an abnormal cervical lymph node, a fine needle aspiration biopsy (FNAB) may be performed in order to obtain a diagnosis. This procedure may be performed in the office or by an interventional radiologist, and ultrasound guidance is frequently employed. It is not uncommon for metastatic lymph nodes to have central necrosis, thus complicating needle biopsy procedures as the necrotic material is generally unhelpful for diagnosis. If a FNAB is nondiagnostic, it may be either repeated or a core needle biopsy can be pursued. Where FNAB typically uses a small gauge needle, a core needle biopsy often uses an 18 gauge or higher bore and thus is able to obtain more cellular material. A core needle is also advantageous if lymphoma is suspected, as it has a higher diagnostic yield compared to FNAB [9]. Excisional biopsies are considered the gold standard for diagnosing lymphoma, but are generally not recommended when metastatic disease is suspected.

13.5.3 Histopathology and Immunohistochemistry

Squamous cell carcinomas of the upper aerodigestive tract are often differentiated into keratinizing or non-keratinizing subtypes, where the latter is associated with HPV-related disease. Comprehensive evaluation of an oropharyngeal squamous cell carcinoma must include testing for HPV or surrogate markers. The tumor suppressor p16 is most commonly used as a surrogate marker to diagnose HPV-related disease, although several other modalities may be used, such as in situ hybridization (ISH) and polymerase chain reaction (PCR). A threshold of 70% or more nuclear and cytoplasmic expression of p16 on immunohistochemistry is recommended by the American Society of Clinical Oncology (ASCO) to diagnose HPV-related squamous cell carcinoma in the oropharynx. Despite the high sensitivity, ease, and cost-effectiveness of p16 testing, it is not considered the gold standard since it is an indirect marker of HPV infection and other pathologic processes may lead to an increase in p16. Thus, in cases where the p16 results are discordant with other information and findings (e.g. a young, non-smoker with p16-negative non-keratinizing oropharyngeal squamous cell carcinoma), further testing with ISH or PCR may be warranted.

13.5.4 Panendoscopy

A panendoscopy refers to the comprehensive physical examination of the upper aerodigestive tract under general anesthesia. This is accomplished by both bimanual examination of the oral cavity and accessible parts of the oropharynx/supraglottis, as well as flexible or rigid endoscopic instruments that can be used to visualize the nasal cavity, nasopharynx, oropharynx, larynx, esophagus, trachea, and mainstem bronchi. A panendoscopy may be performed when a patient has a tumor that is inaccessible for biopsy in the office setting, or if a patient presents with a neck metastasis and there is no obvious primary tumor on examination. Further evaluation under general anesthesia often affords the surgeon the ability to very closely inspect areas that are difficult to examine in the awake patient, determine the extent of the tumor, evaluate for second primary malignancies, and to perform more extensive biopsies. In some patients, deep biopsies of the tongue base and tonsils are required for diagnosis, which can be very challenging outside of the operating room. Performing biopsies in the operating room also gives the surgeon the opportunity to send specimens for frozen section analysis. If a primary tumor is unable to be identified on physical exam or panendoscopy (CUP), the surgeon may elect to do a concurrent tonsillectomy, base of tongue resection, or a combination of the two in an effort to identify the site [10, 11].

13.5.5 Imaging

As with histologic confirmation of disease, imaging of the primary site as well as sites of possible regional and distant metastasis is essential for staging and treatment planning in patients with oropharyngeal cancer. CT and MRI are commonly employed to characterize lesions and metastatic sites in the head and neck. The choice of study depends on the clinical suspicion and questions about what structures may or may not be involved with the tumor. CT has the advantage over MRI for evaluation of bony invasion and is faster and often easier to obtain, whereas MRI has superior soft tissue definition and can demonstrate perineural spread of disease. CT thorax or PET/CT are appropriate to evaluate for distant metastasis, with PET/CT having slightly higher detection rates of distant metastasis compared to CT thorax [12]. In the case of a patient with an unknown primary tumor, PET/CT has demonstrated utility in indicating the source [13].

- Staging (Tables 13.1 and 13.2—OPSCC HPV-vs HPV+)

Table 13.1 AJCC ninth edition TNM staging for the oropharynx (p16/HPV-)

T category	Tx	Primary tumor cannot be assessed
	Tis	Carcinoma in situ
	T1	Tumor 2 cm or smaller in greatest dimension
	T2	Tumor larger than 2 cm, but not larger than 4 cm in greatest dimension
	T3	Tumor larger than 4 cm in greatest dimension or extension to lingual surface of epiglottis
	T4a	Moderately advanced local disease. Tumor invades the larynx, extrinsic muscle of the tongue, medial pterygoid, hard palate, or mandible
	T4b	Very advanced local disease. Tumor invades lateral pterygoid muscle, pterygoid plates, lateral nasopharynx, or skull base or encases carotid artery
N category	Nx	Regional lymph nodes cannot be assessed
	N0	No regional lymph node metastasis
	N1	Metastasis in a single ipsilateral lymph node, ≤3 cm and ENE(−)
	N2a	Metastasis in a single ipsilateral lymph node, 3–6 cm and ENE(−) [a]Metastasis in single ipsilateral node ≤3 cm and ENE(−)
	N2b	Metastasis in a multiple ipsilateral lymph node, ≤6 cm and ENE(−)
	N2c	Metastasis in bilateral or contralateral lymph nodes, ≤6 cm and ENE(−)
	N3a	Metastasis in a lymph node >6 cm and ENE(−)
	N3b	Metastasis in any node and clinically overt ENE (+) [a]Metastasis in single ipsilateral node≥3 cm and ENE (+); or multiple, ipsilateral, contralateral, or bilateral nodes, any with ENE (+) or a single contralateral node of any size and ENE (+)

[a]Denotes pathologic staging

Table 13.2 AJCC ninth edition TNM staging for the oropharynx (p16/HPV+)

T Category	T0	No primary tumor identified
	T1	Tumor ≤2 cm
	T2	Tumor 2-4 cm
	T3	Tumor >4 cm or extension to lingual surface of epiglottis
	T4	Tumor invades larynx, extrinsic tongue muscle, medial pterygoid, hard palate or mandible, or beyond
N category	Nx	Regional lymph nodes cannot be assessed
	N0	No regional lymph nodes metastasis
	N1	One or more ipsilateral lymph nodes (≤6 cm) [a]Metastasis in ≤4 lymph nodes
	N2	Contralateral or bilateral lymph nodes (≤6 cm) [a]Metastasis in >4 lymph nodes
	N3	Lymph node >6 cm

[a]Denotes pathologic staging

13.6 Management of OPSCC

The past several decades have seen numerous significant changes in the treatment for OPSCC. Historically, oropharyngeal tumors were treated surgically via transcervical and transfacial incisions with a mandibulotomy for access. These approaches had a high potential for both disfigurement and oropharyngeal dysfunction, and since it was common for many of these patients to receive adjuvant radiation, these adverse effects were then further compounded. Regarding non-surgical treatment, radiation with or without chemotherapy offers very favorable locoregional control rates, but also has several short- and long-term associated toxicities. Dysphagia and oropharyngeal dysfunction are common with both surgical and non-surgical management of OPSCC, but CRT can also induce significant fibrosis, trismus, mucositis, and xerostomia (which itself can predispose patients to dental caries, periodontal disease, and recurrent infections) depending on treatment site [14]. A dreaded complication of radiation therapy is osteoradionecrosis, which most often occurs in radiated areas of the mandible and can lead to pathologic fractures and chronic infections, both of which are extremely problematic and difficult to treat. The psychosocial impact is enormous no matter what the treatment modality, and depression is highly prevalent within the head and neck cancer patient population [15, 16].

In recognition of the numerous physical and psychosocial side effects of both surgical and non-surgical treatment, the modern paradigm for treatment of OPSCC has paid particular attention to maximizing function and quality of life. The formation of multidisciplinary teams composed of surgeons, radiation oncologists, medical oncologists, speech-language pathologist, and other specialists has allowed for greater discourse and personalized treatment in an effort to identify treatments that achieve both disease remission and retain function and maintain quality of life. This has been particularly important due to several recent changes in both the etiology of disease and treatment options available. HPV-positive OPSCC is not only a demographically different disease from HPV-negative OPSCC, but a biologically distinct disease as well. HPV-positive OPSCC is much more sensitive to chemotherapy and radiation (CRT) regimens compared to HPV-negative OPSCC [17], and thus the former has a much higher survival rate with CRT [18]. Additionally, there have been several technological advances within the surgical and non-surgical realms. The introduction of intensity modulated radiation therapy (IMRT), which allows for more precision in the delivery of radiation, and transoral surgery (TOS), which includes trans oral robotic surgery (TORS) and transoral laser microsurgery (TLM), have both presented new treatment options. These innovations have allowed for more exploration into deintensifying treatment regimens, which is particularly important in HPV-positive OPSCC as these patients are younger, and therefore will have to live longer with the effects of their treatment. Furthermore, there is the concern about a radiation-induced second primary malignancy, which would likely affect a younger cohort considering it may take decades to become apparent.

The introduction of TOS as an option for treatment of selected early stage OPSCC has allowed for some patients to avoid radiation altogether, or be treated with lower dose radiation and still maintain high rates of cure with lower rates of adverse effects and a higher quality of life [19]. TOS is not an option for every patient with OPSCC. The ideal TOS patient has a small (cT1/2) exophytic, lateralized tumor, and limited or no clinical evidence of metastatic disease in the neck. Contraindications to TOS can be divided into vascular, functional, oncologic, and general factors [20] (Fig. 13.2).

Regarding non-surgical treatment, some studies have found that reducing radiation therapy to as little as half of a traditional dosing regimen

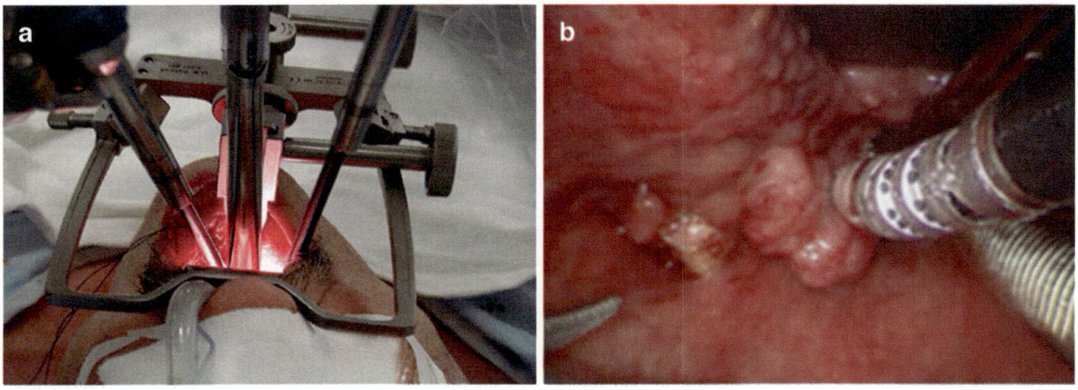

Fig. 13.2 (**a**) Setup for transoral robotic surgery. (**b**) Intraoperative image of transoral robotic resection of left base of tongue tumor

has comparable cure rates with significantly better quality of life metrics [21]. In a comparison of TOS and CRT, TOS did have higher rates of dysphagia, though this was not significant [22]. At this time, CRT is favored as the preferred method of treatment for OPSCC though there are still many questions yet to be answered about which treatment regimen is truly superior. One principal that most will agree on is that triple modality therapy (i.e. surgery with adjuvant CRT) is to be avoided, if possible. Each option has its advantages and disadvantages, and so the decision making process must be patient-centered. At this time, there are several ongoing studies examining cure rates and quality of life metrics for various treatment regimens. This ever-changing landscape and nuance in different regimens highlights the importance of the multidisciplinary care team as well as the vigilance of the participants in keeping up to date with the newest findings.

13.6.1 Management by Clinical Stage

- Definitive RT.
- P16/HPV- T1-2N0–1.
  - P16/HPV + T1-2N0 and T0-2N1 (single node ≤3 cm).
  - Definitive radiation treatment to the primary site, ipsilateral neck, and possibly the contralateral neck (consider for tumors of the tongue base, posterior pharynx, and soft palate).
- Resection of primary and neck dissection.
  - P16/HPV- T1-2N0–1 and T1-4aN0–3.
  - P16/HPV + T1-2N0–1, T0–3N3 or T4N0–3.
  - TOS: Eligible candidates may undergo TLM or TORS for resection of the primary tumor.
  - TOS is rarely a safe option for patients with T3-T4a disease. The majority of cases treated surgically are accessed via open approaches (transfacial and transcervical incisions).
  - Neck dissection: At least an ipsilateral neck dissection is performed. A contralateral neck dissection is considered for tumors of the tongue base, posterior pharynx, and soft palate.
  - Adjuvant RT/CRT may be required for adverse features on pathological analysis.
- Concurrent CRT.
- P16/HPV- T1-2N0–1 and T1-4aN0–3.
- P16/HPV + T0-2N0–1, T0–3N3 or T4N0–3.
- Cisplatin (cetuximab for patients unable to tolerate cisplatin) should be considered for N1 disease, in addition to definitive RT.
- Induction chemotherapy followed by RT or CRT.
- P16/HPV- T1-4aN0–3.
- P16/HPV+ T0-2N1 (single node >3 cm or 2 or more ipsilateral nodes ≤6 cm), T0–3N3 or T4N0–3.
- Unlike the previous options, there is significant disagreement about the propriety of this option. This option is typically considered for very complex cases.
- This option may be considered in the context of a clinical trial.

Top Five Takeaways

1. Distinct anatomic subsites with variations in etiology of OPSCC.
2. Evolving demographic secondary to HPV infections.
3. Role of panenodoscopy in diagnosis of both evident and occult primary lesions.
4. Despite de-intensification trials to reduce impact on QOL metrics, standard of care remains centred on concurrent CRT.
5. Importance of early detection and treatment.

References

1. Chaturvedi AK. A snapshot of the evolving epidemiology of oropharynx cancers. Cancers. 2018;124:2893–6. https://doi.org/10.1002/cncr.31383.
2. Megwalu UC. Oropharyngeal squamous cell carcinoma incidence and mortality trends in the United States, 1973–2013. Laryngoscope. 2018;128(7):1582–8. https://doi.org/10.1002/lary.26972.
3. Gillison ML, Koch WM, Capone RB, et al. Evidence for a causal association between human papillomavirus and a subset of head and neck cancers. J Natl Cancer Inst. 2000;92(9):709–20.

4. Van Dyne E, Henley S, Saraiya M, Thomas C, Markowitz L, Benard V. Trends in human papillomavirus–associated cancers—United States, 1999–2015. MMWR Morb Mortal Wkly Rep. 2018;67:918–24. https://doi.org/10.15585/mmwr.mm6733a2.
5. Cianchetti M, Mancuso AA, Amdur RJ, et al. Diagnostic evaluation of squamous cell carcinoma metastatic to cervical lymph nodes from an unknown head and neck primary site. Laryngoscope. 2009;119:2348–54. https://doi.org/10.1002/lary.20638.
6. Pawlita M, Fakhry C, Koch WM, Westra WH, Gillison ML. Ph D. Case–Control Study of Human Papillomavirus and Oropharyngeal Cancer. 2007.
7. Sullivan BO, Huang SH, Su J, et al. Development and validation of a staging system for HPV-related oropharyngeal cancer by the international collaboration on oropharyngeal cancer network for staging (ICON-S): a multicentre cohort study. Lancet Oncol. 2016;17(4):440–51. https://doi.org/10.1016/S1470-2045(15)00560-4.
8. Marks MA, Chaturvedi AK, Kelsey K, et al. Association of marijuana smoking with oropharyngeal and oral tongue cancers: pooled analysis from the INHANCE consortium. Cancer Epidemiol Biomarkers Prev. 2014;23:160–72. https://doi.org/10.1158/1055-9965.EPI-13-0181.
9. Demharter J, et al. Percutaneous core-needle biopsy of enlarged lymph nodes in the diagnosis and subclassification of malignant lymphomas. Eur Radiol. 2001;11(2):276–83.
10. Civantos FJ, et al. Metastatic squamous cell carcinoma to the cervical lymph nodes from an unknown primary cancer: management in the HPV era. Front Oncol. 2020;10:593164.
11. Maghami E, et al. Diagnosis and management of squamous cell carcinoma of unknown primary in the head and neck: ASCO guideline. J Clin Oncol. 2020;38(22):2570–96.
12. Rohde M, et al. Head-to-head comparison of chest X-ray/head and neck MRI, chest CT/head and neck MRI, and (18)F-FDG PET/CT for detection of distant metastases and synchronous cancer in oral, pharyngeal, and laryngeal cancer. J Nucl Med. 2017;58(12):1919–24.
13. Liu Y. FDG PET/CT for metastatic squamous cell carcinoma of unknown primary of the head and neck. Oral Oncol. 2019;92:46–51.
14. Turner L, Mupparapu M, Akintoye SO. Review of the complications associated with treatment of oropharyngeal cancer: a guide for the dental practitioner. Quintessence Int. 2013;44(3):267–79.
15. Kugaya A, et al. Prevalence, predictive factors, and screening for psychologic distress in patients with newly diagnosed head and neck cancer. Cancer. 2000;88(12):2817–23.
16. Neilson KA, et al. Psychological distress (depression and anxiety) in people with head and neck cancers. Med J Aust. 2010;193(S5):S48–51.
17. Kimple RJ, et al. Enhanced radiation sensitivity in HPV-positive head and neck cancer. Cancer Res. 2013;73(15):4791–800.
18. Fakhry C, et al. Improved survival of patients with human papillomavirus-positive head and neck squamous cell carcinoma in a prospective clinical trial. J Natl Cancer Inst. 2008;100(4):261–9.
19. Ferris RL, et al. Phase II randomized trial of transoral surgery and low-dose intensity modulated radiation therapy in resectable p16+ locally advanced oropharynx cancer: an ECOG-ACRIN cancer research group trial (E3311). J Clin Oncol. 2022;40(2):138–49.
20. Weinstein GS, et al. Understanding contraindications for transoral robotic surgery (TORS) for oropharyngeal cancer. Eur Arch Otorhinolaryngol. 2015;272(7):1551–2.
21. Ma DJ, et al. Phase II evaluation of aggressive dose De-escalation for adjuvant chemoradiotherapy in human papillomavirus-associated oropharynx squamous cell carcinoma. J Clin Oncol. 2019;37(22):1909–18.
22. Nichols AC, et al. Radiotherapy versus transoral robotic surgery and neck dissection for oropharyngeal squamous cell carcinoma (ORATOR): an open-label, phase 2, randomised trial. Lancet Oncol. 2019;20(10):1349–59.

The Larynx

14

Avital Fellner and Daniel Novakovic

14.1 Introduction

The Larynx is a complex-shaped organ located in the anterior part of the neck between the pharynx and the trachea. It extends vertically from C4 to C6 vertebral levels and is structurally comprised of 9 cartilages (3 unpaired and 3 paired) suspended in the anterior neck from the hyoid bone superiorly by way of ligaments and muscles.

The Larynx has four main functions:

- Transmission of gases between upper airways (nasopharynx and oropharynx) and lower airways (trachea, bronchi, and lungs).
- Protection of the lower airways from aspiration of potential harmful materials.
- Cough.
- Voice production.

A. Fellner
Voice Research Laboratory, Faculty of Medicine and Health, University of Sydney, Camperdown, NSW, Australia

Department of Otolaryngology-Head and Neck Surgery, Shamir (formerly Assaf Harofeh) Medical Center, Zerifin, Israel

Affiliated the Faculty of Medicine, Tel Aviv University, Tel Aviv, Israel

D. Novakovic (✉)
Voice Research Laboratory, Faculty of Medicine and Health, University of Sydney, Camperdown, NSW, Australia

Department of Otolaryngology, The Canterbury Hospital, Campsie, NSW, Australia

14.2 Laryngeal Anatomy

14.2.1 Cartilages of the Larynx

14.2.1.1 Unpaired Laryngeal Cartilages

There are three unpaired cartilages which form the main "skeleton" or framework of the larynx, the epiglottis, the thyroid cartilage, and the cricoid cartilage.

The *epiglottis* is a type of elastic cartilage, leaf-shaped, which is attached to the anterior aspect of the inner thyroid cartilage. This structure flattens and closes off the airway during swallowing to prevent aspiration.

The *thyroid cartilage* is the main (hyaline) cartilaginous structure of the larynx. Two thyroid lamina meet in the midline to form a shield-like structure with a triangular notch and bilateral superior and inferior horns, reminiscent to an open book. The (thyroid) angle between the laminae and dimensions of the cartilage differs between males and females. Among males, the average thyroid angle of the cartilage is 95 degrees and with vertical and antero-posterior dimensions usually larger and cartilage thicker in comparison to females which usually have an angle of 115 degree. Due to this angle, the anterior portion of the thyroid cartilage is often easily visible in men as the laryngeal prominence, also known as the 'Adam's apple'.

B. Ashford (ed.), *Head and Neck Surgery for General Surgeons*,
https://doi.org/10.1007/978-981-19-7900-2_14

The *cricoid* is a ring of hyaline cartilage that encircles the top of the trachea in a shape of a signet ring. It attaches to the inferior horns of the thyroid cartilage and articulates with the arytenoid cartilages via paired synovial cricothyroid and cricoarytenoid joints, respectively.

14.2.1.2 Paired Laryngeal Cartilages

The 3 paired sets of cartilages include the arytenoid, corniculate, and cuneiform complex.

The (hyaline) *arytenoid cartilages* are triangular pyramidal in shape with a base sitting on the cricoid cartilage and an apex which articulates with the corniculate cartilage. The anterior vocal process attaches to the vocal ligament and the lateral muscular process attaches to the intrinsic laryngeal muscles which act upon the arytenoid cartilage to move upon the cricoid cartilage affecting vocal fold movement and tension.

The *corniculate cartilages* are small elastic cone-shaped structures, which articulate with the apex of each arytenoid cartilage.

The small, elongated (elastic) *cuneiform cartilages* sit inside the aryepiglottic folds to help strengthen laryngeal structure.

14.2.2 Muscles of the Larynx

Muscles of the larynx are divided into two subgroups – extrinsic and intrinsic:

The *extrinsic laryngeal muscles* sit outside the larynx and are inserted to the only bony structure that supports the larynx from outside the hyoid bone which is strongly bound to the larynx via ligamentous attachments. They act to stabilize and vertically move the larynx. They are divided into the *suprahyoid muscles* (mylohyoid, stylohyoid, digastric, geniohyoid) which elevate the larynx and the *infrahyoid muscles* (omohyoid, thyrohyoid, sternohyoid, sternothyroid) which depress the larynx.

The *intrinsic laryngeal muscles* act on cartilages *within* the larynx. Collectively, these muscles help to control the shape, length, and tension of the vocal folds. They can be broadly divided into adductor and abductor muscle complexes (Fig. 14.1).

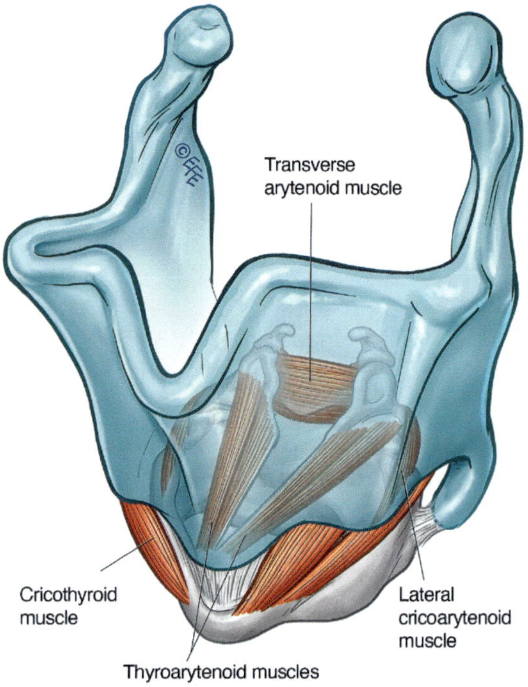

Fig. 14.1 Intrinsic muscles of the larynx—anterior view showing adductor muscles

The adductor muscle complex consists of the thyroarytenoid, lateral cricoarytenoid, transverse, and oblique arytenoid muscles which act to approximate the vocal folds and narrow the laryngeal inlet.

The posterior cricoarytenoid is the primary abductor of the larynx, acting on the arytenoid cartilages to separate and widen the laryngeal inlet. It has a critical role in respiration (Fig. 14.2).

The cricothyroid muscle acts to tile the thyroid cartilage forward on the cricoid, thus lengthening and tensioning the vocal fold and vocal ligament. It is also a weak adductor of the larynx and has separate innervation to the other intrinsic muscles (see below).

14.2.3 Laryngeal Innervation

Laryngeal Innervation is primarily via the superior laryngeal nerve and the recurrent laryngeal nerve, both originating from the inferior ganglion (ganglion nodosum) of the vagus nerve.

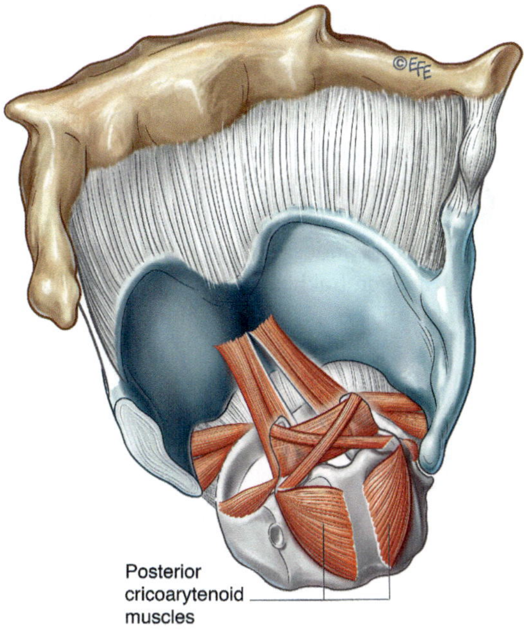

Fig. 14.2 Intrinsic muscle of the larynx—posterior view showing abductor muscles

They are at risk of damage during surgical procedures on or trauma to the neck and mediastinum.

The *superior laryngeal nerve* (SLN) after leaving the inferior ganglion of the vagus passes medial to the internal carotid artery and then divides at the level of the hyoid bone into two branches, external and internal. The *external branch of the superior laryngeal nerve* (EBSLN) contains motor fibres only and passes on the inferior constrictor muscle near the superior thyroid artery to innervate the cricothyroid muscle. It has an intimate relationship with the superior thyroid pedicle. There are two main classifications of this relationship, suggested by Cernea [1] and Friedman [2].

Cernea's describes three variations of the EBSLN in relation to the superior thyroid vessels: Type I EBSLN crosses the superior thyroid vessels at least 1 cm above the plane horizontal to the upper edge of the superior thyroid pole, Type IIa crosses less than 1 cm but above the plane, and type IIb passes less than 1 cm but below the plane of the upper edge of the superior thyroid pole [1, 3].

Friedman's classification is based upon the relationship between the nerve and inferior constrictor: Type I crosses superficial or lateral to the inferior constrictor with the superior thyroid vessels until terminating in the cricothyroid muscle. Type II penetrates the lower portion of the inferior constrictor and terminates in the cricothyroid muscle. Type III penetrates the superior portion of the inferior constrictor and terminates in the cricothyroid muscle [2, 3].

The *internal branch of the superior laryngeal nerve* (ibSLN) originates from the sensory nucleus of CN V, which supplies sensation to the mucosa of the larynx and the pharynx above the true vocal cord, including the epiglottis and the vallecula. It also carries fibres from the Nucleus Solitarius, supplying taste to the vallecula. After the SLN divides, the ibSLN passes alongside the superior laryngeal artery to enter the larynx by piercing the thyrohyoid membrane. The ibSLN provides the primary sensory supply to the larynx required for protective reflexes and coordination of swallowing.

The *recurrent laryngeal nerve* (RLN) is a mixed nerve supplying laryngeal sensation below the vocal folds including the upper oesophageal sphincter and upper trachea, via the sensory nucleus of the trigeminal nerve in the posterior part of the medulla. The motor part of the recurrent laryngeal nerve originates from the Nucleus Ambiguus and supplies all intrinsic muscles of the larynx except the cricothyroid. The nerve begins as part of the vagus nerve at the inferior (nodose) ganglion at the jugular foramen and descends in the carotid sheath towards the mediastinum, with a different trajectory between the right and the left sides of the body.

The right vagus passes anteriorly to the subclavian artery before giving off the RLN which continues posteromedially around the artery and continues superiorly to the larynx via the tracheoesophageal groove in around 65% of cases, but also can pass lateral to the trachea (33% of cases), and rarely anterolateral. Its length is approximately 6 cm [3].

The left RLN leaves the vagus as it passes over the aorta to loop posteromedially under the aorta then continues superiorly towards the larynx via the tracheoesophageal groove (77% of cases), or lateral to the trachea (22%) and rarely anterolateral to the trachea. It is usually twice as long (12 cm), when compared to the right RLN. The nerve branches external to the larynx in 40% of cases within 5 mm of the cricoid cartilage [3].

Both right and left RLN run in or near the tracheoesophageal groove posterior to the thyroid gland, entering the larynx posterior to the cricothyroid joint.

Non-recurrent laryngeal nerve is a rare anatomic variant occurring in around 0.52% of cases [4], more commonly on the right side, with no functional effect but of great importance during thyroid surgery. It passes in a horizontal manner from the vagus nerve in the neck to the area of the cricoarytenoid joint without mediastinal descent. It usually accompanies vascular anomalies of the aorta or subclavian arteries such as situs inversus viscerum [5]. When the RLN cannot be identified at the area of the tracheoesophageal groove, a non-recurrent laryngeal nerve should be sought.

14.2.4 Laryngeal Blood Supply

Laryngeal blood supply is primarily by branches of the external carotid artery and the subclavian artery.

The superior thyroid artery is a branch of the external carotid artery and gives rise to the *superior laryngeal artery*, which enters the larynx together with, immediately inferior to the internal branch of the superior laryngeal nerve, via the thyrohyoid membrane.

The thyrocervical trunk is a branch of the subclavian artery which gives rise to the *inferior thyroid artery* (ITA) and inferior laryngeal artery. The ITA enters the larynx accompanied by the recurrent laryngeal nerve at the inferior border of the inferior constrictor muscle.

Within the larynx, there is a rich vascular anastomosis between the superior and inferior systems. The laryngeal veins run parallel to the arteries with similar names and drain into the internal jugular and subclavian systems.

14.2.5 Laryngeal Lymphatics

The lymphatic drainage of the larynx is divided into three parts. The superior lymphatics accompany the superior thyroid vessels. Similarly, the inferior laryngeal lymphatics accompany the inferior thyroid vessels, both draining to deep cervical lymph nodes. Lymph nodes in the prelaryngeal and pretracheal drain some lymphatics that pierce the cricothyroid membrane.

14.2.6 Mucosal Structures of the Larynx

The mucosal structures of the larynx include the false vocal folds, the ventricles, and the true vocal folds. The true vocal folds have a unique five layer structure giving them their unique vibratory ability. The thyroarytenoid muscle is the deepest layer of the vocal fold. Medial to this, the intermediate and deep layers of the lamina propria contain elastin and collagen to create the vocal ligament. The superficial layer of the lamina propria, also called Reinke's space, contains loose fibrous tissue and gelatinase matrix. The epithelium is comprised of non-keratinizing stratified squamous epithelium.

14.3 Laryngeal Physiology

The vocal folds are a V-shaped structure attached anteriorly to the inner border of the thyroid cartilage and posteriorly to the vocal process of the arytenoid cartilage by the vocal ligament. They open (abduct) to let air pass and close (adduct) to protect the airway and produce cough and phonation.

Normal physiological functions require a complex interplay of nerves and muscles in the larynx coordinated in the brainstem by task-specific subgroups.

The pharyngeal phase of swallow is reflexive during which the suprahyoid muscles act to elevate the larynx and move it anteriorly thus opening the upper oesophageal sphincter. This creates inversion of the epiglottis to cover the laryngeal inlet and at the same time the intrinsic laryngeal muscles act to adduct the vocal folds to prevent aspiration of food bolus or liquids. Disruption of supraglottic sensation or laryngeal adduction can cause impaired swallowing (dysphagia) or aspiration.

Normal respiration is characterized by well-defined phasic laryngeal movements. During inspiration, the larynx lowers and a burst of neural activity via the RLN causes abduction of the arytenoid cartilages via the PCA muscle and widening of the glottic aperture to allow air entry. On expiration, there is slight vocal fold adduction.

Several important factors are required for normal voice production (phonation).

Glottal closure—The vocal folds must meet in the midline, relying on the adductor action of the RLNs which also control vocal fold tension.

Mucosal wave vibration–Subglottic air passes through the closed glottis making the vocal folds vibrate. This relies on the pliability of the mucosa overlying the vocal ligament, specifically the superficial layer of the lamina propria (SLLP) also called Reinke's space.

Furthermore, the SLN lengthens and tightens the vocal ligament causing pitch elevation via action of the cricothyroid muscle.

The degree and pattern of glottal closure are dependent on intrinsic muscle balance or postures which will affect perceived voice quality.

14.4 Clinical Voice Assessment

History gives important clues to the dysphonic patient. Details regarding the duration and onset of the complaint as well as any preceding events such as upper respiratory tract infection, intubation, surgical procedures (especially on the head, neck, or chest), or preceding phonotrauma such as loud shouting may give clues to potential causes of acute onset events.

Where the onset is more gradual and progressive, mucosal lesions and hyperfunctional voice disorders (especially in professional voice users) should be considered.

Alcohol and tobacco consumption are major risk factors for laryngeal cancer, and these as well as age and red flag symptoms such as haemoptysis and neck lumps must be considered.

Phonatory dyspnoea (running out of air when talking), vocal fatigue, and decreased projection as well as pitch disturbances are commonly reported symptoms in addition to perceptual voice changes.

Patient-reported outcome measures (PROMs) of laryngeal and voice function are a cheap and invaluable screening tool. One commonly used instrument is the "Voice Handicap Index 10" questionnaire (VHI-10), which is a validated assessment tool for people with voice problems [6]. A score of above 11 in this questionnaire is considered abnormal voice (maximal score is 40).

Perceptual evaluation of the voice should be performed during the consultation listening for features such as roughness, breathiness, weakness, and strain during conversation along with basic vocal tasks such as counting from one to ten and calling out loud to assess projection. Gliding from low to high on an /i/ is useful for assessing pitch range. Maximal phonation time is a useful clinical measure of glottal insufficiency where the patient is asked to phonate on an /ah/ for as long as possible. A maximal phonation time less than normal (between 20–23 s [7]) may indicate incomplete glottal closure.

14.5 Examination of the Larynx

Indirect laryngoscopy allows office-based visualization of laryngeal structure and function and can be performed by several methods.

1. Transoral mirror examination is a cheap and basic tool that can give information regarding gross vocal fold mobility, making this a useful screening tool. The technique of using a laryngeal mirror requires a headlight and some training.
2. Transnasal flexible laryngoscopy (TFL) using a constant light source is the most common technique for visualization of the larynx, allowing examination of entire upper aero-digestive tract including nasal cavity, nasopharynx, oro-

pharynx, hypopharynx, larynx, and upper trachea in a simple and well-tolerated fashion in an office-based setting. It facilitates accurate assessment of vocal fold structure including masses or mucosal lesions. Vocal fold range of movement and closure can be assessed by asking the patient to say /i/ and then sniff repeatedly several times. Vocal fold immobility is easily recognizable, but hypomobility or asymmetry is more subtle and may give clue to a paresis (partial neurological weakness). Hyperfunctional behaviours can be identified on vocal tasks such as connected speech.
3. Laryngeal Stroboscopy is an advanced endoscopic system that generates an apparent slow-motion view of vocal fold vibration by selectively capturing consecutive phases across successive vibratory cycles, by using short lasting light flashes to illuminate vocal folds at various frequencies. This technique allows evaluation of vocal fold vibration which can unmask subtle vocal fold pathologies, such as vocal fold paresis and scar which could be easily missed by using constant light laryngoscopy. This form of evaluation by Otolaryngologists requires specific equipment and is available in specialized settings.

14.6 Common Laryngeal Pathologies

Laryngeal pathologies include a very wide range of pathologies, but at least one of two physiological concepts are basically interrupted due to those pathologies: the vocal fold closure and the vocal folds' mucosal wave. Laryngeal pathologies can be broadly divided into four main groups: neurological, neoplastic, non-neoplastic mucosal lesions, and functional voice problems.

14.6.1 Neurological Conditions Affecting the Larynx

A wide range of central and peripheral neurological conditions can affect the voice and other laryngeal functions. Vocal fold palsy related to recurrent or superior laryngeal nerve injury is the most common of these and is discussed separately below. Parkinson's disease, essential tremor, and spasmodic dysphonia are common movement disorders presenting with characteristic weak, tremulous, or strained voice quality, respectively. Neurodegenerative disorders such as Amyotrophic lateral sclerosis (ALS) can manifest with voice or swallow changes that precede other symptoms. Other neurological conditions that can affect voice function include cerebrovascular accident, Myasthenia gravis, and multiple sclerosis.

14.6.2 Laryngeal Neoplasms

The squamous mucosa of the larynx can give rise to both benign and malignant neoplasms.

Recurrent Respiratory Papillomatosis (RRP) is a benign proliferation of squamous epithelium in the larynx and vocal folds causing dysphonia with potential to spread into the distal airway. It occurs secondary to infection with HPV 6 or 11 and typically recurs after treatment with a protracted disease course over time.

Leukoplakia represents a whitish lesion or plaque on the vocal fold and warrants investigation as it may indicate malignant or premalignant lesion **Dysplasia** is a premalignant lesion of laryngeal epithelium which is now categorized into high grade or low grade.

Squamous cell carcinoma is the most common malignancy of the larynx, with a wide range of clinical appearances including mucosal thickening, irregularity, ulceration, or impairment of vocal fold mobility.

14.6.3 Non-neoplastic Mucosal Lesions

Vocal fold inflammation (laryngitis) secondary to viral infection is the most common cause of acute dysphonia and is generally self-resolving.Other common mucosal pathologies include vocal fold nodules, which are bilateral mid vocal fold phonotraumatic lesions; vocal fold polyps, polypoid corditis (Reinke's oedema), submucosal cysts, and vocal cord vascular lesions and haemorrhages. Vocal fold granulomas are a hypertrophic inflammatory lesion which usually arise posteriorly from the vocal process or arytenoid cartilage rather than the membranous area and are generally related to laryngopharyngeal reflux. Many other inflammatory conditions can also affect the larynx including fungal laryngitis and autoimmune disorders.

14.6.4 Functional Voice Disorders

Represent dysphonia without any obvious underlying structural or neurological pathology. Primary muscle tension voice disorders are common and represent a hyperfunctional pattern of usage characterized by excessive and inappropriate laryngeal and neck muscle tension [8] causing disturbances in voice quality and pain on phonation. Psychogenic voice disorders (now referred to as functional neurological disorders) also fall into this category presenting with acute aphonia.

14.7 Vocal Fold Palsy

Represents absent (paralysis) or reduced (paresis) vocal fold mobility secondary to neurological weakness affecting the recurrent laryngeal nerves (or superior laryngeal nerves).

Unilateral vocal fold paralysis presents with signs of glottal insufficiency. Typically, patients have a weak and breathy voice with ineffectual cough, inability to perform Valsalva, and severely reduced maximal phonation time. Aspiration of liquids or saliva into the lungs may also occur in some cases and should prompt immediate intervention to reduce the risk of pneumonia.

Vocal fold paresis is a partial neurological weakness which causes a reduced vocal fold mobility. The effect of this impairment is usually very subtle. Moreover, unilateral vocal fold paresis could be asymptomatic. In some cases, the patients complain regarding vocal fatigue or a mild change in voice quality, volume, and projection difficulties, but could present with the same clinical picture as vocal cord paralysis as well.

Bilateral vocal fold palsy typically presents with airway compromise rather than dysphonia. It could cause life-threatening respiratory distress, with dyspnoea and stridor, aspiration due to loss of sensation innervated by the RLN, but also present with only mild hoarseness and cough while drinking fluids, if the vocal fold is in paramedian position. In cases of bilateral RLN injury with respiratory distress—urgent tracheostomy is often needed.

Superior laryngeal nerve injury—external branch superior laryngeal nerve injury could cause problems with volume and projection and also affect pitch range, with a limited high pitch range. Internal branch superior laryngeal injury could cause laryngeal sensation alternation and aspiration.

Vocal fold palsy usually represents LMN pathology with a variety of potential causes including viral infection and local pressure due to neoplasm along the route of the nerve/s or iatrogenic injury.

Malignancy accounts for 17–32% of vocal fold paralysis cases [9, 10] and represents pressure on or direct invasion into the vagus nerve or its recurrent laryngeal nerve branch. Careful clinical examination and imaging along the course of the recurrent laryngeal nerve from skull base to mediastinum is thus imperative where vocal fold paralysis is identified.

Iatrogenic injuries to the laryngeal nerves are considered to account for 30–40% [9, 10] of vocal fold palsies.

Iatrogenic injuries of the larynx and its related nerves include a wide range of surgery which could cause a transient or permanent laryngeal nerve injuries, neck surgeries, such as thyroid, parathyroid resections, cervical esophagostomies, carotid endarterectomies, and orthopaedic anterior approach cervical spine surgeries.

RLN injury due to intubation—RLN injury secondary to tracheal intubation, is a rare complication (less than 1%) in short-term intubation. There are few assumptions regarding the mechanism, which were not proved. Local pressure of the endotracheal tube or the cuff could cause local ischemia and RLN neuropraxia, usually unilateral. The differential diagnosis in those cases is dislocation or subluxation of the crico-arytenoid joint. Older age, longer intubation, and vascular comorbidities are risk factors for this entity [11].

Idiopathic vocal fold hypomobility and immobility is thought to be related to viral infection of the laryngeal nerves, is diagnosed after exclusion of other causes, and is accounted for 10–27% [9, 10] of vocal fold palsies. It may affect a single or multiple nerves, such as other cranial nerves as well.

14.8 Laryngeal Dysfunction in Thyroid Disease

14.8.1 Thyroid Pathology Affecting the Larynx

Hypothyroidism could lead to gradually progressive hoarseness and easily fatigued raspy voice, which is suspected to be related to myxedematous thickening of the vocal cord [12].

Hyperthyroidism, on the other hand, usually does not have a direct effect on voice, although local pressure on RLN, secondary to thyroid gland enlargement, could cause vocal cord palsy. Also, rare cases of hoarseness secondary to stuttering movement of the vocal cords have also been described [13].

Thyroid carcinoma can also invade the recurrent laryngeal nerve and cause dysphonia (paresis or paralysis). The chances of RLN invasion increase when the thyroid carcinoma invades the tracheoesophageal groove, there is a gross extra thyroid extension or pathologic T4 tumours, and also with aggressive histopathology tumour and positive central neck nodes [14]. Local compression on the RLN or displacement of its natural position, which both lead to vocal cord paresis, could be seen also in non-malignant pathologies such as extensive goitre as well as malignancies. Invasion to trachea and thyroid cartilage can be seen in very advanced cases and aggressive histologic variants, such as anaplastic thyroid carcinoma.

14.8.2 Laryngeal Dysfunction After Thyroid Surgery

Overview statement about incidence of voice change in thyroidectomy.

The RLN is highly prone to injuries in a vast range and visualizing intact nerve during surgery is not a guarantee for nerve preservation, since any manipulation around the nerve can cause some damage, from traction, stretch, damage secondary to heat in the surgical field, or nerve resection or sacrifice. All those surgical manipulations could cause paresis or paralysis, in most of the cases temporary, but in some permanent.

Unilateral RLN injury - Transient RLN injury is reported in 1–30% of patients in the literature [15–17] and the recovery time is usually between 4 and 6 weeks but can last 12 months. RLN injury which persists more than 12 months is considered permanent. The rate of permanent RLN damage is between 0.5% and 5% in the literature. Mau and colleagues presented a model that predicts that 86% of patients with UVFP who could be recovered will recover within 6 months, with 96% recovering within 9 months. They also showed that earlier vocal recovery is associated with younger age and the recovery of vocal fold movement [18].

Bilateral RLN injury—bilateral RLN injury post-thyroidectomy and was reported in 0.58% of cases [5, 19]. It could cause life-threatening respiratory distress, with dyspnea and stridor, aspirations due to loss of sensation innervated by the RLN, but also could be only be presented with mild hoarseness and cough while drinking fluids, if the vocal fold is in paramedian position. Most reported cases of bilateral RLN injury are temporal [20].

14.9 Treatment Options and Recovery Outcomes of RLN and SLN Injuries

14.9.1 Recovery Outcomes

The likelihood and timing of spontaneous neurological recovery after RLN and SLN injury depends upon the degree of nerve injury and the distance from the injury to the larynx.

Neuropraxia represents a lower grade injury where the axon is still intact and functional with high chance of recovery of purposeful vocal fold movement within 6–8 weeks.

Axonotmesis represents disruption of the axonal fibres, but the nerve pathway remains intact. Wallerian degeneration and then reinnervation may occur along the nerve sheath and may take up to 6 months. Recovery of voice function may occur in the absence of purposeful movement returning as the adductor and abductor fibres are crossed during the reinnervation which will restore some muscle tone.

Neurotmesis represents complete disruption of the nerve bundle. Recovery will be incomplete and permanent surgical procedures to restore laryngeal function should be considered at an earlier stage.

Treatment of laryngeal dysfunction after RLN injury depends upon the severity of patient symptoms and the likelihood of neurological recovery. Aspiration is an absolute indication for early intervention. Patient-reported outcome measures of voice and swallow offer the best way to assess the impact of the vocal fold weakness upon the patient and treatment is indicated where these are elevated or where vocal demands are not being met by the persons' vocal capabilities

14.9.2 Speech and Language Pathologist (SLP)

Speech and Language Pathologist (SLP) assessment and management can promote rehabilitation of the consequences of nerve injuries, approaching voice, swallowing, and effective cough. The SLP can give the patient tools to evaluate and minimize the risk of aspiration during eating and drinking. They can also help the patient's voice work around the functional limitations of vocal fold palsy and prevent hyperfunctional compensatory behaviours, which could lead to further damage.

14.9.3 Medical Therapy

Medical therapy: Nimodipine, a calcium channel blocker originally used for hypertension and vasospasm, may improve recurrent laryngeal nerve injury recovery after thyroidectomy, apparently due to its ability to reduce cellular apoptosis in injured nerves and to promote nodes of Ranvier's axonal sprouting [21, 22]. The use of Nimodipine for this indication is off label since high-quality evidence is still lacking. Adverse effects may include drowsiness and dizziness, due to its hypotensive effects [23].

14.9.4 Surgical Intervention

In the case of bilateral RLN injury, airway tends to be more affected than voice and surgical procedures to restore adequate airway (such as tracheostomy or endoscopic airway procedure) may need to be considered.

Surgical treatments after unilateral RLN injury are generally directed at bringing the affected vocal fold towards the midline allowing the contralateral vocal fold to meet it and improving glottal closure. These procedures are generally divided into short-term (temporary) or long-term (permanent) procedures and are employed based upon the likelihood of spontaneous recovery.

Injection laryngoplasty with a biocompatible resorbable gel should be considered where recovery of RLN function is likely or possible. Hyaluronic acid gel products which have a 3–6-month duration of effect before resorption are typically used for this purpose. This procedure can be performed under general anaesthesia via direct laryngoscopy, although it can also be done as a minimally invasive office-based procedure in the hands of an appropriately trained ENT surgeon. There is evidence that early injection laryngoplasty improves functional outcomes and patient-related quality of life as well as decreases the need for more permanent surgery in the longer term [24].

Where recovery of RLN function is unlikely—e.g. complete nerve transection or >6 months since injury, permanent surgical procedures should be considered to restore glottal closure. Laryngeal framework surgery (Type I thyroplasty) is the gold standard for such voice rehabilitation and may be performed with an arytenoid adduction procedure where there is arytenoid instability and posterior glottal insufficiency [25].

There is increasing evidence for the role of laryngeal reinnervation as a treatment for persistent vocal fold paralysis especially in younger patients with an unstable arytenoid as this approach may help restore muscle tone [26, 27]. In the event where intraoperative nerve transection is recognized during thyroid surgery, direct nerve repair or non-selective reinnervation using a proximal branch of ansa cervicalis is recommended [28].

14.9.5 Superior Laryngeal Nerve Injury

Management of superior laryngeal nerve injury and dysfunction is less well defined. Speech pathology input is the mainstay while we wait for spontaneous recovery to occur. Surgical procedures to medialize and restore tension of the affected vocal fold may be useful in select patients.

14.10 Current American Thyroid Association (ATA) Guidelines for Voice Assessment

The most updated "American Thyroid Association Management Guidelines for Adult Patients with Thyroid Nodules and Differentiated Thyroid Cancer" [29] strongly recommends some form of voice assessment in every patient prior to thyroidectomy. A history of voice changes/problems should be sought as part of the preoperative assessment along with basic perceptual evaluation of the voice (Table 14.1).

Moreover, the ATA strongly recommended laryngeal exam in the following:

Table 14.1 Preoperative factors which may be associated with laryngeal nerve dysfunction (Haugen et al., ATA Thyroid nodule/DTC guidelines, table 9) [29]

Factor	Symptoms/signs
History	Voice abnormality, dysphagia, airway symptoms, hemoptysis, pain, rapid progression, prior operation in neck or upper chest
Physical exam	Extensive, firm mass fixed to the larynx or trachea
Imaging	Mass extending to/beyond periphery of thyroid lobe posteriorly and/or tracheoesophageal infiltration, or bulky cervical adenopathy along the course of the RLN or vagus nerve

- All patient with preoperative voice abnormalities.
- History of cervical or upper chest surgery, which places the RLN or vagus nerve at risk.
- Known thyroid cancer with posterior extrathyroidal extension or extensive central nodal metastases.

A normal sounding voice does not exclude unilateral vocal cord palsy which can be asymptomatic especially in the case of an old, compensated neural injury. In these cases, damage to the contralateral nerve pathways during thyroid surgery affecting mobility of the healthy vocal fold can result in airway compromise. Identification of pre-existing vocal fold palsy by pre-operative laryngoscopy may alter the surgical approach.

According to the ATA guideline, visual identification of the RLN is required in all cases during thyroid surgery. It is also recommended to actively preserve the external branch of the superior laryngeal nerve during the dissection of the superior pole of the thyroid gland. If the EBSLN could not be identified, the recommendation is to stay close to the thyroid capsule at the superior pole and skeletonize the superior vascular pedicle to decrease the risk of damaging this nerve.

The use of neural stimulation with or without nerve monitoring is only a weak recommendation due to low quality literature evidence. However, the use of intraoperative nerve monitoring is the standard of care for many surgeons and is highly popular due to emerging evidence regarding protective effect from RLN injuries during thyroidectomies [30].

Postoperative voice assessment for all patients is also strongly recommended, as well as formal laryngeal examination if the voice is abnormal. There is evolving evidence for the use of translaryngeal ultrasound in evaluating vocal fold mobility following thyroid surgery [31].

It is important to acknowledge that subtle voice change is common following thyroid surgery and may not be reported by the patient in the early post-operative period. Dysphonia may present as difficulty meeting increasing vocal demands as the patient returns to normal activities. Specialist Otolaryngology assessment of voice function should be sought in these cases.

Top Five Takeaways

1. The Larynx has 4 main functions: transmission of gases between upper and lower airways, protection of the lower airways, cough and voice production.
2. The superior laryngeal nerve and the recurrent laryngeal nerve, both originating from the vagus nerve, innervate the larynx. Their anatomy is very variable bilaterally and between individuals. Familiarization with their routes is extremely important due to their high damage potential during surgical procedures.
3. Clinical voice assessment, including relevant history taking, performing simple vocal tasks, such as maximal phonation time, using PROMs and visualization, usually by transnasal flexible laryngoscopy, is important before thyroid surgeries. It is also highly recommended in some indications by the ATA guidelines.
4. The prevalence of unilateral RLN injuries after thyroid surgeries is between 1 and 30% of patients for transient and recoverable injuries (4–6 weeks).

   The rate of permanent RLN damage (persistent for more than 12 months) is between 0.5% and 5%. Bilateral nerve injury is rare. Ninety-six percent of the patients with UVFP would recover within 9 months.
5. Treatment options for iatrogenic nerve injuries include Nifedipine, SLP assessment and treatment (compensation strategies), short-term surgical intervention such as injection laryngoplasties with biocompatible resorbable gels, or permanent procedures such as type 1 thyroplasty and laryngeal reinnervation.

References

1. Cernea CR, et al. Surgical anatomy of the external branch of the superior laryngeal nerve. Head Neck. 1992;14(5):380–3.
2. Friedman M, LoSavio P, Ibrahim H. Superior laryngeal nerve identification and preservation in thyroidectomy. Arch Otolaryngol Head Neck Surg. 2002;128(3):296–303.
3. Bailey D, Goldenberg D. Surgical anatomy of the larynx. Oper Tech Otolaryngol Head Neck Surg. 2019;30(4):232–6.
4. Henry JF, et al. The nonrecurrent inferior laryngeal nerve: review of 33 cases, including two on the left side. Surgery. 1988;104(6):977–84.
5. Sadiq Z, et al. Non-recurrent laryngeal nerve in thyroid surgery–an important lesson. Br J Oral Maxillofac Surg. 2011;49:S93.
6. Rosen CA, et al. Development and validation of the voice handicap index-10. Laryngoscope. 2004;114(9):1549–56.
7. Maslan J, et al. Maximum phonation time in healthy older adults. J Voice. 2011;25(6):709–13.
8. Andrea M, et al. Functional voice disorders: the importance of the psychologist in clinical voice assessment. J Voice. 2017;31(4):507.e13–22.
9. Myssiorek D. Recurrent laryngeal nerve paralysis: anatomy and etiology. Otolaryngol Clin North Am. 2004;37(1):25–44. v
10. Gowd A, et al. Indications for direct laryngoscopic examination of vocal cord function prior to anterior cervical surgery. Geriatr Orthop Surg Rehabil. 2017;8(1):54–63.
11. Kikura M, et al. Age and comorbidity as risk factors for vocal cord paralysis associated with tracheal intubation. Br J Anaesth. 2007;98(4):524–30.
12. Altman KW, et al. Identification of thyroid hormone receptors in the human larynx. Laryngoscope. 2003;113(11):1931–4.
13. Hari Kumar KV, et al. Voice and endocrinology. Indian J Endocrinol Metab. 2016;20(5):590–4.
14. Nayyar SS, et al. Risk factors predisposing for recurrent laryngeal nerve palsy following thyroid malignancy surgery: experience from a tertiary oncology centre. Eur Arch Otorhinolaryngol. 2020;277(4):1199–204.

15. Rosato L, et al. Recurrent laryngeal nerve damage and phonetic modifications after total thyroidectomy: surgical malpractice only or predictable sequence? World J Surg. 2005;29(6):780–4.
16. Bergenfelz A, et al. Complications to thyroid surgery: results as reported in a database from a multicenter audit comprising 3660 patients. Langenbecks Arch Surg. 2008;393(5):667–73.
17. Jeannon JP, et al. Diagnosis of recurrent laryngeal nerve palsy after thyroidectomy: a systematic review. Int J Clin Pract. 2009;63(4):624–9.
18. Mau T, Pan HM, Childs LF. The natural history of recoverable vocal fold paralysis: implications for kinetics of reinnervation. Laryngoscope. 2017;127(11):2585–90.
19. Zakaria HM, et al. Recurrent laryngeal nerve injury in thyroid surgery. Oman Med J. 2011;26(1):34.
20. Misron K, et al. Bilateral vocal cord palsy post thyroidectomy: lessons learnt. BMJ Case Rep. 2014;2014:bcr2013201033.
21. Mattsson P, et al. Nimodipine promotes regeneration and functional recovery after intracranial facial nerve crush. J Comp Neurol. 2001;437(1):106–17.
22. Rosen CA, et al. Prospective investigation of nimodipine for acute vocal fold paralysis. Muscle Nerve. 2014;50(1):114–8.
23. Lin RJ, Klein-Fedyshin M, Rosen CA. Nimodipine improves vocal fold and facial motion recovery after injury: A systematic review and meta-analysis. Laryngoscope. 2019;129(4):943–51.
24. Vila PM, Bhatt NK, Paniello RC. Early-injection laryngoplasty may lower risk of thyroplasty: A systematic review and meta-analysis. Laryngoscope. 2018;128(4):935–40.
25. Isshiki N, Tanabe M, Sawada M. Arytenoid adduction for unilateral vocal cord paralysis. Arch Otolaryngol. 1978;104(10):555–8.
26. Aynehchi BB, McCoul ED, Sundaram K. Systematic review of laryngeal reinnervation techniques. Otolaryngol Head Neck Surg. 2010;143(6):749–59.
27. Blumin JH, Merati AL. Laryngeal reinnervation with nerve-nerve anastomosis versus laryngeal framework surgery alone: a comparison of safety. Otolaryngol Head Neck Surg. 2008;138(2):217–20.
28. Lee WT, et al. Results of ansa to recurrent laryngeal nerve reinnervation. Otolaryngol Head Neck Surg. 2007;136(3):450–4.
29. Haugen BR, et al. 2015 American Thyroid Association management guidelines for adult patients with thyroid nodules and differentiated thyroid cancer: the American Thyroid Association guidelines task force on thyroid nodules and differentiated thyroid cancer. Thyroid. 2016;26(1):1–133.
30. Bai B, Chen W. Protective effects of intraoperative nerve monitoring (IONM) for recurrent laryngeal nerve injury in thyroidectomy: meta-analysis. Sci Rep. 2018;8(1):1–11.
31. Phung D, et al. Translaryngeal ultrasound in thyroid surgery: state of the art review. ANZ J Surg. 2022;92(3):385–9.

Vascular Access and Control in Trauma of the Neck

15

Paul Ghaly, Jim Iliopoulos, and Mehtab Ahmad

15.1 Background

Given the anatomical complexity of the neck region, management of injuries here can be daunting as they occur in a relatively confined space and on occasion a head and neck or general surgeon may be caught unawares having been called upon to deal with vascular trauma. Such situations include incorrect pre-hospital triage of a patient with unrecognised cervical vessel trauma to a non-trauma unit, or in cases of iatrogenic injury in procedures performed for other reasons.

In comparison to other countries, the incidence of trauma-related vascular neck injuries in Australia remains low. Nevertheless, a sound basis of neck anatomy and familiarity with basic exposure and repair techniques is important for emergency treatment, especially in a rural setting where definitive sub-specialty expertise or endovascular treatments may not always be readily available and the clinical situation does not allow for patient transfer to a specialised service. The incidence of arterial injury within the neck in civilian trauma varies between regions, ranging between 12 and 17% and is associated with significant morbidity and mortality related directly to the injury or its sequelae (cerebral ischaemia, cranial nerve deficit) which may not always be apparent at the time of presentation [1].

Neck injuries have traditionally been classified by mechanism of injury, namely blunt trauma, penetrating trauma, and strangulation injury. In the context of arterial injury, strangulation often presents in a manner similar to blunt trauma and for the purposes of this chapter will be grouped together. No consensus international guidelines exist for the management of penetrating neck injuries with most of the available literature focused on the traditional zonal approach. Vascular injuries in the neck include complete or partial occlusion, transection, dissection, pseudoaneurysm, or arteriovenous fistula formation. The latter two are often late presentations of an injured vessel. Typically, vascular injuries in the neck predominately involve the carotid arteries (80%) and/or the vertebral arteries (43%) [2].

15.2 Zonal vs. No-zonal Presentation and Classification of Cervical Neck Trauma

First described in 1969 by Monson et al., the assessment and management of vascular cervical injuries has been traditionally tailored to a

P. Ghaly · J. Iliopoulos · M. Ahmad (✉)
Department of Vascular Surgery, Liverpool Hospital, SWSLHD, Liverpool, NSW, Australia
e-mail: Jim.Iliopoulos@health.nsw.gov.au; Mehtab.Ahmad@health.nsw.gov.au

B. Ashford (ed.), *Head and Neck Surgery for General Surgeons*,
https://doi.org/10.1007/978-981-19-7900-2_15

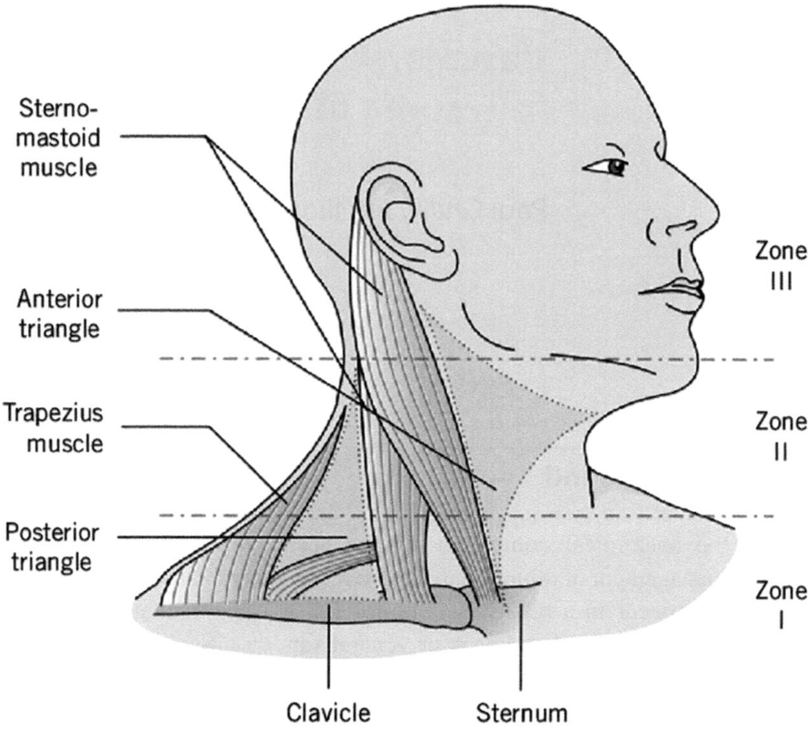

Fig. 15.1 Anatomical zones of the neck

zonal approach with the neck divided into thirds (Fig. 15.1). Zone I refers to the most caudal aspect of the neck, from the sternal notch and clavicles to the cricoid cartilage. Zone II continues cephalad from the cricoid cartilage to the angle of the mandible and Zone III refers to the most cephalad portion of the neck from the point above the angle of the mandible to the base of the skull [2, 3]. In cases of penetrating injuries, management principles differ depending on the injured zone, and traditionally, this approach has advocated surgical exploration of all presentations with surgical approach dictated by the zone injured as the risks of missing a critical injury were deemed to be high. This fear has not been borne out by the review literature however, where a traditional exploratory approach has been found to result in half of patients having no significant injury found [4]. A 'no zonal approach' where haemodynamically stable patients can be evaluated with radiographic studies in combination with trauma-protocol-driven serial examinations irrespective of the zone of injury is becoming increasingly popular with advancements in diagnostic and treatment modalities [5].

15.3 Vascular Head and Neck Anatomy

The head and neck region receives its blood supply from the carotid and vertebral arteries. The right common carotid artery (CCA) arises from the bifurcation of the brachiocephalic trunk which itself originates from the aortic arch. The left CCA arises directly from the aortic arch (Fig. 15.2). There are anatomical variants to this configuration, the most common of which (occurring in 8–25% of the general population) is the 'bovine arch' where the brachiocephalic trunk shares a common origin with the left CCA [6]. Travelling laterally to the trachea and the oesophagus (which courses posterior to the trachea), the CCA bifurcates into the internal and external carotid arteries (ICA and ECA, respectively) at the level of the fourth cervical vertebra. A surface landmark for this is between the hyoid

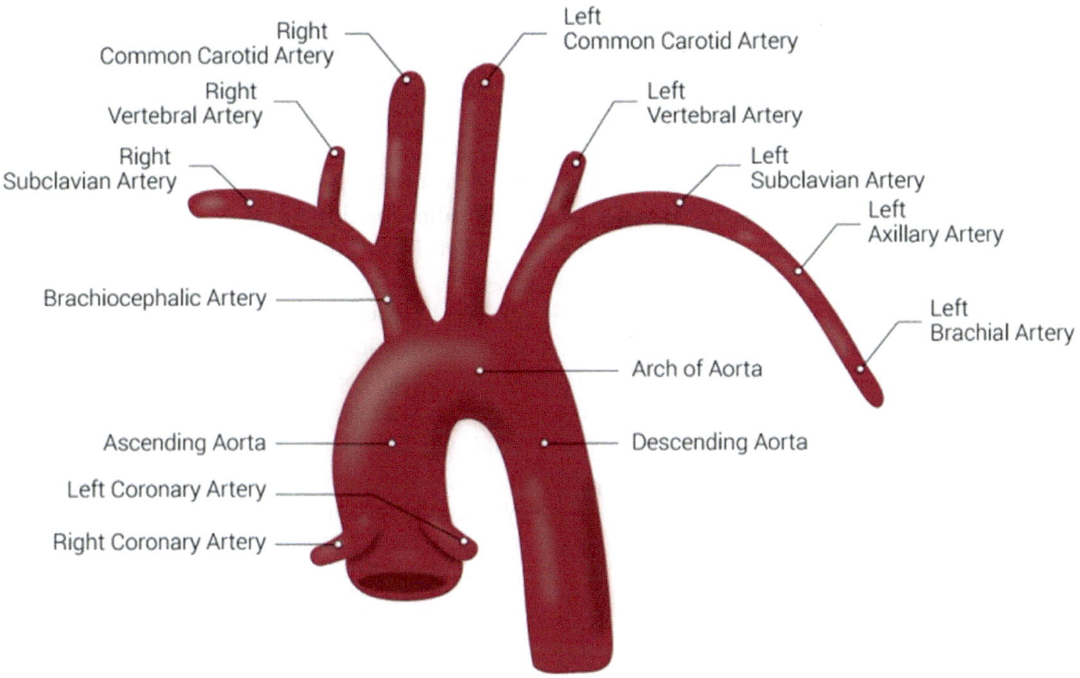

Fig. 15.2 Aortic arch and its anatomy

bone and thyroid cartilage. The normal configuration is for the external carotid artery to branch laterally; however, caution must be taken in the trauma setting, which may distort the usual anatomical orientation. In this setting, identifying the vessel with branches can be utilised as another landmark, as the internal carotid gives no branches in the neck while the superior thyroid artery (the first branch of the ECA) is commonly encountered at the level of the bifurcation extending antero-medially. The paired ICAs are the main bloody supply to the intra-cranial cavity where it bifurcates into the anterior and middle cerebral arteries at the Circle of Willis. The ECAs supply the extra-cranial structures of the head and neck via six-paired branches: superior thyroid artery, ascending pharyngeal artery, lingual artery, facial artery, occipital artery, and posterior auricular artery and terminates in the parotid gland where it divides into the maxillary artery and superficial temporal artery.

Each of the carotid arteries is encompassed in the carotid sheath, a derivative of all three layers of the deep cervical fascia. In many cases this sheath is often quite a nebulous structure and not clearly defined. The contents of the sheath include the internal jugular vein (IJV) and vagus nerve. The vein lies laterally, the CCA medially, and the vagus nerve in between and behind the two. Behind the vagus nerve lies the sympathetic trunk. A variable amount of deep cervical lymph nodes is also found here and can be safely excised to improve the view of the surgical field. At the upper margin of the sheath, the 9th–11th cranial nerves can be seen, with the hypoglossal an important landmark for the extent of a neck incision. It gives off the ansa cervicalis which innervates the infrahyoid muscles and has a variable course but is usually found lying anteriorly on the carotid artery. If needed, it can be readily divided to increase exposure.

15.4 Initial Assessment and History

The initial management of all neck vascular injuries is centred on Advanced Trauma Life Support (ATLS) principles. The exsanguinating patient experiences several physiological changes as a result of volume loss to include hypothermia, coagulopathy, and metabolic acidosis which in combination can be lethal and resuscitative measures should try to mitigate and reverse the effects of these. A quick and succinct history of the mechanism of injury (e.g. penetrating vs blunt), obvious injuries sustained, vital signs, and treatment received, is required. A more detailed patient history can be conducted once stability is achieved. Prompt examination of the neck is recommended. In urgent cases where patient instability from other injuries precludes time for formal assessment and imaging, infiltration of a short-acting local anaesthetic, e.g. 1% lignocaine, can be used within an emergency department (ED) setting for assessment of breach of the platysmal layer requiring mandatory exploration in theatre [2].

15.5 Clinical Examination

When faced with a penetrating neck injury, immediate consideration should be given to the airway. Two main immediate issues should be addressed: airway protection and cervical spine stabilisation or clearance. Approximately 8–11% of all penetrating neck injuries have associated airway compromise [2]. Cervical spine stabilisation is not routinely required for penetrating neck injuries, but is mandatory in cases of blunt force trauma (e.g. motor vehicle accidents). Additionally, careful examination for injury to the aerodigestive tract (oral, pharyngeal, laryngeal, or tracheal) should be conducted. Signs of aerodigestive tract injury include voice hoarseness, stridor, dyspnoea, subcutaneous emphysema, bubbling from the wound, and haemoptysis.

A collection of 'hard' signs have been determined to be an absolute indication for surgical exploration, bypassing any pre-operative imaging other than an ED chest X-ray to exclude the presence of a haemo/pneumothorax. Hard signs include [1–3, 5]:

- Decompensated haemodynamic shock.
- Pulsatile bleeding or expanding hematoma.
- Audible bruit or palpable thrill.
- Airway compromise.
- Bubbling from the wound.
- Subcutaneous emphysema.
- Stridor.
- Hoarseness.
- Swallowing difficulties.
- Neurological deficits.

The absence of hard signs does not exclude underlying injury and ultimately surgical exploration depends on the hemodynamic status of the patient. Other signs such as minor haemorrhage, mild hypotension, minor haemoptysis or hematemesis, non-expanding hematoma, dysphonia, or dysphagia are referred to as 'soft' signs and generally these patients can be taken for further imaging evaluation prior to transfer for operative intervention if indicated [1–3, 5].

If vascular injury in the neck is suspected, the traditional zonal approach is helpful to engaging the relevant surgical subspeciality.

Zone I vascular injuries may require cardiothoracic surgical input as haemorrhage control may require a sternotomy or thoracotomy for proximal control. Zone II arterial injuries require consultation with vascular surgeons as common or internal carotid arterial injuries may require repair during neck explorations. Surgical management of zone II injuries will be the focus of this chapter. Zone III injuries require neurosurgical or neurointerventional consultation as proximal and distal control may require access to the base of skull and intra-cranial portion of the carotid arteries [2].

Venous injuries are generally low risk and self-tamponade without major haemorrhage owing to the low-pressure nature of the venous system and can be controlled with basic haemorrhage control principles, i.e. pressure and elevation.

15.6 Investigations

The increase in advancements and accessibility of computed tomography with contrast angiography (CT-A) has led it to become the imaging modality of choice for the evaluation of trauma-related neck injuries, providing a high sensitivity (90%) and specificity (100%) for detecting vascular and other injuries in the neck [3]. Multiplanar reformatting software additionally allows for detailed assessment of structures and precise identification of extra- and intra-luminal injury. It is the authors' belief that CT-A is the investigation of choice in such cases due to the relative ease of image acquisition and reliability of results. Other options for the assessment of suspected vascular injuries in the neck include duplex ultrasound and magnetic resonance angiography (MR-A), but these are often not available and in the case of ultrasonography, are limited mostly to Zone 2 injuries in addition to pitfalls associated with inter-user variability. Conventional angiography may be required if metallic debris results in too much artefact obscuring the injury and should be considered in Zone III injuries where embolisation or stenting is anticipated [2, 3].

15.7 Surgical Management Including Risks

Vascular injuries in all zones of the neck can be difficult to manage due to complex anatomy in a relatively confined space. Additional injuries in the context of trauma can make clinical evaluation challenging and a high index of suspicion must also be raised for concomitant aerodigestive and cranial nerve damage when dealing with a vascular injury. Expectation for the need to repair additional anatomical structures lying adjacent to the vessels must be anticipated early in the treatment pathway and it is prudent to remember that injuries can often traverse more than one zone.

Appropriate, timely investigations in the form of non-invasive imaging (namely contrasted CT angiography [CTA] with reformatting of images) in sufficiently stable patients should be performed whenever possible prior to exploration. This is particularly important in suspected Zone 1 and 3 injuries where surgical access is most challenging and may require involvement of cardiac and neurosurgeons or endovascular techniques for definitive repair.

Advances in endovascular techniques mean a pure-endovascular or a combined hybrid approach is required, to control haemorrhage within Zones 1 and 3. Endovascular techniques can preclude the need for sternotomy in proximal pathology and base of skull dissection in distal lesions by use of Fogarty balloon catheters to control haemorrhage or covered stent graft deployment across an injured vessel. Vessels amenable to treatment by endovascular treatment include the distal ICA, subclavian, proximal common carotid, and vertebral arteries. An additional benefit of endovascular surgery is that it can often be performed under local anaesthesia, allowing for real-time assessment of a patient's neurological status in theatre.

15.8 Principles of Vascular Surgery in Cases of Penetrating Neck Trauma

As with all vascular procedures, the mainstay of surgical access is to gain proximal (inflow) and distal (outflow) control. In an emergency setting, focus should be on damage control techniques to stop haemorrhage and restore circulation. This is particularly challenging in cervical vascular trauma because familiar haemorrhage control techniques such as vessel ligation or embolisation can have serious implications (e.g.: cerebral ischaemia), particularly when dealing with injury to the (internal) carotid circulation.

In anticipation of vessel repair, skin preparation and draping should additionally allow access to the proximal thigh (for possible great saphenous venous conduit harvesting) and chest (if the need for a sternotomy arises). In cases where open surgical repair is required, Zone 1 injuries require proximal control in the chest, proximal and distal control for Zone 2 injuries is achieved within the neck, and although proximal control for Zone 3 injuries is in the neck, distal control requires access to the base of skull.

In cases where surgical expertise limits the potential for repair, temporary shunting can be

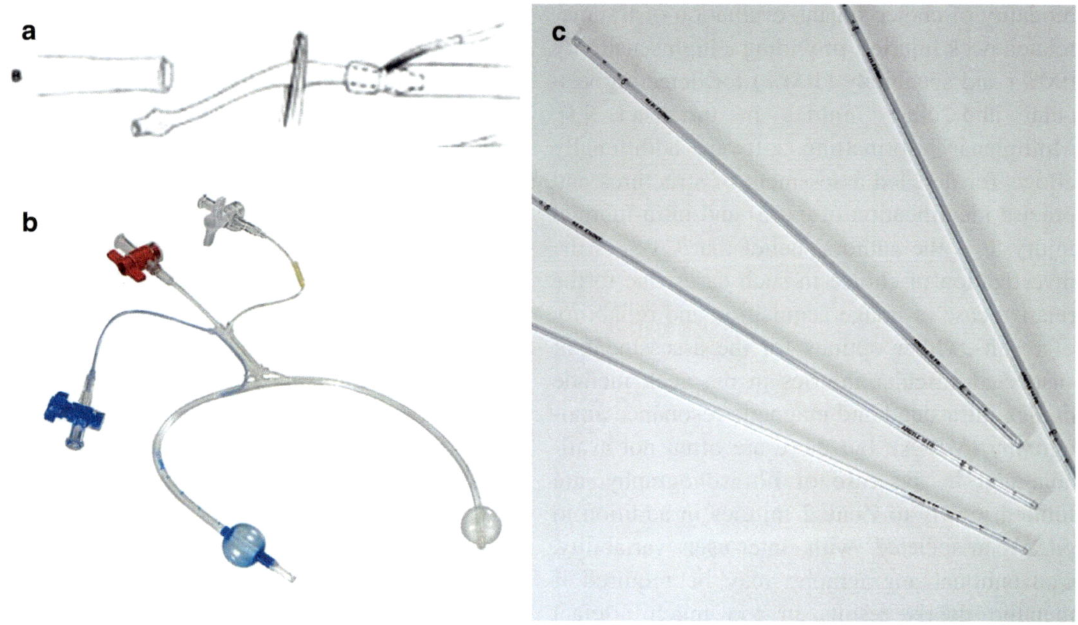

Fig. 15.3 Shunt types. (**a**) Javid® Shunt (Bard Peripheral Vascular Inc., Tempe, Ariz, USA). A long and tapered shunt with smooth tips. The ends are typically clamped following insertion. (**b**) Pruitt-Inihara® Shunt (Horizon Medical, Santa Ana, Calif, USA). A 3-way shunt in the form a T-shape with balloons at the tube ends. Balloons are inflated gently following insertion and gently fixed externally with a silastic sling. The T-port allows for removal of air and embolic particles as well as infusions and pressure monitoring. (**c**) Argyle® Shunt (Kendall Healthcare Products, Mansfield, Mass, USA). A typical carotid kit includes four sizes (8, 10, 12 and 14 Fr) with radiopaque markers for X-ray verification

used as a measure to stabilise a patient prior to transfer of care to a place where specialist vascular surgeons involvement can take place. Temporary vascular shunting (TVS) come in many forms, but the most commonly used ones include the Javid® (Bard Peripheral Vascular Inc., Tempe, Ariz, USA), Pruitt-Inihara® (Horizon Medical, Santa Ana, Calif, USA), Sundt® (Integra Plansboro, NJ, USA) or Argyle® (Kendall Healthcare Products, Mansfield, Mass, USA) tubular prosthesis (Fig. 15.3). Once proximal and distal control has been achieved, a Fogarty balloon catheter should be passed both ways to clear the lumen of any clot and flushed with heparinised saline (a solution comprised of 25,000 IU/L) and an approximately sized TVS inserted up to 2 cm both proximally and distally. The shunt is secured in place by tying two heavy gauge sutures externally to the proximal and distal insertion points. Shunt sizing should avoid mismatch as too large a shunt can cause excessive intimal damage, and too small a shunt is more likely to thrombose. Skin closure can be performed over the top while waiting for transfer to an appropriate service and the patient should be anticoagulated in the absence of contraindications until TVS removal [7].

15.9 Immediate Control of a Vascular Injury

Mortality from penetrating neck injuries in 50% of cases is the result of exsanguination [8]. Direct pressure can be used to control a situation but in cases of extremis where this is insufficient, emergency control with the use of a Foley balloon catheter can be used as a temporising measure ahead of definitive surgery. A large calibre catheter is passed into the projection tract of the injury prior to balloon inflation with >15 mL of water. The catheter is then pulled back until the balloon meets resistance prior to the catheter being clamped and the neck wound sutured tightly around it to provide tamponade control [2].

15.10 The Carotid Arteries

15.10.1 Zone 1 Exposure

Zone 1 injuries occur in 18% of penetrating neck trauma and proximal control is achieved in the chest either via a median sternotomy or anterolateral thoracotomy [9]. Endovascular techniques to attain proximal control can be performed via a femoral approach with deployment of a large compliant balloon or Fogarty balloon catheter. This is often a temporising adjunct while a sternotomy is performed to gain direct visual control of a vessel, at which point the catheter is exchanged for a direct clamp on the injured vessel.

15.10.2 Zone 2 Exposure

As Zone 2 is the most commonly injured area of the neck in trauma (occurring in 47% of cases), familiarity with exposure of the vessels here should be part of a head and neck surgeons' expertise [2, 9]. Due to the ease of access and ability to directly visualise the vessels, traditional teaching has suggested that penetrating injuries in Zone 2 should always be surgically explored, although this paradigm is changing in high-volume trauma centres where a 'no zonal' approach to managing neck trauma is the growing trend. This strategy, however, is best undertaken by those clinicians who regularly encounter such injuries and are confident in their expectant clinical examination and management skills [2].

Positioning: Standard operative setup for exploration of the neck vessels includes positioning the patient supine, with careful hyperextension of the neck in cases where the cervical spine has been cleared prior to surgery. This can be achieved using a 'split' table allowing elevation of the torso (reverse Trendelenburg) during dissection to decrease venous pressure, placing the head on a head-ring, with support (e.g.: using a gel pad or rolled towel) placed vertically between the shoulder blades. If unilateral access only is required, rotation of the head ≥45° allows easy access to the carotid artery. Nasotracheal intubation is useful as it allows better access, particularly in cases where there is a high carotid bifurcation.

Skin preparation: As a minimum, skin preparation and draping should leave the sternal notch, angle of the mandible, and inferior aspect of the pinna exposed, as surface landmarks.

Incision and dissection: Although there has been some debate in recent times about the type of incision (transverse vs. oblique), there is no documented difference in mortality or morbidity between groups [10, 11]. It is the authors' opinion that an oblique incision provides safe and easy access to all unilateral structures without the challenging limitations accessing a high carotid bifurcation from a transverse incision. For immediate bilateral access, a collar incision starting 2 cm above the sternal notch with extension obliquely up both sternocleidomastoids can be performed.

1. The skin is incised from 2 cm above the sternal notch along the anterior border of the sternocleidomastoid muscle (SCM) towards the mastoid process. At the level of the angle of the jaw, it should be curved posteriorly to avoid injury to the parotid gland.
2. The incision is deepened through skin and subcutaneous fat to the platysma, which is incised longitudinally in line with the incision. The greater auricular nerve (GAN) is encountered at the superior aspect of the incision, superficial to the platysma, and can be safely divided (patients are left with a numb earlobe post-operatively which often regresses with time). If encountered, the external jugular vein can also be ligated and divided. The SCM is then lifted from surrounding tissues along its length anteriorly.
3. The next structure encountered is the internal jugular vein, which lies laterally in the carotid sheath and dissection is continued in an ante-

jugular manner, which is the authors' preferred approach to the vessels*. Although venous tributaries in the neck can be variable, an important one is the common facial vein which is usually located at the level of (and serves as a landmark for) the carotid bifurcation. It, as with all venous tributaries in the neck, can be safely ligated and divided.

*A retro-jugular approach can be used, but most commonly in re-do surgery, where care must be taken not to injure the sympathetic trunk lying behind the vagus, or the accessory nerve in the upper margins of the incision.

4. As with all vascular procedures, the mainstay of vascular access is to gain proximal (inflow) and distal (outflow) control. Attention should thus turn to the common carotid artery at the base of the incision to gain proximal control. Surrounding tissue should carefully be dissected off the artery, which can be controlled by passing a Mixter or Lahey forceps behind the vessel and using a double-looped silastic string for control. Rough manipulation of the CCA and ICA can result in distal embolisation of plaque or clot resulting in intra-operative cerebrovascular accident.
5. Dissection should then continue along the anterior border of the CCA, leading to the bifurcation and the ECA. Just beyond the origin of the ECS, the STA is seen. Both can be controlled with double-looped silastic strings.
6. Dissection of the ICA should start distally, working back towards the bifurcation and control should be sought at a disease-free distal point with a single-looped silastic string clipped on either side to avoid unnecessarily tenting the artery up. It is the authors' view that more proximal dissection towards the carotid bulb should then take place after systemic heparinisation (50 iu/kg) even in cases of trauma unless other injuries preclude its administration. Bradycardia and hypotension may occur when dissecting around the carotid sinus, a baroreceptor found at the base of the ICA, which can be controlled with injection of 1 mL 1% lidocaine into the peri-vascular tissue. The hypoglossal nerve, which courses between the ICA and IJV, should be sought at the upper margin of the wound and directly visualised to avoid iatrogenic injury.

15.10.3 Zone 3 Exposure

Haemorrhage from Zone 3 injuries occurs in 19% of penetrating neck injuries and bleeding here can be catastrophic. Access to this region and the base of skull is challenging even when adjunctive manoeuvres such as subluxation of the mandible and division of the posterior belly of the digastric muscle are performed. It is the authors' opinion that in the modern era of surgery, procedures in this region are best performed using endovascular techniques; however, in extremis it may be possible to achieve proximal and distal control with size 3 or 4 Fogarty catheters while a decision for repair is made. The help of neurosurgeons to access the base of skull or neurointerventional colleagues should be sought to aid both decision making and operative technique.

15.11 The Vertebral Arteries

Exposure of the vertebral arteries in the modern era is uncommon with the advent of endovascular techniques. Pre-operative imaging is vital to plan how best these vessels should be approached, but death from isolated vertebral arterial haemorrhage is uncommon (4%) and if necessary, ligation can be performed with a post-procedural stroke rate of up to 5% [12, 13].

The paired arteries are located deep within the neck and course within the transverse processes of the cervical vertebrae for much of their length. As a result, direct access to all but the most proximal section of either vessel as it arises from the subclavian artery requires involvement of experienced neurosurgeons. The proximal vertebral arteries, before they enter the C6 transverse foramen, can be achieved through a transverse supraclavicular incision or a vertical anterior cervical approach. When accessing the left vertebral origin, care should be taken to avoid injury to the thoracic duct and the recurrent laryngeal nerve on the right.

15.12 The Subclavian Arteries

Traumatic injuries to the subclavian arteries are associated with a high pre-hospital mortality of up to 80%, and of those who survive transfer to hospital, 15% die in the peri-operative period [14]. Open surgical access is achieved via a median sternotomy, but the use of a remote occlusion balloon placed via the femoral or brachial arteries should be considered to attain proximal control. Primary ligation of the subclavian artery can be considered in times of extremis as the upper limb rarely suffers from ischaemia due to an embryologically well-collateralised upper limb arterial supply.

15.13 Venous Injuries in the Neck

Additional venous injuries are commonly associated with cervical arterial trauma due to the close proximity of the internal and external jugular veins. In contrast to injuries to the iliac veins and inferior vena cave, venous injuries in the neck are reasonably easier to access and control without significant long-term sequalae. The venous system of the neck is of low-pressure and injured jugular vessels will often tamponade or occlude, but if required, can be surgically ligated without consequence [15]. If primary repair is a feasible option, haemorrhage can be controlled with the application of pressure on either side of the vessel rent and either side of the vein picked up in allis forceps to lift it out of the wound bed. Repair with a 5/0, 6/0 or equivalently sized prolene suture can then be performed.

15.14 Principles of Vascular Surgery in Cases of Blunt Neck Trauma

Blunt cerebrovascular vascular injury (BCVI) presents a clinical challenge as it is often occult and difficult to diagnose due to the relative paucity of external symptoms and signs. Most injuries are diagnosed after signs of cerebral ischaemia become apparent, resulting in a neurological morbidity of up to 80% and associated mortality of 40% [16]. The modified Denver criteria identify patients at particular risk of BCVI to include those involved in high energy transfer mechanisms with Le Fort II or III midface fractures, base of skull fractures, cervical spine fracture, subluxation or ligamentous injury at any level, near hanging with anoxic brain injury, seat belt abrasion, or any other soft tissue injury to the anterior aspect of the neck causing swelling or Glasgow coma scale score < 6 indicating severe traumatic brain injury [17]. Clinical signs suggestive of BCVI include obvious haemorrhage from the neck, nose or mouth, cervical bruit, expanding haematoma, focal neurological deficit, cerebrovascular accident seen on CT brain, or neurological signs incongruous with CT head findings [17].

Treatments for BCVI can be stratified and graded to help guide management, with the Blunt Carotid Arterial Injury Grading scale being a useful tool in common use [18]. As a general guide, however, non-flow limiting intimal disruptions and dissections seen at the time of trauma can be managed with serial clinical examination, interval imaging, and close follow-up. Anti-platelet agents should be commenced to help stabilisation of the vessel wall, and the patient should be examined for signs of distal embolisation of clot at which point mechanical thrombectomy or anticoagulation may also be considered. Late, occult features of an injured vessel include development of a pseudoaneurysm, which may be managed via endovascular deployment of a covered stent graft if anatomically suitable, or primary repair with *aneurysmorrhaphy* or placement with an autologous venous, or prosthetic (ePTFE) interposition graft, but these procedures should be performed by those with the training and expertise to undertake them.

Top Five Take Away Points

1. Priorities incorporate ATLS principles securing the airway, maintaining ventilation, controlling haemorrhage, and treating shock.

2. Zones 1 and 3 are challenging zones for vascular access, exposure, and control. A multidisciplinary approach including the involvement of vascular, cardiothoracic, and neurosurgeons/neuro-interventional surgeons must be anticipated and sought early.
3. Temporising measures with the use of shunts and balloon occlusion catheters can be used.
4. Clinicians should have a high index of suspicion for blunt cerebrovascular injuries (BCVI) in those patients who have had high-energy transfer injuries.
5. Venous injuries can be treated centrally with endovascular-covered stents, and distally can be ligated if encountered intra-operatively.

References

1. Beard JD, Gaines PA, Loftus I. Vascular and endovascular surgery E-book: companion to specialist surgical practice. Elsevier Health Sciences; 2013.
2. Nowicki JL, Stew B, Ooi E. Penetrating neck injuries: a guide to evaluation and management. Ann R Coll Surg Engl. 2018;100(1):6–11.
3. Newton K. Penetrating neck injuries: Initial evaluation and management In: Grayzel J, ed. UpToDate, Waltham, MA. Accessed 5 Dec 2021: UpToDate; 2021.
4. Apffelstaedt JP, Müller R. Results of mandatory exploration for penetrating neck trauma. World J Surg. 1994;18(6):917–9. discussion 20
5. Tisherman SA, Bokhari F, Collier B, Cumming J, Ebert J, Holevar M, et al. Clinical practice guideline: penetrating zone II neck trauma. J Trauma. 2008;64(5):1392–405.
6. Müller M, Schmitz BL, Pauls S, Schick M, Röhrer S, Kapapa T, et al. Variations of the aortic arch - a study on the most common branching patterns. Acta Radiol. 2011;52(7):738–42.
7. Hornez E, Boddaert G, Ngabou UD, Aguir S, Baudoin Y, Mocellin N, et al. Temporary vascular shunt for damage control of extremity vascular injury: a toolbox for trauma surgeons. J Visc Surg. 2015;152(6):363–8.
8. Burgess CA, Dale OT, Almeyda R, Corbridge RJ. An evidence based review of the assessment and management of penetrating neck trauma. Clin Otolaryngol. 2012;37(1):44–52.
9. Demetriades D, Theodorou D, Cornwell E, Berne TV, Asensio J, Belzberg H, et al. Evaluation of penetrating injuries of the neck: prospective study of 223 patients. World J Surg. 1997;21(1):41–7; discussion 7–8
10. Kazimierczak A, Rybicka A, Rynio P, Gutowski P, Wiernicki I. Cosmetic effects of skin-crease camouflage incision versus longitudinal incision following carotid endarterectomy. Wideochir Inne Tech Maloinwazyjne. 2018;13(1):102–10.
11. Deck M, Kopriva D. Patient and observer scar assessment scores favour the late appearance of a transverse cervical incision over a vertical incision in patients undergoing carotid endarterectomy for stroke risk reduction. Can J Surg. 2015;58(4):245–9.
12. Reid JD, Weigelt JA. Forty-three cases of vertebral artery trauma. J Trauma. 1988;28(7):1007–12.
13. Thomas GI, Anderson KN, Hain R, Merendino KA. The significance of anomalous vertebral-basilar artery communications in operations on the heart and great vessels: an illustrative case with review of the literature. Surgery. 1959;46:747–57.
14. Demetriades D, Rabinowitz B, Pezikis A, Franklin J, Palexas G. Subclavian vascular injuries. Br J Surg. 2005;74(11):1001–3.
15. Kumar SR, Weaver FA, Yellin AE. Cervical vascular injuries: carotid and jugular venous injuries. Surg Clin North Am. 2001;81(6):1331–44, xii–xiii
16. Davis JW, Holbrook TL, Hoyt DB, Mackersie RC, Field TO Jr, Shackford SR. Blunt carotid artery dissection: incidence, associated injuries, screening, and treatment. J Trauma. 1990;30(12):1514–7.
17. Geddes AE, Burlew CC, Wagenaar AE, Biffl WL, Johnson JL, Pieracci FM, et al. Expanded screening criteria for blunt cerebrovascular injury: a bigger impact than anticipated. Am J Surg. 2016;212(6):1167–74.
18. Bromberg WJ, Collier BC, Diebel LN, Dwyer KM, Holevar MR, Jacobs DG, et al. Blunt cerebrovascular injury practice management guidelines: the Eastern Association for the Surgery of Trauma. J Trauma. 2010;68(2):471–7.

Maxillofacial Trauma for the General Surgeon

16

Peter Aquilina

Oral and maxillofacial trauma is frequently a component of major trauma. In theatres of war, such injuries can account for a disproportionate volume of casualties and subsequent consumption of resources and effort. This chapter will not provide detailed protocols for the definitive management of patients with maxillofacial and dental trauma. It is designed to aid the general surgeon in the initial management of these patients, potentially in a remote setting, prior to transfer to a larger centre for definitive care.

16.1 Emergency Management of the Patient with Isolated or Concomitant Maxillofacial Trauma

The early management of trauma as per the ATLS/EMST protocols apply to the patient with maxillofacial injuries; however, the presence of trauma to the face does introduce some dilemmas [1–3]. In particular, there can be a conflict between the management of the airway and the ATLS protocols regarding the management of actual or potential c-spine/thoracic/lumbar spine and pelvic trauma.

All trauma to the maxillofacial region puts the airway at risk to a variable degree. This risk can evolve from being low at initial presentation to being high as oedema and haematomas for example develop (Fig. 16.1). Patients with facial injuries invariably prefer to sit up and lean forward to allow blood to drain from their mouth. When patients are prevented from doing this when restrained with a spine board and a rigid cervical collar/head box, the patient's ability to maintain their airway is restricted (Fig. 16.2a–c). This situation is further exacerbated by the risk of vomiting [1, 3] which is frequently seen in this cohort of patients due to the common presence of alcohol [4], and the effect of swallowing blood arising from the facial injuries. Vomiting occurring in a patient restrained as above can lead to aspiration or airway loss.

The presence of fractured or avulsed teeth also poses a potential risk to the airway. Thorough suctioning of the mouth and upper airway should be done, and any missing teeth or fragments of teeth should be accounted for. If a tooth is missing, or a fragment from a tooth has been fractured off and is unacounted for, chest films need to be obtained to exclude aspiration of these fragments.

Aids to airway management may be useful in some situations. Guedel airways are poorly tolerated and may precipitate vomiting [1, 2]. Nasopharyngeal airways are better tolerated, and despite common opinion, they are associated with a low risk of cranial intubation [5]. A poten-

P. Aquilina (✉)
The University of Sydney School of Medicine, Sydney, NSW, Australia

B. Ashford (ed.), *Head and Neck Surgery for General Surgeons*,
https://doi.org/10.1007/978-981-19-7900-2_16

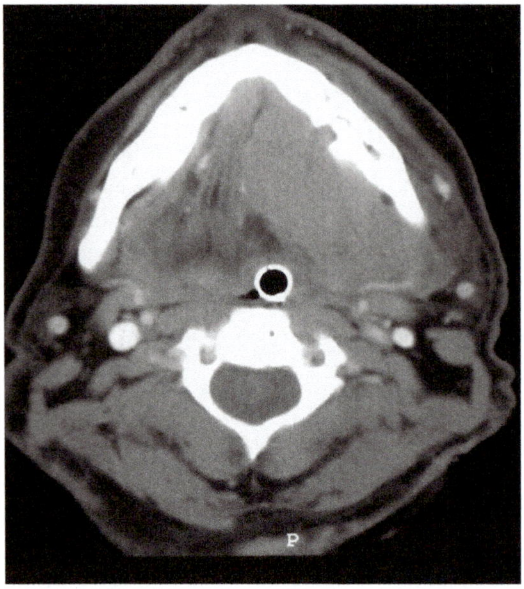

Fig. 16.1 CT scan axial view of a sublingual haematoma compromising airway patency. Note the ETT tube

tial problem with nasopharyngeal airways is their association with epistaxis. Bag and mask ventilation is commonly utilized but can be difficult in the presence of facial fractures due to altered anatomy and the presence of bleeding.

Early clearance of spine and pelvic injuries is imperative to allow patients with facial trauma to sit up if able. Alternatively, consideration needs to be given to early definitive airway management. The preferred definitive airway is an oral endotracheal tube [2]. Concerns with potential spinal cord injury occurring during intubation in the presence of a c-spine injury are valid but unlikely to occur if manual in line stabilization is used [6]. Nasal intubation is not associated with an increased risk of cranial intubation [7] but is seldom used due to the increased technical difficulty.

Emergent surgical airways are rarely required. Needle cricothyroidotomy can be used as a tempo-

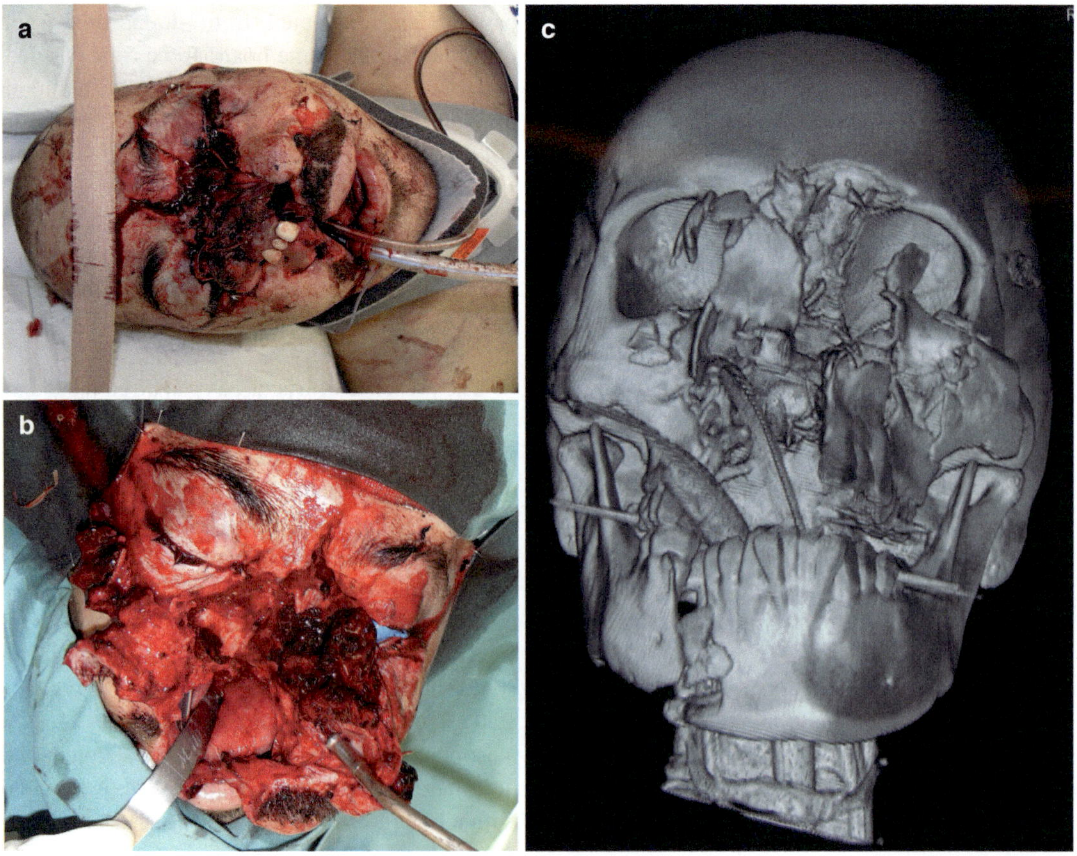

Fig. 16.2 (**a**) A patient after a high speed motorbike accident with spinal precautions in situ. Not the presence to grass and foreign material in the wound. (**b**) The same patient with the extent of the facial disruption shown. (**c**) The 3D CT reconstruction of this patient demonstrating significant skeletal disruption

rizing measure. Surgical cricothyroidotomy is the preferred surgical airway in a trauma setting [8].

16.1.1 Basic Dental Anatomy

There are normally 32 adult teeth (secondary) and 20 deciduous (primary teeth). There may be more or less teeth present due to congenital absence, loss due to dental disease, previous trauma or extraction for orthodontic reasons and the presence of supernumerary (additional teeth) teeth. Each tooth has three basic layers: an inert outer enamel layer, a layer of dentine and an inner dental pulp.

Each tooth is supported within the bony alveolar processes (alveolus) of the maxilla and mandible by the periodontal ligaments. The neurovascular and lymphatic supply to the dental pulp of each tooth enters primarily via the apical foramen(s) at the end of each root. Disruption of this supply can result in inflammation or necrosis and infection of the dental pulp. Teeth are richly innervated with branches from the mandibular and maxillary trunks of the trigeminal nerve and noxious stimuli can result in exquisite pain.

Teeth can be individually named (i.e., upper left central incisor) but internationally the most commonly used identification system is the FDI (World Dental Federation) system. In this system, the dental arches are divided into four quadrants starting at the upper right, which is denoted quadrant 1, and moving in a clockwise fashion (looking at the patient) to the upper left, which is denoted quadrant 2, the lower left, which is denoted quadrant 3, and the lower right which is denoted quadrant 4. Within each quadrant, there are normally eight teeth. These teeth are numbered 1–8 commencing at the central incisor and proceeding posteriorly in a sequential fashion to the third molar tooth. It is thus able to identify a tooth by giving the quadrant it is in and the number it is in that quadrant. For example, the lower right second molar is the seventh tooth in the lower right quadrant and is designated as tooth 47.

16.1.2 Dentoalveolar Injuries

The detailed management of these dental injuries is beyond the scope of this chapter and early referral to a dentist is indicated. Nonetheless, there are steps that can be taken to maximise patient recovery from these injuries. The following applies to the adult dentition (permanent teeth). Deciduous teeth should not routinely be replanted due to the risk of damage to the underlying and developing permanent teeth.

16.1.2.1 Classification

1. *Isolated tooth injury*
   (a) Ellis class I: Trauma is restricted to the enamel only. The dentine layer is not exposed.
   (b) Ellis Class II: There is a fracture of both enamel and dentine, however the dental pulp is not exposed.
   (c) Ellis class III: There is a fracture of the tooth involving all three layers and exposing the pulpal tissues.
   After accounting for any lost tooth structure and where required excluding aspiration, the initial management of these injuries is supportive whilst waiting for definitive dental review. Analgesia and antibiotic coverage may be indicated. Large portions of tooth should be kept as a dentist may use them as a part of a repair.
2. *Subluxation*
   Provided the tooth is not mobile, no acute management is required. If the tooth is mobile, splinting of the tooth until dental review occurs is indicated. Temporary splinting can be achieved by moulding aluminium foil around the mobile tooth and the adjacent teeth.
3. *Intrusion*
   If the tooth is not mobile, no acute management is required prior to referral.
4. *Extrusion*
   The tooth should be pushed back into the socket and then a temporary splint placed until dental review occurs. Infiltration with

local anaesthetic can assist; however, infiltration is less effective in the mandible compared to the maxilla due to the increased thickness of bone between the tooth socket and the bone surface. Obtaining reliable local anaesthesia of the mandibular teeth requires the use of a nerve block technique to anaesthetise the inferior alveolar nerve.

5. *Avulsion*
   Avulsion of an adult tooth is a dental emergency [9]. The tooth should be handled by the crown and the root should not be touched. The reason for avoiding handling of the root is to maximise the survival of periodontal ligament cells on the root surface which are required for successful replantation. If the tooth is dirty, it should be gently rinsed in milk or saline without scrubbing or manipulating the surface of the root. Replant the tooth as soon as possible without removing the blood clot in the tooth socket [9]. Teeth replanted within 15 min of avulsion have the best prognosis [10]. If replantation is not immediately possible, store the tooth in cool milk. Periodontal ligament cells will remain viable for up to 6 h when stored this way [10]. Alternatives to milk such as saliva or saline can be used, but the survival of the periodontal ligament cells in these cases is only about an hour. It is important to not rinse the tooth with water or store the tooth in water. Following replantation, a temporary aluminium foil splint should be applied, and urgent dental review organised. Antibiotic treatment should be commenced. Doxycycline is preferred as it has documented efficacy in reducing the risk of root resorption post replantation [10]. In children younger than 8 with a developing dentition, or in patients in which tetracyclines are contraindicated, amoxicillin can be used. The use of a chlorhexidine mouth wash 8 hourly is also recommended.
6. *Root fractures*
   These have a poor long-term prognosis. If the remaining tooth portion is mobile, it can be splinted with aluminium foil as described above.
7. *Dentoalveolar fractures*
   These are fractures of the alveolar bone. The teeth contained within the bone segment may be uninjured. Treatment pending maxillofacial review is supportive, consisting of analgesia, antibiotics, and splinting, if possible, to minimize movement. Gentle reduction under local after administration of local anaesthesia may be performed if it is judged that a segment is significantly displaced.

16.1.3 Maxillofacial Injuries

Maxillofacial injuries often accompany dental trauma and one may be indicative of the presence of the other. Equally, a fracture of the bony skeleton of the face should also be taken as a strong indicator of the likelihood of both head injury (closed or open) or of injury to the cervical spine. The facial skeleton comprises multiple bones and is arbitrarily divided into the areas we have outlined below. In clinical practice, it is common to have fractures of multiple regions. In this section, we outline the various components of the facial skeleton and the associated soft tissues and discuss the acute management of injuries to these tissues.

1. Frontal sinus.
2. Orbits.
3. Zygoma.
4. Nasal bones.
5. Maxilla.
6. Mandible.
7. Soft tissue.
   (a) Eyelids.
   (b) Lips.
   (c) Tongue.
   (d) Oral mucosa.
   (e) Facial skin.

16.1.3.1 Frontal Sinus

Relevant Anatomy

The frontal sinus has an outer table covered by skin and an inner table forming the anterior wall of the anterior cranial fossa (Fig. 16.3). It is drained via the nasofrontal ducts into the nose.

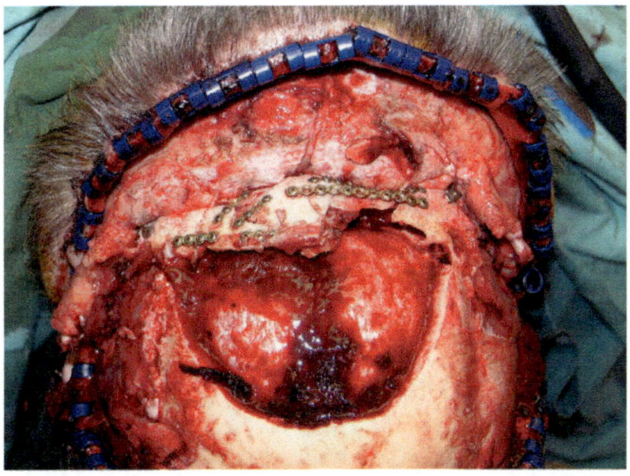

Fig. 16.3 Intra-operative view of reconstruction of the anterior frontal sinus table demonstrating the relation between the frontal sinus and the brain

Investigations

1. Clinical examination directed towards cranial pathology.
2. CT scan with fine (0.75–1.0 mm) cuts.

Management

The presence of an anterior table fracture indicates that significant energy was involved in the injury and intracranial pathology should be looked for. Definitive treatment is complex and varies depending on the status of the posterior table and the functional status of the nasofrontal ducts. Brief debridement and closure of soft tissue is indicated prior to referral to definitive maxillofacial surgical care.

16.1.3.2 Orbital Fractures

Relevant Anatomy

The bony orbit contains and protects the globe and its associated structures. The roof of the orbit forms the floor of the frontal sinus and the anterior cranial fossa. The optic nerve and its supporting structures enter via the optic canal in the greater wing of the sphenoid bone. Several important structures enter the orbit via the superior orbital fissure including the trochlear nerve (Cranial Nerve IV), the oculomotor nerve (CNIII) and the abducens nerve (CN VI). Injury to the superior orbital fissure and its contents is seen in high energy injuries and should prompt further investigation for other injuries.

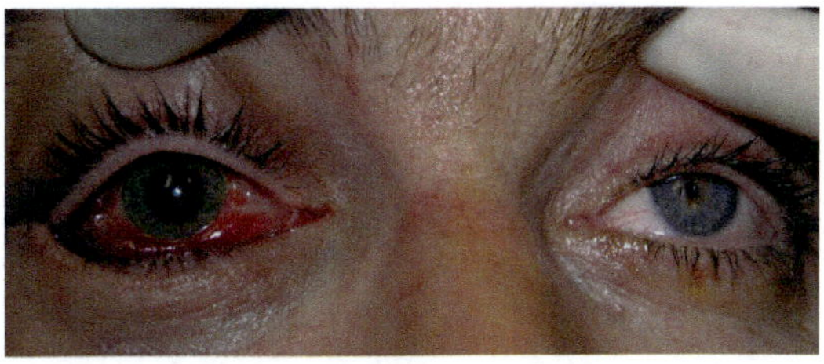

Fig. 16.4 A dilated and non-responsive right pupil post fracture of the right orbit

The floor of the orbit forms the roof of the maxillary sinus. The inferior orbital nerve, a branch of the ophthalmic division of the trigeminal nerve travels through the floor, variably encased in bone, to exit via the infraorbital foramen on the anterior maxilla where it supplies a portion of the skin of the cheek and lateral nose with sensation.

Investigations

Clinical examination to determine the presence of vision-risking injuries is mandatory. Wherever possible, assessment of visual acuity should be performed and recorded. Pupillary size and response, including direct and consensual reflexes should be documented (Fig. 16.4). The globes must be visualised to exclude the presence of globe injury (Fig. 16.5).

The function of the extra-ocular eye muscles should be determined by assessing the range of motion of the eyes, noting any restriction in movement and diplopia.

Pupillary responses can be abnormal secondary to cranial pathology, injury to the oculomotor nerve, the presence of opioids or mydriatics, and injury to the optic nerve. The cause of an abnormal pupillary response must be determined and managed appropriately.

Diplopia is usually due to mechanical restriction of one or more of the extra-ocular muscles due to their entrapment in fracture lines or due to oedema. Rarer but more urgent causes of diplopia are retinal detachment or lens dislocation. Diplopia due to mechanical restriction of globe movement disappears on covering either eye. Diplopia that persists on covering an unaffected eye is a significant clinical finding that warrants opthalmological review.

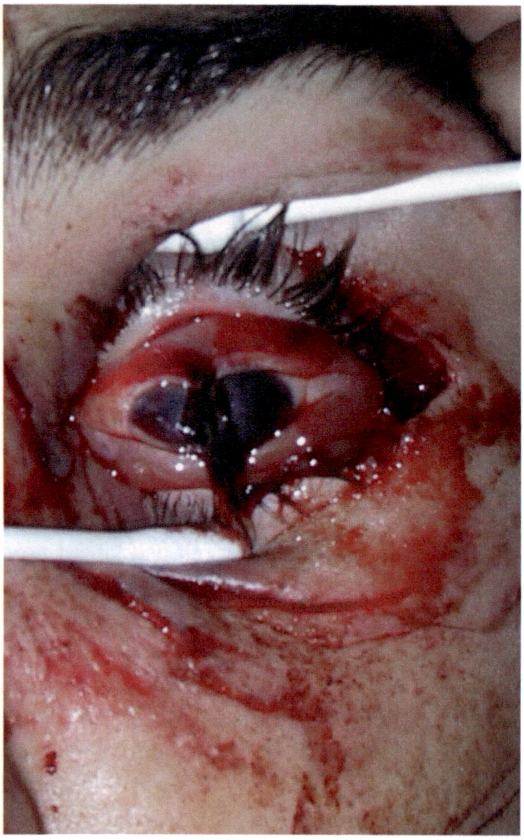

Fig. 16.5 Globe trauma occurring in the presence of a fracture of the left orbit

A CT scan of the facial skeleton including the orbits should be obtained.

Management

General supportive care is indicated prior to definitive maxillofacial surgery care. Patients should be advised not to blow their nose in order to avoid the development of surgical emphysema.

Management should be directed to addressing conditions that threaten vision. Specific findings of note include

(a) Globe trauma. Trauma to the globe needs urgent opthalmological review.

(b) Retrobulbar haemorrhage.

Retrobulbar haemorrhage is a compartment syndrome of the orbit. It is marked by pain, proptosis, decreasing visual acuity and altered pupillary response. It is a vision-threatening emergency requiring urgent management.

Management includes medical treatment aimed at reducing orbital pressures and surgical management directed at increasing orbital volume.

Medical management aims to decrease compartment pressure within the orbit and consists of high-dose steroids, acetazolamide and mannitol.

Emergent surgical management consist of lateral canthotomy and cantholysis to allow the orbital contents to come forward, thus increasing the effective volume (and reducing the compartment pressure) of the orbit.

(c) Lens dislocation warrants ophthalmological advice.

(d) Retinal detachment warrants ophthalmological advice.

(e) Hyphaema (Fig. 16.6) (blood in the anterior chamber) warrants ophthalmological advice.

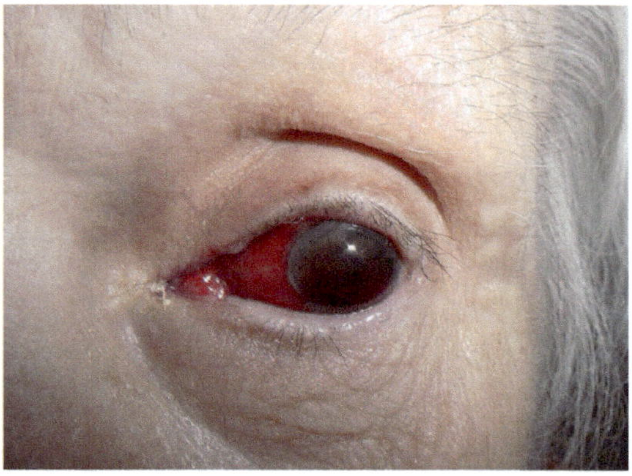

Fig. 16.6 Hyphaema

Definitive management depends on the degree of anatomical disruption, the amount of functional impairment and patient preference. It may involve open reduction and internal fixation and/or orbital floor reconstruction. In patients with no functional deficit, some patients choose to accept a cosmetic defect rather than have corrective bone reconstructive surgery.

16.1.3.3 Zygoma

Unless it is an isolated arch fracture, fractures of the zygoma always involve the orbit as the zygomatic bone forms part of the orbital skeleton. As such, acute management should be directed to orbital injuries as outlined above.

16.1.3.4 Nasal Bones

Injuries to the nasal bones are common and rarely pose significant acute issues. Occasionally severe epistaxis can occur requiring posterior nasal packing or the use of a proprietary device such as a "Rapid Rhino" (Smith and Nephew).

16.1.3.5 Maxillary Fractures

Relevant Anatomy

There are two maxillary bones on either side of the midline. They contribute to the orbital skeleton superiorly, the nasal anatomy medially and the dentition inferiorly. The maxillary sinuses are located within the maxillary bones. The maxillary bones are richly innervated and have an excellent blood supply.

The two maxilla join at the midline to form a significant portion of the middle third of the face. The maxilla and its associated structures sit on the anterior skull base which is at an approximate 45° slope.

Maxillary fractures are traditionally classified as le Fort level fractures I, II and III, based on the level of the fracture; however, this is not particularly useful in an acute setting and pure discrete Le Fort fractures are rarely seen (Fig. 16.7).

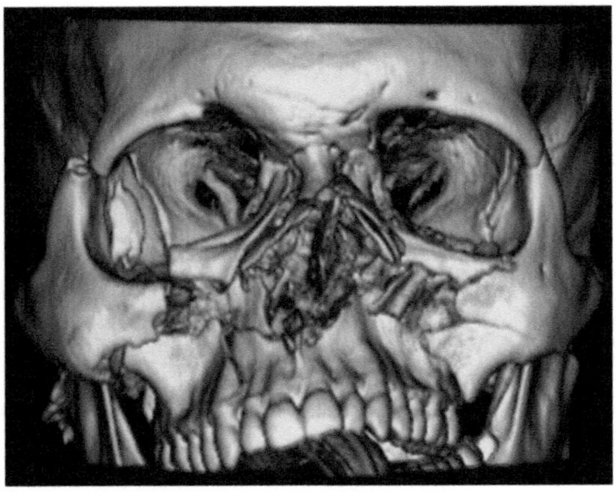

Fig. 16.7 Maxillary fractures involving several le Fort levels as well as extending to the ZMC and orbits

Investigations

Clinical examination may reveal malocclusion and the maxilla may be mobile.

CT scans are required with fine cuts.

Management

Unless the airway is affected, or there is associated orbital injury, management in the acute setting is supportive. Rarely, the maxilla may be displaced down the slope of the anterior cranial base resulting in airway compromise. If this occurs, the maxilla can be reduced by inserting two fingers via the mouth behind the posterior choanae and pulling anteriorly whilst maintaining spinal precautions.

Definitive management in displaced fractures usually involves open reduction and internal fixation. In some edentulous patients, surgical reduction can be avoided, and the changed skeletal relationship can be corrected by adjusting or making the patient a new denture.

16.1.3.6 Mandibular Fractures

Relevant Anatomy

The mandible is an arch-shaped bone that articulates with the skull bilaterally at the temporomandibular joints. The inferior alveolar nerves enter the body of the mandible bilaterally at the lingual foramen, travel through the body of the mandible and exit via the mental foramen to become the mental nerve. The inferior alveolar nerve is a sensory branch of the mandibular division of the trigeminal nerve and supplies sensation to the majority of the mandible and its teeth. The lingual nerve supplies the lingual mucosa of the mandible with sensation.

Structural weak points of the mandible occur at the condylar necks, the mandibular angles and the parasymphyseal areas. Common patterns of fractures are an angle fracture with contralateral parasymphyseal fracture and a condylar neck fracture with a contralateral parasymphyseal fracture. If a patient presents with an isolated parasymphyseal, angle of mandible or condylar fracture, the above fracture patterns should be excluded (Figs. 16.8 and 16.9).

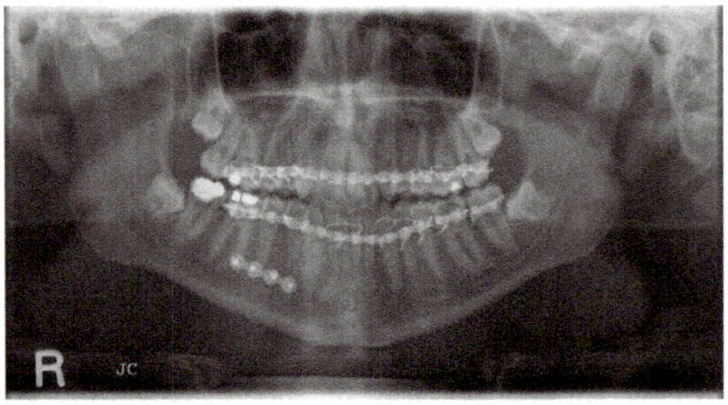

Fig. 16.8 An OPG radiograph (orthopantomogram) showing a typical right parasymphysis and left subcondyar fracture pattern. The right parasymphysis fracture has been reduced and internally fixated, the left subcondylar fracture has had a closed reduction

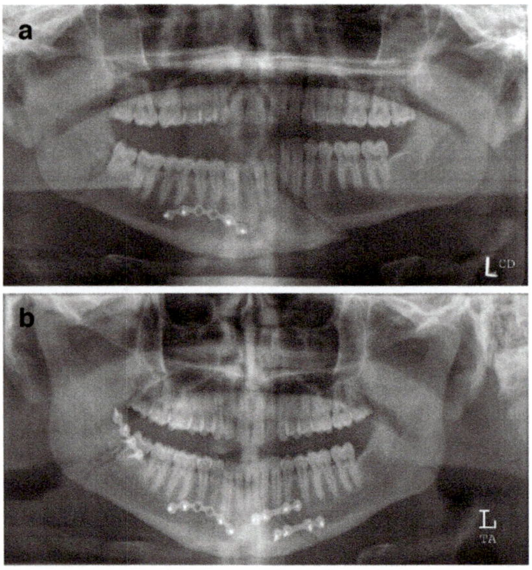

Fig. 16.9 An OPG showing a typical right angle and left parasymphysis fracture pattern. Note the previously treated right parasymphyseal fracture

Investigations

Clinical examination may show a malocclusion (Fig. 16.10). Paraesthesia of the lower lip is common secondary to involvement of the inferior alveolar nerve. The presence of a sublingual haematoma is very suggestive of an underlying fracture. Plain films at 90 degrees are sufficient (OPG and PA mandible), however a CT scan is commonly obtained.

Management

Airway control and supportive treatment are required prior to definitive care with a maxillofacial surgeon. Definitive treatment can range from ORIF

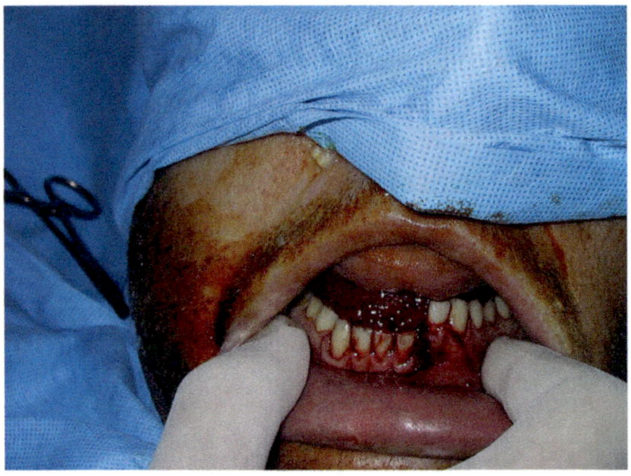

Fig. 16.10 The clinical presentation of the patient in Fig. 16.9. Note the obvious malocclusion with an occlusal step, and the sublingual haematoma. The presence of a sublingual haematoma is almost pathognomic of a mandibular fracture

to observation with a soft diet. The use of intermaxillary wire fixation (IMF, MMF) has largely been discarded in modern management with the use of internal fixation predominating care.

16.1.3.7 Soft Tissue

Soft tissue lacerations are commonly seen, and many can be managed under local anaesthesia using the basic surgical principles of haemostasis, layered closure, accurate soft tissue apposition and tensionless closure. Fine, non-resorbable sutures should be used on the skin and removed within 5 days to minimise suture marks. Minimal debridement of soft tissue should be practiced as tissue that would be non-viable on the extremities may well retain vitality on the face due to the rich vascular supply.

Relevant Anatomy

The face has a rich anastomosing vascular supply and copious bleeding from facial lacerations is common. The facial nerve branches are at risk of injury as are the parotid ducts (Figs. 16.11 and 16.12).

Particular care should be taken in the management of lacerations involving the eyelids and the lips.

(a) Eyelids

The anatomy of the eyelids is complex. Lacerations of the eyelids are not suitable for

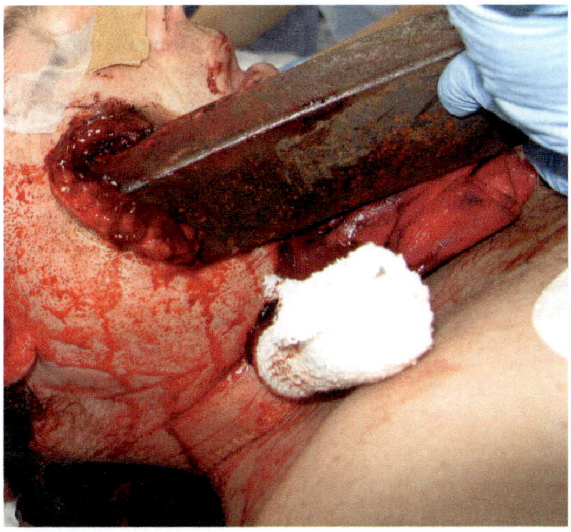

Fig. 16.11 A patient with soft tissue trauma sustained during an industrial accident. The injury would be expected to damage the parotid duct and facial nerve branches

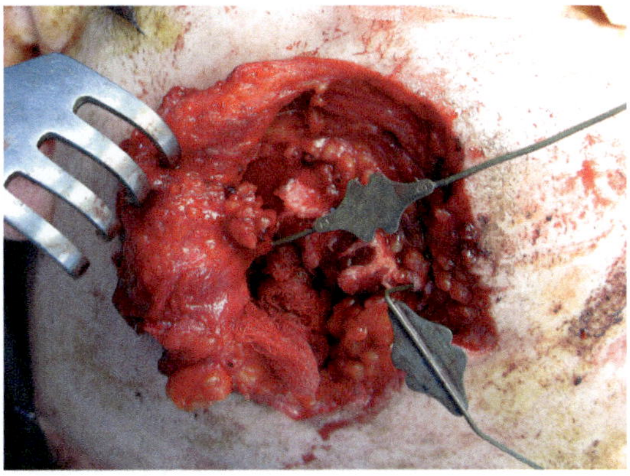

Fig. 16.12 The intraoperative view of the patient in Fig. 16.11 showing lacrimal probes in the ends of the severed parotid duct prior to microsurgical anastomosis

non-specialist repair and referral should be made to an oculoplastic or maxillofacial surgeon.

(b) Lips

Care should be exercised in repairing lip lacerations, especially if the injury involves the vermillion border. Accurate apposition of the vermillion border is required, and this is facilitated by the use of magnification. Careful coaptation of the transected orbicularis muscles if involved is also required. A full thickness laceration of the lip will necissitate closure of the mucosa, muscle and skin. Wounds contaminated with gravel or other foreign matter should be thoroughly debrided. Tooth fragments are sometimes seen in adjacent soft tissues and need to be removed. Plain radiographs and CT scans can often show retained soft tissue foreign bodies, however they cannot be relied upon completely.

(c) Tongue

The tongue is very vascular and muscular. Lacerations may bleed significantly. Repair under local anaesthetic is possible; however, it requires patient co-operation in order to reduce movement of the tongue. Deep tissue bites with 3/0 suture material are required.

Top Five Takeaways

1. Maxillofacial trauma is common.
2. Oral and maxillofacial trauma is often associated with head and spinal injury.
3. Beware of the potential for acute or delayed airway embarrassment in patients with maxillofacial injuries.
4. Retrobulbar haemorrhage due to an orbital injury is a surgical emergency.
5. Dental Practitioners are a good source of advice and help with dental trauma.

References

1. Perry M. Advanced Trauma Life Support (ATLS): can one size fit all? Part 1: Dilemmas in the managment of the mulitply injured patient with coexisting facial injuries. Int J Oral Maxillofac Surg. 2008;37(3):209–14.
2. Perry M, Morris C. Advanced trauma life support (ATLS) and facail trauma: cna one size fit all? Part 2: ATLS, maxillofacial injuries and airway dilemmas. Int J Oral Maxillofac Surg. 2008;37(4):309–20.
3. Tuckett J, Lynham A, Lee G, Perry M, Harrington U. Maxillofacial trauma in the emergency department: A review. Surgeon. 2014;12(2):106–14.
4. Elledge RO, Elledge R, Aquilina P, Hodson J, Dover S. The role of alcohol in maxillofacial trauma - a comparative retrospective audit between two centres. Alcohol. 2011;45(3):239–43.
5. Bahr W, Stoll P. Nasal intubation in the presence of frontobasal fractures: A retrospective study. J Oral Maxillofac Surg. 1992;50(5):445–7.
6. McLeod A, Calder I. Spinal cord injury and laryngoscopy - the legend lives on. Br J Anaesth. 2000;84(6):705–9.

7. Arrowsmith J, Robertshaw H, Boyd J. Nasotracheal intubation in the presence of frontobasal skull fracture. Can J Anaesth. 1998;45(1):71–5.
8. Salvino C, Dries D, Gamelli R, Murphy-Macabobby M, Marshall W. Emergency cricothyroidotomy in trauma victims. J Trauma. 1993;34(4):503–5.
9. Ceallaigh P, Ekanaykaee K, Beirne C, Patton D. Diagnosis and managment of common maxillofacial injuries in the emergency department.Part 5: dentoalveolar injuries. Emerg Med J. 2006;24(6):429–30.
10. Therapuetic Guidelines (digital). (2021, 11 23). Tooth avulsion (knocked-out tooth). www.tg.org.au

17 Odontogenic Infections and Deep Neck Collections

Gary R. Hoffman, Ashim N. Adhikari, and Olivia G. I. Hoffman

17.1 Introduction

The neurocranium, sub-cranial viscero-cranium and cervical spine collectively provide a framework of structural support and protection for a variety of complex anatomical structures that are condensed into a small space.

A number of surgical and medical specialties lay claim to the diagnosis and management of a wide range of diseases, deformities, defects and disorders that afflict the musculoskeletal and soft tissue components of the head and neck.

While such subspecialties idiosyncratically manage their respective pathologies, it is incumbent for all surgeons who operate in the head and neck to have both a working knowledge of, as well as a capacity to manage, both superficial and deep neck space infections.

G. R. Hoffman (✉)
Departments of Oral and Maxillofacial Surgery and Head and Neck Surgery, John Hunter Hospital, Newcastle, NSW, Australia

School of Medicine, University of Newcastle, Newcastle, NSW, Australia

A. N. Adhikari
Department of Oral and Maxillofacial Surgery, John Hunter Hospital, Newcastle, NSW, Australia

O. G. I. Hoffman
School of Medicine, University of Melbourne, Melbourne, VIC, Australia

17.2 Infection

In its broadest sense, infection is arguably the most common pathological denominator that can affect any of the resident tissues and organs of the head and neck. Infection can be defined as the damage that results from the invasion by and growth of pathogenic microorganisms within host tissues. In doing so, they also have the capacity to both activate and overwhelm the host's innate and acquired immune defences.

The microorganisms that are responsible for the damage can be classified as either bacterial, viral, fungal or parasitic. For the purposes of this dissertation, the infections that are discussed are bacterial in origin.

Although a wide variety of pathogenic bacteria exist, they enlist remarkably common strategies to cause their local, regional and systemic effects. These comprise an array of virulence factors, which uphold their intrinsic ability to adhere to (adhesins), invade into (invasins), counter innate host immune defences (elaboration of coat proteins and superoxide dismutases), multiply within and spread throughout, causing primary cytotoxic damage (production of destructive proteolytic enzymes) to host tissues and organs.

These processes are modified by host anatomical factors and resistance capacity. The latter is impaired by poorly or uncontrolled intercurrent systemic disease.

B. Ashford (ed.), *Head and Neck Surgery for General Surgeons*,
https://doi.org/10.1007/978-981-19-7900-2_17

17.3 Sepsis and Septic Shock

The body's ultimate response to the progression of uncontrolled infection is sepsis. Sepsis is a life-threatening condition that arises when the physical, biochemical and pathological contributions to the host response become dysregulated and result in injury to its own tissues and organs (e.g., pulmonary injury/acute respiratory distress syndrome, hypoperfusion and acute tubular necrosis/acute renal failure, ischemia and gastrointestinal ulceration and disseminated intravascular coagulation).

Physiologist, Carl Wiggers, stated that "Shock not only stops the machine, but it wrecks the machinery." For clinical operationalisation, the organ dysfunction due to infection is qualified by an increase in the sequential (sepsis related) organ failure assessment (SOFA) score of two points or more. At the bedside, a *quick* SOFA (qSOFA) score can be used, where any two of respiratory rate ≥22 breaths/minute, altered mental status or systolic blood pressure ≤100 mm Hg are suggestive of sepsis.

Septic shock is a subset of sepsis in which profound circulatory, cellular and metabolic abnormalities conspire to increase the risk of mortality over sepsis alone. This is characterised by serum lactate ≥2 mmol/L and the requirement for vasopressor support in order to maintain a mean arterial pressure ≥65 mmHg, despite adequate fluid resuscitation.

17.4 Aetiology and Microbiology

Many contemporary authors have reiterated the concepts espoused by renaissance philosopher-diplomat, Niccolò Machiavelli in his sixteenth century treatise entitled *Il Principe*, where he prophetically identified two fundamental tenets of sepsis in annotating that, "Hectic fever, at its inception, is difficult to recognise but easy to treat; left unattended, it becomes easy to recognise and difficult to treat." It is that philosophy that underpins the subsequent discussion in this chapter.

Severe infections, as a cause of serious illness or death, have been recorded in the spoken and written word since antiquity.

As a subset, deep neck space infections are usually polymicrobial and generally caused by the resident bacteria that populate the oral cavity and upper aerodigestive tract. These bacteria are a mixture of aerobic, facultative or strict anaerobic organisms, with deeper infections more likely to involve anaerobes.

Implicated bacteria from the oral cavity include *Streptococcus viridans* and subsequent colonisation with anaerobes such as *Septostreptococci*, *Fusobacteria*, *Prevotella*, *Porphyromonas* and *Actinomyces* species. Aerodigestive bacteria include *Streptococcus pyogenes*, *Staphylococcus aureus* and *Haemophilus influenza*, with *Klebsiella* and *Pseudomonas* playing a role in immunocompromised hosts. Many of these organisms are able to produce beta-lactamase and, in turn, inhibit the action of a broad range of conventional antibiotics.

Although there are many causes of head and neck infection, those of odontogenic origin continue to remain some of the most common, followed by those of the pharyngotonsillar origin [1, 2], and contribute to a significant proportion of those that present as deep neck space infections encountered in clinical practice.

Odontogenic infections arise as a result of episodes of either dental pulp necrosis (and a resultant periapical abscess secondary and most commonly to dental decay – but also any process that exposes the dental pulp: attrition, erosion, abrasion and trauma), periodontal disease (chronic gingivo-periodontal pathos) or pericoronitis. A rising cause of related infections also include osteonecrosis of the jaws resulting from either therapeutic radiotherapy or pharmacotherapy (anti-resorptive or immune-modulation/suppression).

Non-odontogenic causes include a variety of acute conditions de novo or arising as exacerbations of chronic pathology such as otitis media, mastoiditis, sinusitis, pharyngitis, tonsillitis, sialadenitis, thyroiditis, infected brachial cleft and thyroglossal duct anomalies, suppurative cervical lymphadenitis, post-surgical or traumatic head and neck wounds.

They are typically diagnosed by thorough history-taking and clinical examination.

17.5 Anatomy

Once odontogenic infection has spread beyond the confines of the jaws, it is essentially anatomical factors that play a key role in the clinical presentation of disease.

In its simplistic presentation, if the suppurative exudate discharges above muscular attachments in the lower jaw or below muscular attachments in the upper jaw, the resultant presentation is that of an acute alveolar or vestibular abscess (parulis/gum boil). This may devolve into a chronic state and present as an intra-oral sinus tract, and for that matter, if the path of least resistance is relatively short, it may present as an extra-oral submental, submandibular or facial sinus tract.

Infections can spread more broadly via lympho-haematogenous dissemination and/or direct extension via fascial layers, into the deep recesses of the head and neck, with direct extension being the most common route of spread.

Retrograde flow through the veins that drain the mid-face in association with the abundance of anastomoses that exist between intra- and extra-cranial structures, may predispose to haematogenous spread, leading to serious complications such as cavernous sinus thrombophlebitis and cerebral abscess [3]. Haematogenous spread can also cause bacterial endocarditis and infection of distant sites, including prosthetic implants.

Lymphadenitis in the regional draining basin often resolves with treatment of the primary infection. Occasionally, this results in fibrosis or suppuration and lymphadenopathy may be persistent. Other causes of lymphadenopathy, including neoplasia, need to be ruled out.

Landmark papers by Grodinsky and Holyoke [4], who used dyed gelatin injections to determine the path of least resistance between fascial planes, Williams and Guralnick [5], who described the anatomical basis of managing Ludwig's angina (a life-threatening cellulitis of the submental and bilateral sublingual and submandibular spaces), and Granite [6], who summarised the literature on the potential interfascial spaces of the head and neck, with periodic supplementation by a variety of sporadic anatomical studies [7] and case reports are fundamental to an understanding of both the spread into and occupancy of deep neck spaces. This work is further supplemented by Flynn [8], who has published extensively on odontogenic infections, and described the likely routes of spread, based on causative teeth, and the approach for draining their associated collections. This information is summarised in Table 17.1 [3, 8] and depicted in anatomical drawings and imaging in Fig. 17.1.

These anatomical spaces are potential in nature, until they are occupied by an inflammatory exudate, and, in addition, are able to freely communicate. The severity of an infection can be linked to the anatomical location of the affected spaces due to their effect on local structures, including the airways and vital structures such as the orbital contents, intracranial contents, carotid sheath and mediastinum as well as their ability to spread into these spaces.

As such, submandibular and masticator space infections would be considered moderate risk, for their ability to induce trismus and spread to high-risk spaces such as parapharyngeal, retropharyngeal and pretracheal. Infection spreading within the so-called "danger space" (prevertebral space), mediastinum or intracranially would be considered very high risk.

Table 17.1 Spaces involved in deep neck space infections, their contents, communications, likely causes and surgical approaches to draining them

Space	Location	Contents	Communicating spaces	Likely aetiology	Surgical approaches for incision and drainage
Buccal	Between buccinator/buccopharyngeal fascia and skin	Buccal fat pad, parotid duct, facial vessels	Pterygomandibular, submasseteric, superficial temporal	Upper premolars and molars, lower premolars	Intraoral Transcutaneous
Submasseteric	Between mandible and masseter	Masseteric vessels	Superficial temporal, pterygomandibular, buccal	Lower third molars, mandibular angle fracture	Intraoral Transcervical
Pterygomandibular	Between mandible and medial pterygoid	Mandibular nerve and vessels	Deep temporal, sublingual, parapharyngeal, peritonsillar, submandibular, submasseteric, buccal	Lower third molars, mandibular angle fracture	Intraoral Transcervical
Submandibular	Between mylohyoid and superficial layer of deep cervical fascia posteriorly	Submandibular gland, facial vessels	Sublingual, submental, buccal, parapharyngeal	Lower molars	Transcervical
Sublingual	Between floor of mouth mucosa and mylohyoid	Submandibular gland and duct, sublingual gland, lingual and hypoglossal nerves, lingual vessels	Contralateral sublingual, submental, submandibular, parapharyngeal	Lower premolars and molars, trauma	Intraoral Transcervical
Submental	Between mylohyoid and superficial layer of deep cervical fascia anteriorly	Anterior jugular veins	Sublingual, submandibular	Lower anterior teeth, symphyseal fracture	Transcervical
Parapharyngeal	Between pharyngeal constrictors and buccopharyngeal fascia anteriorly and medial pterygoid and parotid posteriorly	Divided by styloid process Anterior: Styloid muscles Posterior: Carotid sheath, IX, XI, XII	Retropharyngeal, submandibular, sublingual, pterygomandibular, peritonsillar, along carotid sheath	Upper and lower molars, tonsils, infection in adjacent spaces	Intraoral Transcervical
Retropharyngeal	Between pharyngeal constrictors and prevertebral fascia	Loose connective tissue	Parapharyngeal, mediastinum	Spread from parapharyngeal	Transcervical
Infraorbital	Between canine fossa and muscles of facial expression	Infraorbital nerves and vessels	Buccal	Upper anterior teeth (especially lateral incisor)	Intraoral
Deep temporal	Between temporal bone and temporalis	Maxillary vessels, mandibular nerve, pterygoid plexus	Pterygomandibular	Upper molars	Intraoral Transcervical
Superficial temporal	Between temporalis and temporoparietal fascia	Temporal fat pad, facial nerve	Submasseteric	Upper and lower molars	Intraoral Transtemporal

Adapted from Bridgeman [3] and Flynn [8]

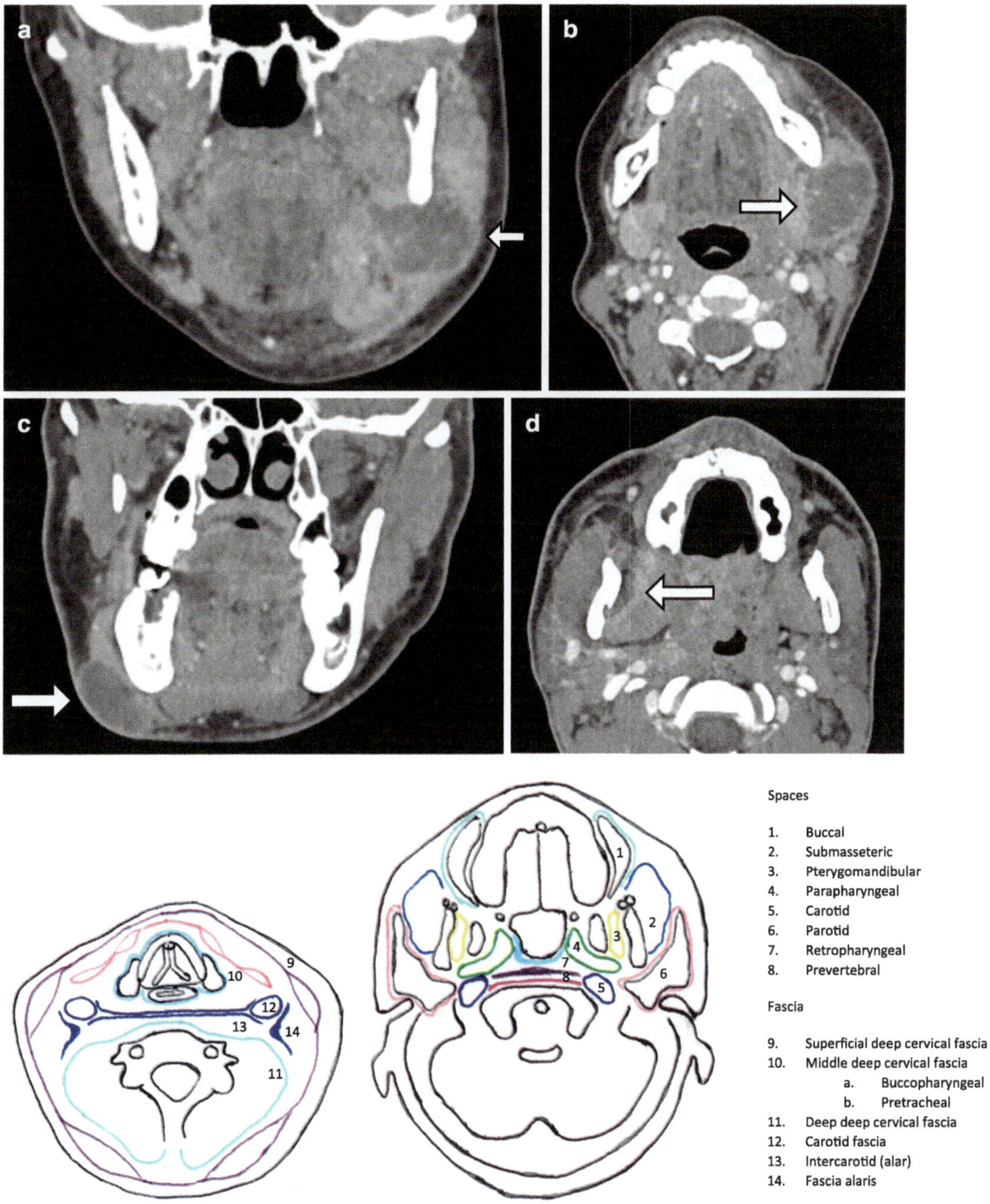

Fig. 17.1 Anatomy and computed tomography of deep neck space infections. Anatomical drawings adapted from Feigl [7], Granite [6], and Grodinsky and Holyoke [4]. Computed tomography scans of deep neck space infections: (**a** and **b**) show a submandibular abscess from the same patient, (**c**) buccal space abscess, (**d**) pterygomandibular abscess causing inflammation of the medial pterygoid muscle and resulting in trismus

17.6 Diagnosis—Management

17.6.1 Clinical Assessment and Work-Up

Patients with deep neck space infections most commonly present with odynophagia, dysphagia, fever, neck pain, neck swelling, trismus and dysphonia. Additional symptomology may result from their direct effect on adjacent structures and is discussed later in this chapter. The signs and symptoms of deep neck space infection are summarised in Table 17.2.

The most sensitive clinical features to detect moderate to high-risk infections are swelling, lymphadenopathy and trismus [9] (Fig. 17.2). The most specific features to differentiate between moderate to high-risk and low-risk infections are: dysphonia, floor of mouth elevation, dyspnoea, dysphagia or odynophagia, trismus, fever and tachypnoea [9].

The teeth most likely to cause moderate- to high-risk infections are the mandibular second and third molars as they drain directly to the submandibular and masticator spaces and can readily spread to the parapharyngeal space.

Miller et al. [10] showed that clinical assessment alone was only 63% accurate (55% sensitive and 73% specific) in identifying a drainable collection of 2 mL or more in deep neck space infections. Contrast-enhanced computed tomography (CT) alone was only 77% accurate (95% sensitive, 53% specific). Combining both of these modalities lead to 89% accuracy with 95% sensitivity and 80% specificity. This highlights the importance of CT as an adjunct to clinical assessment as 40% of the purulent collections on CT were not identified on clinical examination.

Table 17.2 Signs and symptoms of deep neck space infection

Signs	Symptoms
Neck swelling	Neck pain
Fever	Odynophagia
Trismus	Dysphagia
Pharyngeal wall medialisation	Dyspnoea
Dysphonia facial swelling	Otalgia
Oral swelling	Sialorrhea/drooling
Tongue elevation	
Floor of mouth swelling	
Pharyngeal wall medialisation	

Ban et al. [11] developed a prediction tool for the likelihood of finding purulent discharge at incision and drainage and stated that any three of the following was 81.4% accurate in predicting pus (79.5% sensitive, 82.8% specific):

1. Peripheral rim enhancement on CT.
   (a) Also a > 2.45 mL hypodense area on CT.
2. CRP > 41.25 mg/L.
3. ESR > 56.5 mm/h.
4. Neutrophil to lymphocyte ratio > 8.02.

17.6.2 Treatment

In their work on Ludwig's Angina, Williams and Guralnick [5] stated that the fundamental tenets of the management of deep neck space infections are: "to establish an adequate airway, to relieve tension, to secure drainage and to combat the infection by supplementary measures." Adoption of these principles, lead to a drop in mortality of 54–10% in 3 years. Notably, such improvement occurred prior to the use of penicillin, the first true antibiotic, and highlights the role of securing the airway and surgical egress in managing these infections. Modern medical care has further reduced the mortality from Ludwig's Angina to 4%.

We expand on these tenets by outlining the following additional steps:

1. Identify the presenting problem (i.e., infection and spaces involved).
2. Attempt to identify the cause (e.g., odontogenic or pharyngotonsillar).
3. Determine the severity.
   (a) Airway.
   (b) Spaces involved.
   (c) Duration and progression.
   (d) Host factors.
   (e) Determine setting of care (inpatient, intensive care or outpatient).
4. Supportive medical care (including antibiotics, fluid resuscitation and nutrition).
5. Treat surgically.

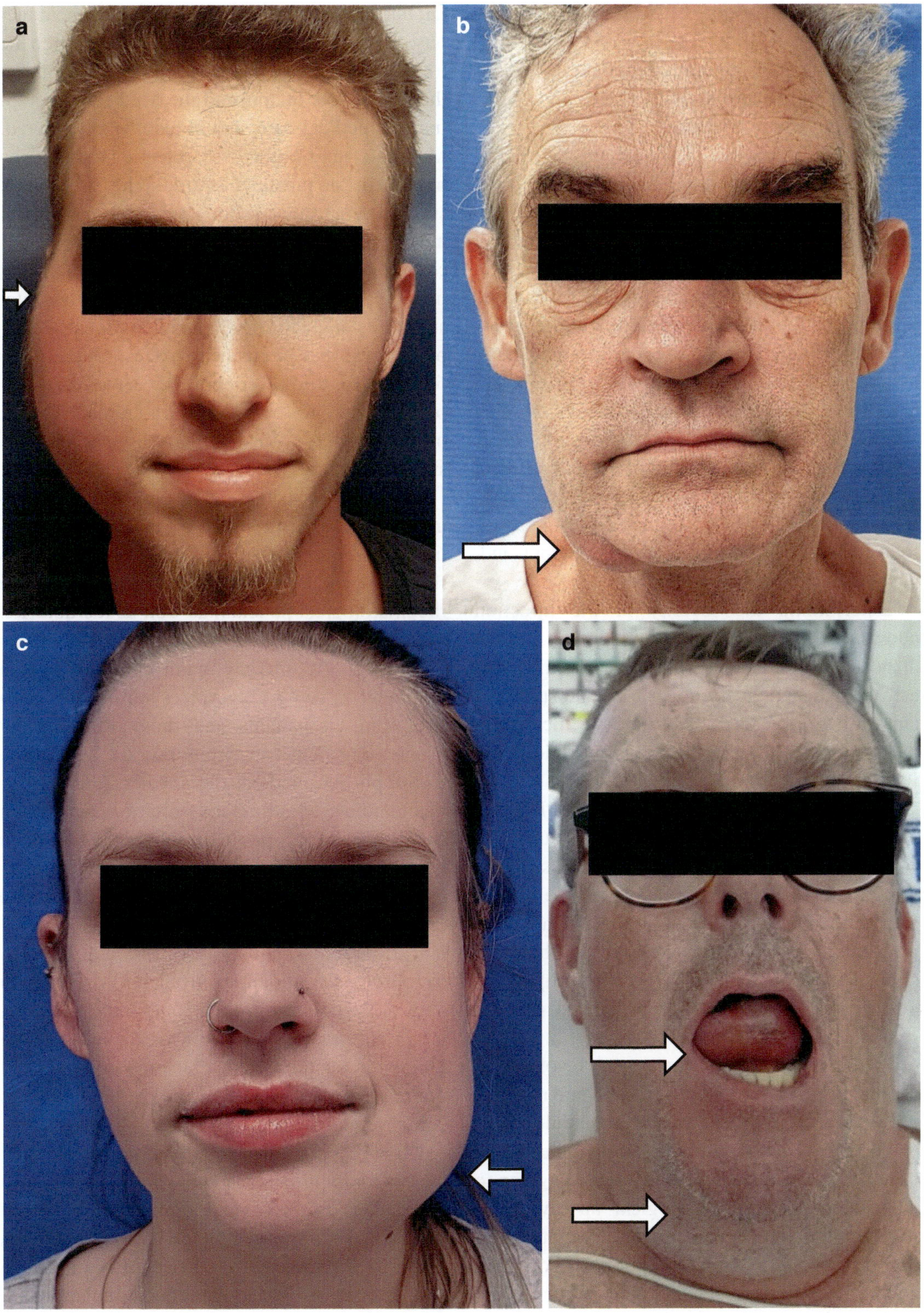

Fig. 17.2 Clinical photographs of deep neck space infections. Clinical photographs of deep neck space infections: (**a**) temporal space infection, (**b**) buccal space infection, (**c**) submandibular space infection, (**d**) Ludwig's Angina affecting the bilateral submandibular, sublingual and submental spaces with elevation of the floor of mouth and tongue

   (a) Removal of the cause (tooth, tonsil or other).
   (b) Drain any suppurative exudate.
   (c) Debride necrotic tissue.
6. Evaluate and re-evaluate.
   (a) Identify causes of treatment failure and adjust (i.e., changing antibiotics).

As is customary in all aspects of medical and surgical care, the identification of the presenting problem (and the spaces involved) can be achieved by the undertaking of a thorough clinical history, selection of appropriate diagnostic imaging (CT scan) and the requesting of relevant blood tests. Orthopantomogram X-rays are also helpful in the assessment of odontogenic infections as they are less susceptible to metal artefact and show the teeth and potential causes of pulp necrosis more clearly. Identification of the cause follows from this but is not always obvious and, in some instances, cannot be found.

Determining the severity of the infection allows for appropriate determination of patient disposition (outpatient, inpatient or intensive care) and ideal delivery of care. The most important of these steps is to determine whether or not the airway is at risk and this is a clinical decision. Inability to lay flat, tripoding and stridor are late signs of impending airway obstruction. Patients with impending airways should not be put in the CT scanner until their airway has been secured. Similarly, they should not be transferred to another health facility for definitive management until their airway has been secured. Thorough clinical assessment includes flexible nasopharyngolaryngoscopy to assess oedema and pharyngeal wall medialisation.

In the stable patient, the spaces involved on CT and their proximity to the airway and muscles of mastication can help predict potential airway challenges. Often trismus will necessitate awake fibre-optic intubation with consideration given to the establishment of a surgical airway being required in more difficult cases. Although aspiration of purulent exudate is a potential consideration, safely securing the airway is paramount.

The anatomical spaces closest to the teeth are considered low-risk spaces (i.e., vestibular, palatal, buccal, infraorbital) as well as the subcutaneous space. These low-risk spaces can often be treated in the outpatient setting under local anaesthetic, but host factors and the need for any supportive medical care should also be considered. Moderate- and higher-risk infections should be treated in an inpatient setting. The sublingual, submental and masticator spaces are considered moderate risk for their ability to spread to adjacent spaces and induce trismus. High-risk spaces include those that affect the airway or other vital structures including the parapharyngeal, retropharyngeal and pretracheal spaces. Once infection involves the prevertebral space, mediastinum, or has gone intra-orbital or intra-cranial, the risk of morbidity and mortality increases significantly.

Host factors such as diabetes mellitus, malnutrition, alcoholism, active malignancy and immune compromise in its broadest sense (including organ transplant, chemotherapy and rheumatological patients) as well as the duration and rate of progression of the infection can further affect the severity with more aggressive treatment being required in immune-compromised patients and those with rapidly progressing signs and symptoms.

Supportive medical therapy starts at assessment and includes fluid resuscitation, nutritional support and appropriate antibiotics. Most deep neck space infections are sensitive to penicillins, but there is a growing trend to microbial production of beta-lactamase. It is also important to note that whilst ampicillin and metronidazole cross the blood-brain barrier, clindamycin does not. The use of steroids in pharyngotonsillar infections has been shown to help reduce length of hospital stay, pain and trismus, but their use in odontogenic infections is controversial.

Fu et al. [12] showed that the most significant factors for requiring an admission to the Intensive Care Unit (ICU) from odontogenic infections were lower third molar involvement, dysphagia and a CRP >150 mg/L. All patients admitted to ICU in their study were identified as having mandibular infections, submandibular swelling and trismus.

Once the airway has been addressed and secured as required, the patient should be treated surgically by incision and drainage, establishing a dependent path of drainage, with copious irrigation of the infected spaces and removal of the cause, whether that involves a dental extraction, tonsillectomy or other. A swab should be sent for culture in moderate or higher-risk infections. Often, a passive drain is left in the infected spaces to allow for ongoing discharge of suppuration. Surgery is the mainstay of treating these conditions, and if there is an opportunity to manage the condition surgically prior to initiation of supportive medical therapy, it should be taken. Supportive medical therapy often precedes surgical treatment by way of logistics.

Post-operatively, the patient needs to be re-evaluated to determine resolution of the infection or the potential need for further surgery or a change in antibiotics. It is important to follow-up on microscopy and sensitivity results to ensure appropriate antibiotics delivery, while lack of improvement after 3 days may warrant a repeat CT scan to determine if there are any undrained loculations, extension of infection, retained foreign bodies, previously undiagnosed neoplasia or other potential causes of treatment failure.

17.7 Specific Deep Neck Space Infections

17.7.1 Actinomycosis

Actinomycosis is caused by the resident oral bacteria *Actinomyces israelii* and leads to purulent collections and sinus tract formation. Patients present with firm swelling associated with the jaws, discolouration of the overlying skin and fistulous tracts that discharge yellowish material, which, on microscopy reveals "sulfur granules," representing clumping of these bacterial colonies and is one of the hallmarks of this disease.

Actinomycosis is usually preceded by dental infection, dental procedures or other trauma. The infection localises to the soft tissues and after removal of the causative agent (i.e., tooth extraction), a prolonged course of antibiotics (usually penicillin) is required. This course includes 2–6 weeks of intravenous antibiotic therapy (occasionally via peripherally inserted central catheter) and is usually followed by several months of oral therapy. Unlike in other odontogenic infections where removal of the causative agent and incision and drainage of purulent material, along with antibiotics, often resolves fistulae, these may need to be excised in actinomycosis.

17.7.2 Necrotising Fasciitis

Necrotising fasciitis (NF) is a rapidly destructive infection which primarily affects muscles, fascia and subcutaneous fat. The viability of the overlying skin is compromised by thrombosis of the supporting dermal capillary network. Altered sensation or severe pain disproportionate to the clinical presentation may herald the onset of the condition.

Local subcutaneous duskiness, oedema and crepitus is the prodrome for the development of bullae, ecchymosis and necrosis in the associated skin. Features of systemic toxicity may become evident and lead to the development of sepsis, shock, organ failure and death.

The majority of cervico-facial presentations of NF are due to odontogenic causes with additional contributions from pharyngeal subsites. NF may also arise in post-operative or post-traumatic settings. Involvement of the mediastinum can occur from contiguous spread.

The microbiology is broadly classified as either being Type I (polymicrobial: *Staphylococcus*, *Streptococcus*, *Haemophilus vibrio*, *Escherichia*, *Bacteroides*), Type II (monomicrobial: Group A β-haemolytic *Streptococcus* (*pyogenes*) or methicillin resistant *Staphylococcus*), Type III (gas gangrene – *Clostridium*) or others (Type IV – *Vibrio*/fungal). Advancing age and immune compromise (including diabetes mellitus) underpin Type I presentations.

A laboratory risk indicator for necrotising fasciitis (LRINEC) score exists and may be useful to support a diagnosis. Imaging can be useful in delineating gas pockets in the affected tissue, but acquisition should not delay surgical treatment.

Once the diagnosis is considered, treatment must not be delayed and involves proportionate debridement of necrotic skin and subcutis. For patients in whom the clinical diagnosis is equivocal, a limited skin incision is made in the affected skin. Due to poor adherence of necrotic fascia to skin, a finger can be pushed through the necrotic tissue resulting in the release of purulent exudate and dishwater-coloured fluid.

For established NF, aggressive surgical debridement is the mainstay of treatment. The initial incision is placed to facilitate the excision of all necrotic skin. Debridement should be radial and extended until healthy, bleeding tissue is encountered both at the periphery and depth. Multiple tissue cultures and biopsies should be undertaken. The resultant wound should be repeatedly and copiously irrigated with diluted 0.25% sodium hypochlorite, and hydrosurgery can be enlisted to remove debris and reduce the bioburden.

Once debridement is completed, antiseptic dressings are applied. The patient will require supportive intensive care, broad spectrum antibiotics, fluid and nutritional support; and may require repeated returns to the operating room until a viable tissue bed is achieved. Repair may be facilitated by vacuum assisted wound closure, or skin grafting.

17.7.3 Descending Mediastinitis

Descending necrotising mediastinitis (DNM) is a life-threatening condition that affects the intrathoracic connective tissues that support the intrapleural space and intrathoracic viscera. Although mediastinitis most often occurs either secondary to oesophageal breach or occasionally following sternotomy, descending presentations typically arise from septic odontogenic or oropharyngeal subsites.

Spread from the neck occurs along fascial planes (pre-tracheal, visceral-perivascular, retropharyngeal-prevertebral) into the deep recesses of the neck, and thereafter to the mediastinum. This is generally thought to be via contiguous spread aided and abetted by gravity as well as the increased negative intrathoracic pressure that is generated during inspiration.

The clinical manifestations of mediastinal sepsis include fever, chest pain, dysphagia, stridor and perhaps the resultant trismus that accompanies deep neck space infection.

The causative bacteria are a mixed and polymicrobial population, most often consisting of Group A and B haemolytic *Streptococci* (*milleri*, *viridans*, *pyogenes*), *Staphylococci* (*aureus*, MRSA, *epidermidis*), *Klebsiella*, *Haemophilus*, *Bacteroides*, *Fusobacterium* and *Peptostreptococcal* groups.

The mediastinal pathology manifests as interstitial oedema, pericardial-pleural effusion, abscess, gas pockets and necrosis (air-fluid levels, loss of fat plane definition and rim enhancement as identified on CT).

Various classifications have been proffered to define the degree of mediastinal involvement. These generally demarcate a superior-inferior boundary at the level of the carina (T4), and an antero-posterior boundary in the mid-sagittal plane. The extent may be segmental or total. For anterior-superior involvement, a suprasternal transcervical-mediastinal approach may be sufficient to establish drainage. If not, and certainly for more extensive mediastinal involvement, transthoracic approaches are better and include thoracotomy or video-assisted thorascopic (via right-left parasternal or subxiphoid portals).

Treatment includes incision, drainage and debridement and can be supplemented by the undertaking of a pericardial window or lung decortication and the placement of a chest drain.

17.7.4 Ludwig's Angina

First described by Wilhelm Frederick Von Ludwig in 1836, Ludwig's angina is an acute onset, severe, rapidly progressive, bilateral spreading cellulitis, simultaneously involving sublingual, submental and submandibular spaces – filling the anterior cervical spaces, raising the floor of mouth and causing glossoptosis, leading to acute upper airway obstruction.

It is characterised, by pain, fever, trismus, dysphonia, dysphagia, elevation and displacement of the tongue and anterior floor of mouth with an inability to swallow saliva and indurated, brawny bilateral neck swellings that may be phlegmon or abscess. Patients are often unable to lie flat, and sit up in the tripod position. Up to a third of patients have a defined medical co-morbidity. An overwhelming majority of Ludwig's Angina cases are odontogenic in origin, although sialadenitis and soft and hard tissue trauma may also be implicated.

Later, concerning features on clinical assessment include stridor and cyanosis with the offending microbiology being similar to other deep neck space infections of an odontogenic origin. Again, the principles of securing the airway and surgical management of these spaces with supportive medical care have reduced the mortality of this condition to 4% in modern practice.

17.7.5 Lemierre's Syndrome

Described by André Lemierre in 1936, anaerobic post-anginal sepsis, in which previously well adolescent/young adult patients develop a pharyngotonsillar infection that results in internal jugular vein thrombophlebitis with septic emboli can be fatal. The causative organism is usually fusobacterium necrophorum.

The condition usually starts with a sore throat, fever and general malaise, progressing to extreme lethargy, rigors, swelling and tenderness along the sternocleidomastoid with a neck mass, pain and stiffness. The septic emboli most frequently travel to the lungs and large joints. As the condition progresses, patients develop pleuritic chest pain, dysphonia and dyspnoea with occasional haemoptysis and involvement of the neural structures associated with the carotid sheath, including Horner's syndrome. It is also important to consider retrograde venous flow and extension into the dural venous sinuses, leading to cerebral abscesses.

The mainstay of treatment is again surgical management of the cause of the infection, drainage of the affected spaces and the institution of supportive therapy, including antibiotics. The use of anticoagulation is controversial; however, ligation and resection of the affected part of the internal jugular vein is sometimes indicated.

17.8 Periorbital and Orbital Cellulitis

Although quite distinct entities, these conditions have overlapping clinical features and can be difficult to differentiate. They are inflammation and infection of the eyelids and pre-septal structures or orbital and post-septal structures and one can lead to the other. Classification of these infections suggests a continuum of disease ranging from pre-septal cellulitis, post-septal cellulitis, subperiosteal abscess and intraorbital abscess to cavernous sinus thrombosis.

Preseptal cellulitis is often caused from odontogenic infections spreading from the canine space, facial trauma, cutaneous infections and dacryocystitis. Orbital cellulitis is most commonly caused by a direct extension from the ethmoid sinuses but may spread from a preseptal infection or result from a penetrating injury or orbital surgery.

Clinical features include periorbital erythema and oedema with tenderness of the eyelids and post-septal extension leads to proptosis, chemosis, painful ophthalmoplegia, decreased visual acuity and a reduced pupillary response. Further progression can lead to autonomic nerve injury, optic neuritis, optic atrophy, superior orbital fissure or orbital apex syndrome, blindness, meningitis and cerebral abscess.

Additional surgical considerations include time to theatre, especially if there are signs of visual impairment or raised intra-ocular pressure as an orbital compartment syndrome can lead to permanent blindness. Intra-orbital collections are typically subperiosteal on the medial and superior walls of the orbit, reflecting their predominantly sinogenic aetiology and can be accessed transnasally with an endoscope or via a transcaruncular incision.

17.9 Cavernous Sinus Thrombosis

This is a septic (or aseptic) thrombosis of abrupt onset, usually due to spread from an antecedent infection located in the mid-facial "danger area," drained by the angular veins, most commonly from the nose, sino-nasal tract, dentition, periorbita or middle ear. The cavernous sinus received blood from the superior and inferior ophthalmic veins, is connected bilaterally across the midline and drains into the superior and inferior petrosal sinuses. As such, further extension can lead to cerebral abscess.

This infection is life-threatening, with a mortality rate of 20%, and requires immediate recognition and treatment as ongoing venous congestion and retinal haemorrhage can cause loss of vision and bilateral involvement can rapidly follow if left untreated.

Patients present with periorbital oedema and chemosis, headaches, photophobia and proptosis with any of the structures that travel within the cavernous sinus being affected. These include the cranial nerves III, IV and VI, leading to ophthalmoplegia, pupil dilation and loss of the accommodation reflex, as well as cranial nerves V1 and V2, leading to loss of the corneal reflex and loss of sensation along their dermatomal distributions.

The microbiology is most often *Staphylococcus aureus*, reflecting the predominantly nasal furuncle source of these infections, followed by *Streptococci* and Gram-negative anaerobes, reflecting oral cavity sources.

Additional considerations in the management of cavernous sinus thrombosis include a prolonged course of IV antibiotics for 6–8 weeks and heparin infusion offering a mortality benefit. The use of corticosteroids is controversial. Complications include blindness (can be bilateral), meningitis, cerebral abscess, epilepsy and Addisonian crisis from pituitary involvement.

17.10 Deep Neck Space Infection Pearls

Improved access to medical and dental care and the widespread availability of antibiotics has reduced the incidence of severe head and neck infections in Western populations. However, occasions of significant morbidity and mortality still occur. It is vital that all clinicians consider the salient features of these infections and their management:

1. Antecedent dental treatment or dental pain, recent peritonsillar pathology or coryza.
2. Critical symptoms include fever, stridor, trismus and a dusky, indurated swelling.
3. The bacteria are usually mixed polymicrobials with several virulence factors.
4. Thorough understanding of fascial planes, potential spaces and their interconnections underpinning propagation and collection are integral to appropriately predicting and surgically managing these infections.
5. Patient factors such as diabetes and immunocompromise exacerbate disease.
6. Management of the airway is first priority, including intubation or tracheostomy.
   (a) A raised, firm floor of mouth may be a sign for impending airway compromise.
7. Surgical treatment includes early incision, drainage, debridement (removal of the cause, drainage of purulent exudate, excision of necrotic tissue) via cervicotomy and/or thoracotomy.
8. Medical treatment includes the early institution of empirical combination antibiotic therapy (broad spectrum) and the adoption of appropriate stewardship following the results of culture and sensitivity, as well as nutritional, fluid and supportive intensive care.
9. Cross-sectional imaging is essential to accurately diagnose and define the extent of deep head and neck collections.

Delay in diagnosis and delay or improper surgical and medical management (including of the airway) are contributing factors to poor outcomes. Poor management of the airway remains a leading cause of death in these patients.

Always maintain a high index of suspicion and be ready to enlist multidisciplinary care where indicated, including general surgery, oral and maxillofacial surgery, ear, nose and throat surgery, cardio-thoracic surgery, neurosurgery, anaesthetics, intensive care physicians and infectious disease physicians.

A useful mnemonic for remembering some of these salient features is the 4Ts and 4Ds:

- Teeth, tonsils, trismus, tachypnoea.
- Dysphonia, dysphagia, diabetes (and other immunocompromise)
  and don't forget the airway!

References

1. Marioni G, Staffieri A, Parisi S, Marchese-Ragona R, Zuccon A, Staffieri C, et al. Rational diagnostic and therapeutic Management of Deep Neck Infections: analysis of 233 consecutive cases. Ann Otol Rhinol Laryngol. 2010;119(3):181–7.
2. Velhonoja J, Lääveri M, Soukka T, Irjala H, Kinnunen I. Deep neck space infections: an upward trend and changing characteristics. Eur Arch Otorhinolaryngol. 2020;277(3):863–72.
3. Bridgeman A, Wiesenfeld D, Newland S. Anatomical considerations in the diagnosis and management of acute maxillofacial bacterial infections. Aust Dent J. 1996;41(4):238–45.
4. Grodinsky M, Holyoke EA. The fasciae and fascial spaces of the head, neck and adjacent regions. Am J Anat. 1938;63(3):367–408.
5. Williams AC, Guralnick WC. The diagnosis and treatment of Ludwig's angina: a report of twenty cases. N Engl J Med. 1943;228(14):443–50.
6. Granite EL. Anatomic considerations in infections of the face and neck: review of the literature. J Oral Surg Am Dent Assoc 1965. 1976;34(1):34–44.
7. Feigl G, Hammer GP, Litz R, Kachlik D. The intercarotid or alar fascia, other cervical fascias, and their adjacent spaces – a plea for clarification of cervical fascia and spaces terminology. J Anat. 2020;237(1):197–207.
8. Flynn TR. Odontogenic infections. Oral Maxillofac Surg Clin N Am. 1991;3(2):311–29.
9. Weyh A, Busby E, Smotherman C, Gautam S, Salman SO. Overutilization of computed tomography for odontogenic infections. J Oral Maxillofac Surg. 2019;77(3):528–35.
10. Miller WD, Furst IM, Sàndor GKB, Keller MA. A prospective, blinded comparison of clinical examination and computed tomography in deep neck infections. Laryngoscope. 1999;109(11):1873–9.
11. Ban MJ, Jung JY, Kim JW, Park KN, Lee SW, Koh YW, et al. A clinical prediction score to determine surgical drainage of deep neck infection: a retrospective case-control study. Int J Surg. 2018;52:131–5.
12. Fu B, McGowan K, Sun H, Batstone M. Increasing use of intensive care unit for odontogenic infection over one decade: incidence and predictors. J Oral Maxillofac Surg. 2018;76(11):2340–7.

18 Regional Flaps for Head and Neck Reconstruction

Nitisha Narayan and Sinclair Gore

Regional flaps for reconstruction of the head and neck region come from the chest wall, scalp, face, neck and oral cavity. When planning reconstruction, attention is paid to the relevant anatomy, landmarks for flap harvest and the blood supply of the chosen flap. The flap size and design is then tailored to fit the defect. Consideration is given to the donor site morbidity; some donor site defects close directly while others may need skin grafts or undermining of the skin for closure.

In all cases general complications like bleeding, haematoma, seroma, delayed healing, wound breakdown and partial or complete flap necrosis may occur. Oher complications listed are specific to the individual flaps.

In this chapter, we have summarised the most important regional flaps available for head and neck reconstruction with key points pertaining to indications, relevant anatomy, flap design, harvest, management of the donor site and specific complications.

N. Narayan (✉) · S. Gore
Oxford University Hospital, Oxfordshire, UK
e-mail: Nitisha.Narayan@ouh.nhs.uk

18.1 Flaps from the Thorax

18.1.1 Pectoralis Major Flap

18.1.1.1 Background and Scope of Reconstruction

The pectoralis major flap, described by Ariyan in 1979, has played a central rolein reconstruction of head and neck defects [1]. Advantages of this flap include easy harvest, abundant soft tissue volume, large skin paddle, relative versatility, vascular reliability and short operating time. Its current applications include:

- Use as a "salvage flap" in cases with flap failure or complications (e.g., pharyngocutaneous fistula and carotid rupture),
- Use in primary procedures in patients with neck/laryngeal/pharyngeal defects who are excessively high-risk candidates for free flap reconstructions,
- Use in situations where bulky flaps are needed for volume restoration.

18.1.1.2 Anatomical Considerations

The Pectoralis Major flap is a type V Mathes and Nahai flap [2]. The flap blood supply is based on the thoracoacromial trunk and the sternal perforators of the internal mammary artery (Fig. 18.1). The thoracoacromial trunk has four described branches called the humeral, pectoral, clavicular and acromial branches. The muscle has sternal

B. Ashford (ed.), *Head and Neck Surgery for General Surgeons*,
https://doi.org/10.1007/978-981-19-7900-2_18

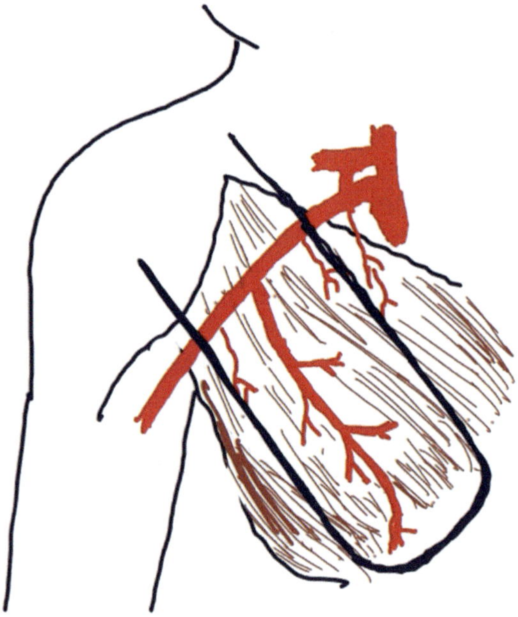

Fig. 18.1 Pectoralis major myocutaneous flap based on the pectoral branch of the thoracoacromial artery

and clavicular heads and it inserts onto the lateral lip of the bicipital groove. It is the sternal head that is typically taken as a flap, with or without a skin paddle.

18.1.1.3 Landmarks and Flap Design

The surface markings of the vascular pedicle are made by drawing a line from the ipsilateral acromion to the xiphisternum and another line vertically from the midpoint of the clavicle to intersect the first line. This is known as Ariyan's point and is where the vascular pedicle enters the deep surface of the muscle. The skin paddle of the flap is positioned over the pectoralis muscle along the course of the pectoral branch of the thoracoacromial artery.

18.1.1.4 Flap Harvest

Flap elevation commences with defining the skin paddle (if included as a myocutaneous flap) and islanding this on the muscle. If no skin paddle is included simple incision over the muscle is used. If included the skin paddle may be sutured to the underlying pectoralis muscle with sutures if there is concern about shearing injury to the myocutaneous perforators. However, the external aspect of the muscle has been defined division of the distal and medial muscle fibres permits dissection between the pectoralis minor and pectoralis major muscles. The flap vascular pedicle is found on the undersurface of the upper half of the pectoralis major muscle towards its lateral border. The pectoralis major muscle is divided lateral to the pedicle while keeping the pedicle in view, thereby freeing it from the humerus. Once dissected off the chest, the flap is passed into the neck through a subcutaneous tunnel created superficial to the clavicle. The tunnel is made wide enough to permit easy delivery of the flap into the neck without any compression. The flap is inset into the defect. Suction drains are placed in the neck and chest and the wounds are closed in layers. This flap has also been modified as a folded or tubed flap for circumferential pharyngeal defects.

18.1.1.5 Donor Site Considerations

The donor site may be closed primarily with mobilisation of fasciocutaneous flaps. If a large skin paddle is used and closure is difficult, local flaps or skin grafts may be used to facilitate wound healing.

18.1.1.6 Potential Complications

- Excessive flap bulk.
- Thoracic wall deformity.
- Functional impairment of the shoulder girdle.
- (Partial) skin paddle necrosis.
- Neck movement restriction due to flap insetting constraints.

18.1.2 Deltopectoral Flap

18.1.2.1 Background and Scope of Reconstruction

The deltopectoral flap was first described by Bakamjian [3]. This original 'workhorse' flap is a fasciocutaneous flap that provides thin, pliable skin which is ideal for reconstructing defects in the neck. This flap was popular in the 1960s, but its popularity gradually faded out with the advent of pedicled myocutaneous flaps and perforator-based microvascular free flaps. It was primarily used for:

- Reconstruction of anterior neck and lower face defects.
- Tracheostome reconstruction.
- Circumferential pharyngeal defects.

18.1.2.2 Anatomical Considerations

The flap is based medially and is supplied by the first three or four parasternal perforators from the internal mammary artery. It is raised in a subfascial plane to within 2–3 cm of the sternal margin. Beyond the medial (proximal) axial component of the flap, the lateral extent over the deltoid muscle is based on a random pattern blood supply. As such, this extension should be limited to a 1:1 base-to-length ratio beyond the axial chest wall section.

18.1.2.3 Landmarks and Flap Design

The flap is designed by estimating the arc of rotation needed to reach the defect and is oriented parallel to the clavicle over the deltoid. It is harvested in a lateral-to-medial fashion.

18.1.2.4 Flap Harvest

The deltopectoral fascia is incorporated into the flap and dissection is performed in subfascial plane. The flap is transposed on a broad base. Care should be taken to keep at least 2 cm from the lateral border of sternum to avoid injury of the perforating vessels. For neck or lower face defects, the skin between the defect and donor site may be de-epithelialised allowing one-stage reconstruction. Alternatively, the skin bridge can be left intact with the distal flap inset over the intact neck skin. In staged reconstruction of circumferential pharyngeal defects, the flap may be used for posterior wall reconstruction in the first stage leaving a pharyngostome. The anterior walls may be reconstructed separately with a pectoralis major flap. After a few weeks, the base of the flap is divided permitting closure of the neopharynx. For augmentation of an end-tracheostome with a short tracheal remnant, deltopectoral flaps may be inset to augment the posterior tracheal wall in a one-stage reconstruction.

18.1.2.5 Donor Site Considerations

The donor site often needs split skin graft reconstruction.

18.1.2.6 Potential Complications

- Neopharynx fistula and stricture formation.
- Poor donor site aesthetic outcome.
- Partial flap necrosis.

18.1.3 IMAP Flap

18.1.3.1 Background and Scope of Reconstruction

The internal mammary perforator (IMAP) flap introduced by Morain et al. in 2006 is a modification of the deltopectoral flap, allowing the flap to be completely islanded, resulting in a better donor site [4]. This flap has effectively replaced the deltopectoral flap in reconstructing the following defects:

- Inferior or lateral tracheostomal defects.
- Replacement of bulky myocutaneous flaps which obstruct the tracheostome.
- Small- to moderate-sized anterior neck defects.

18.1.3.2 Anatomical Considerations

The IMAP is based on the dominant internal mammary perforator vessels (typically a single artery and two venae commitantes) within either the second or third intercostal space.

18.1.3.3 Landmarks and Flap Design

The IMAP vessels are located in the first five intercostals spaces, less than 20 mm from the lateral edge of the sternum. The second IMAP is the most constant and reliable. Mean arterial diameter ranges from 0.85 mm to 1–1.5 mm. A handheld Doppler is used to confirm and mark the location of the perforator artery. Once the perforator is marked, the flap is designed transversely towards the axilla or obliquely across the chest wall. The medial limit is the sternum (midline). Flaps up to 10 cm width can be raised reliably and the resultant donor sites can often be closed primarily.

18.1.3.4 Flap Harvest

The superior and inferior incisions are made down to the pectoralis fascia, and subfascial dissection is carried out from lateral to medial until 4–5 cm from the sternal border. From this point, dissection is performed using fine scissors until the perforator vessels are identified and dissected to the pedicle origin which is usually 1–2 cm lateral to the edge of the sternum. The flap is then islanded. If needed, additional pedicle length can be achieved by division of the pectoralis major muscle, intercostals muscles and excision of the second costal cartilage. The flap is transposed to reconstruct the defect by dividing the narrow skin bridge between the donor site and neck defect. Alternatively, the flap can be de-epithelialised and tunneled under the skin bridge.

18.1.3.5 Donor Site Considerations

The donor defect is closed primarily over suction drains after undermining.

18.1.3.6 Potential Complications

- Flap vascularity impairment due to twisting of the pedicle.

18.1.4 Trapezius Muscle Flap

18.1.4.1 Background and Scope of Reconstruction

Since the description by Baek et al. in 1980, the pedicled lower trapezius musculocutaneous flap has been a standard flap in head and neck reconstruction. Its applications include reconstruction of

- The oropharynx, buccal mucosa, cheek and anterior neck.
- The temporal fossa.
- The integument overlying the cervical spine.

18.1.4.2 Anatomical Considerations

The trapezius muscle is classified as a Mathes and Nahai type II vascular pattern with a dominant pedicle and additional minor pedicles. The upper part of the trapezius muscle is supplied by branches of the occipital artery; the middle and lateral parts are supplied mainly by the superficial cervical artery (the superficial branch of the transverse cervical artery) and the lower part is supplied by the dorsal scapular artery. It originates from the occiput, superior nuchal line and spinous processes of C7-T12 and inserts to the clavicle and scapula.

18.1.4.3 Landmarks and Flap Design

Upper Trapezius Myocutaneous Flap: The anterior margin of the flap follows the border of the trapezius muscle and is parallel to the posterior border. Flap is usually 6–10 cm wide and can be up to 30 cm long. It is based on the occipital artery.

Lower Trapezius Myocutaneous Flap: This flap is based on the transverse cervical artery (traditionally) and dorsal scapular artery (more recent descriptions). This flap is designed at right angles to the lateral border of the trapezius muscle just below the tip of the scapula with an elliptical skin paddle. This enhances the reach of the flap, which is pivoted at the level of the base of the spine of the scapula capturing the fasciocutaneous perforators of the dorsal scapular system.

18.1.4.4 Flap Harvest

Upper Trapezius Myocutaneous Flap: The distal part of the flap is fasciocutaneous, two large muscular perforators are divided at this stage. Nerve supply to the trapezius is carefully preserved. At the neck shoulder junction, the plane of dissection changes to submuscular. Three perforators supply the proximal part of the flap, at least one may be divided to improve flap mobility. Flap may be delayed if longer length required to reach the tip of the nose.

Lower Trapezius Myocutaneous Flap: After the incision around the skin paddle of the flap has been made, it is continued as a vertical incision from the upper limit of the flap toward the posterior triangle of the neck. This vertical incision is at the midpoint between the scapula and the spinous processes of the vertebrae. The inferior portion of the trapezius muscle is included in the elevation of the flap by its detachment medially from the spinous processes of T10 and its paraspinous perforators. In elevating the skin paddle laterally, it is important to include the fascia overlying the latissimus dorsi muscle and then to dissect from lateral to medial under this fascia. The attachment of the trapezius muscle to the scapula and clavicle is preserved [5].

18.1.4.5 Donor Site Considerations

The upper trapezius flap donor site often needs a split skin graft; the lower flap defect can usually be closed directly.

18.1.4.6 Potential Complications

- Shoulder weakness/stiffness.

18.2 Flaps from the Neck

18.2.1 Supraclavicular Flap

18.2.1.1 Background and Scope of Reconstruction

In 1949, the first clinical application of a flap from the shoulder was performed by Kazanjian and Converse. In 1983, Lamberty and Cormack described the supraclavicular axial patterned flap. Beginning in the 1990s, Pallua et al. popularised its use as the supraclavicular island flap. Its applications include

- Anterior neck defects (including burn contracture reconstruction).
- Laryngopharyngeal and tracheostomal defect reconstruction.
- Lateral face and ear reconstruction.

18.2.1.2 Anatomical Considerations

The supraclavicular flap is a fasciocutaneous flap based on the supraclavicular artery which is a branch of the transverse cervical artery. Less frequently, it may arise from the suprascapular artery, which may be smaller. The supraclavicular artery mean diameter varies from 1.1 to 1.5 mm, its pedicle length ranges from 1 to 7 cm and it is present in 80 percent of cases [6].

18.2.1.3 Landmarks and Flap Design

Bolsters are placed under the shoulder site to improve exposure. The neck and the arm are prepared to the elbow. The vascular source of the flap arises from the lateral neck bordered by the clavicle and the sternocleidomastoid and trapezius muscles. Confirming a vascular doppler signal tangential to the clavicle is useful to guide where the pedicle emerges from the neck to perfuse the angiosome overlying the deltoid muscle. A 6–7 cm wide elliptical island flap is designed over the anterior deltoid and supraclavicular region with the proximal part of the flap designed to include the previously identified pedicle (Fig. 18.2).

18.2.1.4 Flap Harvest

The flap is dissected from distal to proximal in a subfascial fashion toward the pedicle using electrocautery. Once proximate to the acromion, fine dissection proceeds to lift the flap off the acromion and clavicle, sometimes including periosteum to minimise the chance of pedicle injury. Typically, the flap extends as far as the deltoid insertion although the distal part of the flap may be trimmed until healthy bleeding tissue is noted. The flap can be partially de-epithelialised to facilitate it being tunneled under intact neck skin. It can transposed for external cutaneous replacement or can be 'turned over' for aerodigestive tract reconstruction.

18.2.1.5 Donor Site Considerations

A donor site up to 7 cm wide over the deltoid can usually be closed directly over a suction drain. Although the skin may be tight upon closure this typically stretches well over time leaving very little long term functional donor site morbidity.

18.2.1.6 Potential Complications

- Distal flap necrosis.
- Temporary restriction in shoulder function due to tension on skin closure.

18.2.2 Submental Flap

18.2.2.1 Background and Scope of Reconstruction

The submental island flap was first described in 1992 by Martin et al. as a submental artery regional flap for soft-tissue head and neck reconstruction. It has the advantages of thinness, pli-

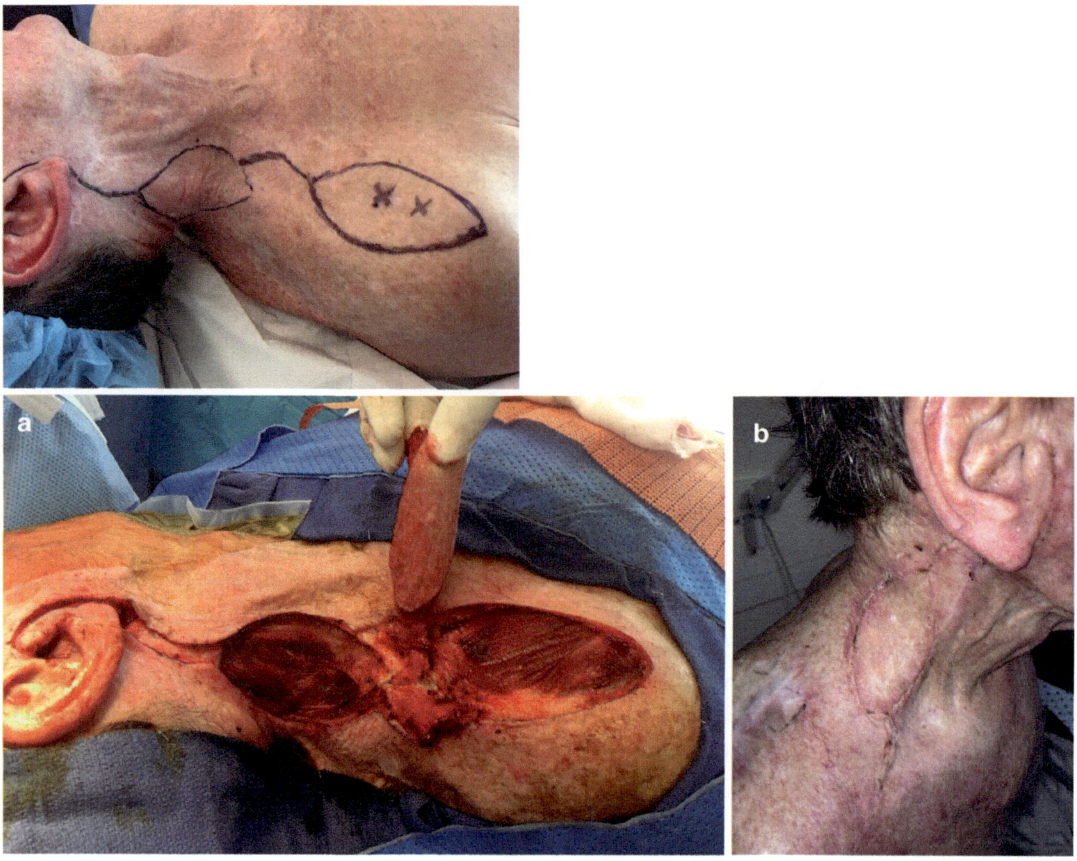

Fig. 18.2 Landmarks right supraclavicular flap for recurrent metastatic neck disease. Supraclavicular flap (**a**) mobilisation and (**b**) and post-operative

ability and versatility in design shared by the radial forearm free flap [7]. It also provides an excellent colour match for the head and neck region, can be raised with ease and has an acceptable donor site. It can be used as a cutaneous, myocutaneous, fasciocutaneous, or osteocutaneous flap. It should be used with caution in the presence of metastatic disease in the neck (given the usual requirement to dissect effected nodal basins) and it is contraindicated in the setting of previous radiotherapy, ligation of the facial artery, or prior ipsilateral neck surgery. Its uses include reconstruction of

- Facial and neck skin defect.
- Intraoral defects.
- Maxillofacial defects (reverse submental artery flap).

18.2.2.2 Anatomical Considerations

The flap is based on the submental vessels which are branches of the facial artery. The marginal mandibular branch of the facial nerve is in proximity and must be preserved, including the anterior belly of digastric in the flap increases the chance of preserving adequate flap vascularity.

18.2.2.3 Landmarks and Flap Design

A pinch test is performed to delineate the maximal width of the skin paddle under the mandible in the midline that will allow primary closure to be possible. The submental island is planned within this according to the size of defect. The surface marking of the origin of the submental artery is a point 5.5 (4–7) cm anterior to the angle of the mandible and 7 (3–15) mm from the mandibular border.

18.2.2.4 Flap Harvest

The inferior incision is performed first, and the ipsilateral submandibular salivary gland is approached after dissection through skin, subcutaneous tissue and platysma. Care is taken to preserve both the facial artery and vein. The vascular tributaries to the submandibular gland are carefully identified and ligated as close as possible to the gland. The skin paddle is then dissected in the subplatysmal plane starting at the contralateral side of the symmetrical ellipse. The dissection plane is superficial to the anterior belly of the digastric muscle on the contralateral side. On the ipsilateral side, the anterior belly of digastric is identified, its common tendon is sectioned and the muscle is then included in the flap. The attachment of the anterior belly of the digastric muscle to the mandible is divided and the superior incision is completed to raise the flap. The pedicle is defined proximally towards the submandibular gland; the facial vessels are ligated distal to the origins of the submental vessels, allowing the flap to be freely mobile. The flap is then transposed and sutured into place.

18.2.2.5 Donor Site Considerations

Directly closed under the mandible over a drain.

18.2.2.6 Potential Complications

- Lower branch facial nerve weakness.
- Aesthetic outcome can be unpredictable.

18.3 Flaps from the Scalp Region

18.3.1 Temporo-Parietal Fascia Flap

18.3.1.1 Background and Scope of Reconstruction

The temporoparietal fascia flap (TPFF) is the thinnest flap described here and is the only pedicled fascial flap routinely used in the head and neck. It is highly vascular and pliable and therefore conforms to a wide variety of defects [8]. It also gives a robust scaffold for covering cartilage or bone grafts with minimal donor site contour defect. These properties make it extremely versatile. As a pedicled flap, it may be used to reconstruct the following defects:

- Auricular defects (congenital and acquired).
- Orbital exenteration defects.
- Soft tissue augmentation for facial contour defects in the setting of previous trauma or hemifacial microsomia.
- Hair-bearing flap reconstruction of lip or brow defects using an interpolated or tunneled design (uni- or bi-pedicled) in a staged manner.
- Skull base defects.

18.3.1.2 Anatomical Considerations

The temporoparietal fascia (TPF) is a thin layer of connective tissue immediately deep to the hair follicles. It is continuous with the occipitofrontalis and galea and the superficial musculoaponeurotic system (SMAS) below the zygomatic arch. The branches of the facial nerve run on its deep surface whilst the superficial temporal vessels run on its external surface. It is separated from the deep temporal fascia (DTF) by a loose areolar layer. The blood supply of the TPF flap comes from the superficial temporal artery. It travels with the vein anterior to the root of the helix, gives anterior and posterior branches in the temple and goes on to ramify on the surface of the TPF. The auriculotemporal sensory nerve which lies posterior to the artery provides sensation to the scalp and is often divided during elevation of the flap.

18.3.1.3 Landmarks and Flap Design

The lower skin incision is placed anterior to the ear, in the preauricular crease. Numerous scalp access incisions may be used allowing for wide exposure of the flap under the scalp skin and follicles.

18.3.1.4 Flap Harvest

In the scalp, the skin is elevated just deep to the hair follicles avoiding injury to the vessels. After the anterior and posterior flaps are developed in the scalp and the pedicle is identified anterior to the ear, the area of the desired flap is marked and incised. The anterior margin of the flap should be placed posterior to the path of the frontal branch of the facial nerve. The flap is raised easily off the deep temporal fascia. At the root of the helix, the flap may be narrowed dramatically to allow optimal movement.

18.3.1.5 Donor Site Considerations

Closed directly with a suction drain.

18.3.1.6 Potential Complications

- Alopecia.
- Scalp wound breakdown.

18.3.2 Temporalis Muscle Flap

18.3.2.1 Background and Scope of Reconstruction

The temporalis muscle flap (first described by Lentz in 1895) is a robust pedicled flap which is commonly used for reconstruction after oncological resections or craniofacial surgery [9]. It is thin, has reliable vascularity, is easy to access and gives minimal donor site morbidity. It is used in the following situations:

- Orbital reconstruction.
- Facial reanimation.
- Reconstruction of defects in the lateral and posterior pharyngeal wall.
- Reconstruction of the hard and soft palate and the retromolar trigone.

18.3.2.2 Anatomical Considerations

The temporalis muscle originates from the temporal fossa and inserts onto the coronoid process and the anterior border of the ramus of the mandibule. The muscle lies between the deep temporal fascia and the temporal fossa of the lateral skull, and courses beneath the zygomatic arch, elevating and retracting the mandible. It is a type III (Mathes and Nahai) muscle supplied by the anterior and posterior deep temporal arteries which are branches of the second part of the internal maxillary artery. It enters the muscle on its medial surface and is therefore protected when dissection is performed in the subperiosteal plane. Motor innervation is supplied by the deep temporal nerves from the mandibular branch of the trigeminal nerve.

18.3.2.3 Landmarks and Flap Design

A hemi-coronal incision is made with extension inferiorly into the preauricular region.

18.3.2.4 Flap Harvest

The scalp is elevated from superior to inferior in the subaponeurotic plane directly on the deep temporal fascia, reaching the upper margin of the superficial temporal fat pad and finally the zygoma. The periosteum is elevated from the zygomatic arch and the scalp flap elevation is completed. Maintaining the attachment of the superficial temporal fat pad protects the temporal branch of the facial nerve and prevents hollowing. The scalp flap is further elevated from the preauricular region anteriorly over the length of the zygoma to the orbital rim. Removal of the zygomatic arch facilitates elevation of the temporalis muscle flap, provides extra length, facilitates coronoid resection and reduces trauma to the flap and the temporomandibular joint during flap delivery into the oropharynx. Most tissue defects require the full length of the temporalis muscle for reconstruction but may not need the full width. Therefore, the anterior one-third of the muscle is often not elevated, minimising any significant hollowing of the temporal region. The paired internal maxillary vessels are identifiable when the flap has been elevated to a level below the zygoma. The flap is typically 12–16 cm wide and 0.5–1.0 cm thick. The flap can reach the oral cavity and the pharynx. Because of its axial blood supplies, the flap can also be split into anterior and posterior portions to cover adjacent defects, such as the palate and tonsillar fossa.

18.3.2.5 Donor Site

The scalp incision closes directly over a drain.

18.3.2.6 Complications

- Facial nerve injury.
- Temporal hollowing.
- Hair loss.
- Trismus.

18.3.3 Washio Flap

18.3.3.1 Background and Scope of Harvest

Transferring retroauricular tissue on a temporal pedicle was first described by Washio and popularised by Maillard and Montandon. The Washio retroauricular temporal flap provides thin skin and, if required, cartilage that can be adapted for various defects [10]. The flap has largely been replaced by the paramedian forehead flap for nasal reconstruction because of its versality and ability to cover larger defects including total nasal reconstruction.

18.3.3.2 Anatomical Considerations

The retroauricular temporal flap relies upon rich anastomoses between the superficial temporal and posterior auricular vessels. It is an axial pattern flap with a random pattern distal extension. The prerequisites are a palpable superficial temporal artery and no evidence of scarring in the temporoparietal region. The tip of the flap can be designed with retroauricular skin, ear cartilage and subcutaneous tissue from the mastoid region as required.

18.3.3.3 Landmarks and Flap Design

The first step in planning the flap is to palpate the superficial temporal artery in the upper pre-tragal region. This point is marked and the distance from this point to the defect is measured; this distance is then projected onto the temporoparietal scalp to design the flap.

18.3.3.4 Flap Harvest

The flap is raised in the subgaleal plane. If some or all of the flap is being taken from the posterior aspect of the pinna, it is important that sufficient deep tissue is raised from the retroauricular sulcus to include the posterior auricular artery which sends branches to the tissues on the posterior aspect of the pinna. Once the flap is raised, it is transferred to the defect and inset. The temporal component of the flap may be tubed or the raw surface may be skin grafted to make the weeks between stages more manageable.

18.3.3.5 Donor Site Considerations

The secondary defect in the scalp should be grafted with thin split skin grafts to prevent periosteal desiccation and skull exposure. The secondary defect in the retro-auricular area should be skin grafted with thicker split skin graft or a full thickness skin graft.

18.3.3.6 Potential Complications

- Alopecia.
- Numbness of the scalp.

18.4 Flaps from the Face

18.4.1 Paramedian Forehead Flap

18.4.1.1 Background and Scope of Reconstruction

The forehead flap has been mentioned in ancient Indian, Italian and Greek texts and has been extensively described by Gillies, Millard and Converse. More recently, Burget and Menick have popularised its applications in nasal reconstruction.

18.4.1.2 Anatomical Considerations

The forehead is a multilaminar structure comprising of skin, subcutaneous tissue, frontalis muscle, and a thin areolar layer overlying periosteum. When a paramedian forehead is raised, the supratrochlear vessels pass over the periosteum at the supraorbital rim extend vertically upward within the frontalis muscle to lie subcutaneously at the hairline. It is both a myofascial and an axial flap.

18.4.1.3 Landmarks and Flap Design

The flap is commonly planned in reverse using a template from the defect from the ipsilateral paramedian forehead (Fig. 18.3a).

18.4.1.4 Flap Harvest

Traditionally, the upper forehead skin is transferred in stages. At the first stage, the skin island is raised with frontalis muscle. Some surgeons choose to include periosteum inferiorly although this does not add vascular benefit to the flap. Distally, the flap may be thinned partially such that the transferred skin is inset into the recipient site. A skin graft may be used to line the pedicle to reduce the need for dressings during the period of flap transfer. In a two-stage procedure, the pedicle is divided at least 3 weeks later, permitting final inset of the skin flap. At this time, the base of the pedicle is re-inset to the brow, aiming for a smooth contour in the brow and neat linear closure in the lower forehead. In such a setting, aggressive thinning of the skin flap (to improve the aesthetic contour of the final result) or use of the flap to 'turn over' to create nasal lining is not possible. To overcome these problems, the technique of forehead flap transfer has been modified to a three-stage technique which ensures an optimal blood supply, a thin covering flap, controlled shaping and the possibility of nasal lining being created separate to the external nasal covering. In this setting, the flap is raised and thinned at an intermediate operation, whilst the pedicle is only divided at a third stage after another period of at least 3 weeks between the second and third stages. Adding an intermediate stage gives the ability to improve aesthetic results and minimise the need for later revisions. Prior to planned reconstruction of larger defects, the forehead tissue may also be expanded. This technique expands the surface area of skin that can be harvested whilst permitting acceptable forehead skin closure [11].

18.4.1.5 Donor Site Considerations

The forehead donor site can be closed directly or should be left to heal by secondary intention (Fig. 18.3b). Such a defect should not typically be skin grafted as this invariably leads to a poor aesthetic outcome and one that is worse than secondary intention healing would give.

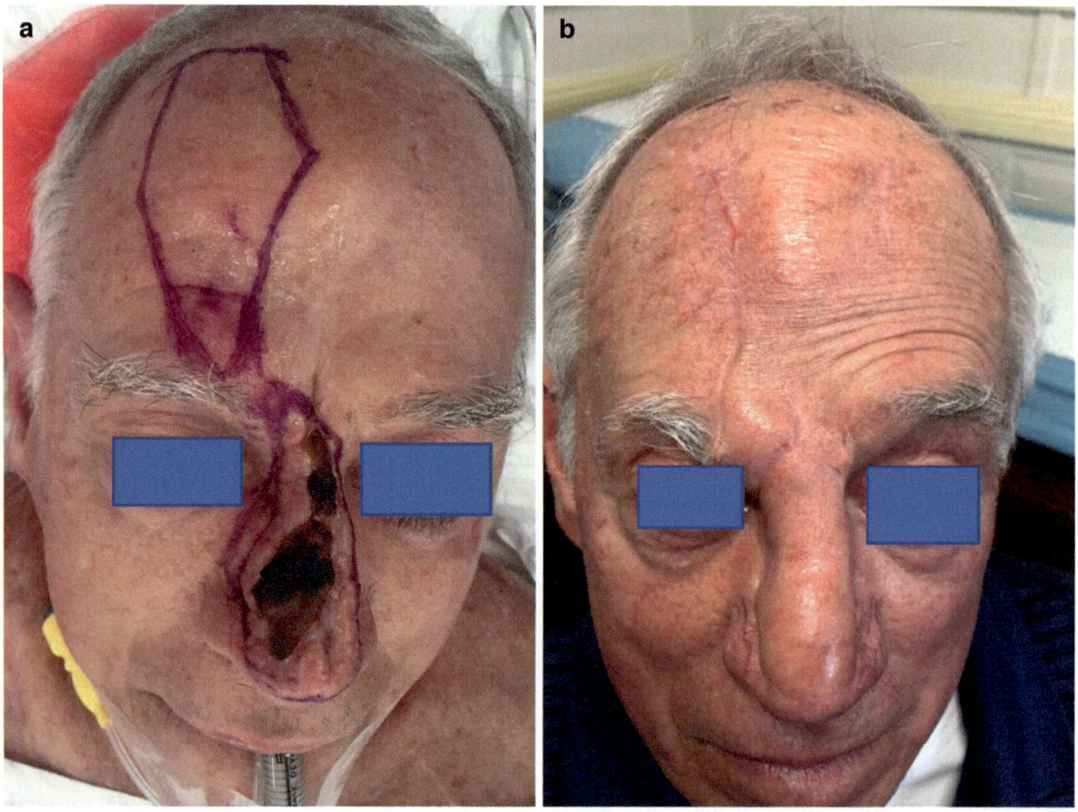

Fig. 18.3 Paramedian forehead flap for nasal defect. (**a**) Flap design. (**b**) Healed donor site (by secondary intention) and inset at 4 months

18.4.1.6 Potential Complications

- Venous congestion (possibly requiring treatment with leeches).
- Altered scalp sensation above the flap.
- Temporary partial obstruction of vision due to flap pedicle positioning.
- Donor site aesthetic issues related to scar healing and forehead contour.

18.5 Flaps from the Oral Cavity

18.5.1 Facial Artery Musculomucosal Flap

18.5.1.1 Background and Scope of Reconstruction

The FAMM flap, originally described by Pribaz, is an axial flap based on the facial artery which comprises mucosa and submucosa from the intraoral cheek, buccinator muscle and the deepest part of the labial orbicularis muscle [12]. Its applications include

- Reconstruction following tumour excision in the oral cavity or oropharynx.
- Closure of perforations or fistulas of the oral cavity.
- Osteoradionecrosis reconstruction.

18.5.1.2 Anatomical Considerations

The flap can be designed with an inferior pedicle with anterograde flow in the facial artery or with a superior pedicle with retrograde flow. As such, it is a type 3 Mathes and Nahai flap. It is versatile providing a wide arch of rotation, a superior or inferior pivot depending on the defect location, and a good aesthetic result with no skin incision.

18.5.1.3 Landmarks and Flap Design

The facial artery crosses the mandible 2.5 cm anterior to the angle of the mandible is palpable in most patients at this point. As it ascends in the cheek, its path can be marked using a doppler device. When designing the flap mucosal paddle, the location of Stenson's duct papilla should be identified and not included in the flap. A silk stitch is inserted at lip commissure to provide traction. Orientation of the flap paddle horizontally may result in less trismus than a vertically or obliquely oriented paddle.

18.5.1.4 Flap Harvest

The flap margins are infiltrated with adrenaline-containing local anaesthesia to facilitate dissection. The initial dissection commences anteriorly, 1 cm behind the commissure. The flap is raised with the mucosa, submucosa and buccinator muscle until the facial artery and vein are identified. Once the vessels are identified and preserved, the remainder of the flap is raised.

18.5.1.5 Donor Site Considerations

The donor site can usually be subtotally or completely closed directly using absorbable sutures. Temporary restricted mouth opening improves with regular physical therapy once initial healing is underway.

18.5.1.6 Potential Complications

- Partial flap necrosis.
- Trauma to the pedicle from the teeth.
- Trismus.
- Long-lasting cheek tightness.

18.5.2 Buccinator Flap

18.5.2.1 Background and Scope of Reconstruction

The buccinator flap is another musculomucosal flap variant harvested from cheek mucosa. It was initially described by Bozola with a posteriorly-based blood supply to the buccinator muscle deriving from the buccal artery [13]. It is mostly used for reconstructing palatal defects and lengthening the palate as part of speech surgery following cleft palate repair.

18.5.2.2 Anatomical Considerations

The buccinator muscle originates from the pterygomandibular raphe and blends with the orbicularis oris muscle anteriorly. It extends between the maxillary vestibule superiorly and the mandibular vestibule interiorly. It lies between the oral mucosa and the facial artery and vein. Its blood supply is posteriorly-based from the buccal branch of the maxillary artery.

18.5.2.3 Landmarks and Flap Design

Stensen's duct pierces the buccinator muscle slightly above its centre. Therefore, only half of the buccinator muscle and overlying mucosa can be used for reconstruction. The flap is designed as an ellipse with the upper margin of the flap sited just below the duct orifice. Relocation of Stensen's duct can add more mucosa if a larger flap is required.

18.5.2.4 Flap Harvest

The flap is harvested taking mucosa, buccal fat and part of the buccinator muscle. It is not dependent on the facial artery and vein from which it is separated. Incorporation of the inferior buccal branch makes the blood supply more reliable. Islanding the flap to increase flap mobility is a variant. Bite blocks are required to protect the pedicle. A second stage may be needed to divide the pedicle and provide a smooth flap inset.

18.5.2.5 Donor Site Considerations

Primary donor site closure is possible in defects less than 2.5 cm in width. Larger donor sites can be managed with buccal fat pad mobilisation or masseter flap transposition and subsequent secondary re-epithelialisation. When the pedicle is divided at a second stage, the donor site may need a z-plasty to avoid scar contracture.

18.5.2.6 Potential Complications

- Partial necrosis of flap.
- Trauma to the pedicle from the teeth.
- Trismus.
- Long-lasting cheek tightness.

Table of key details of regional flaps in head and neck reconstruction

Flap	Type of flap	Blood supply	Described by	Uses
Pec major	Myocutaneous Ty5 M&N	Pectoral branch of thoracoacromial artery, perforators internal mammary artery	Ariyan	Ant neck, tracheostome, pharyngeal defects
Deltopectoral	Fasciocutaneous	First three or four branches of the internal mammary artery	Bakamjian	Ant neck, tracheostome, pharyngeal defects
IMAP	Fasciocutaneous	2,3rd perforator from IMA	Moraine	Small ant neck defects, tracheostome
Supraclavicular	Fascioutaneous	Supraclavicular branch of transverse cervical A	Kazanjian, Converse, Pallua	Ant neck, lateral face, ear, laryngo-pharyngeal
Trapezius	Ty2 M&N- myocutaneous	Upper-occipital A Lower-transverse cervical artery (traditionally) and dorsal scapular artery (more recent)	Baek	Pharynx, ipsilateral tonsil, buccal mucosa, cheek and anterior neck, temporal fossa Posteriorly, op mid-neck or mastoid region
Submental	Axial fasciocutaneous	Submental branch of facial Artery	Martin	Intra/peri-oral and mandibular defects
TPF	Axial fascia only	Superficial temporal artery	Monks	Orbit, facial, skull base, ear
Temporalis	Ty 3 M&N muscle flap	2 Branches off deep temporal artery	Lentz	Facial animation, LTM (Labbe), fill orbit/skull defect
Washio	Axial fasciocutaneous	Anastomoses between the superficial temporal and posterior auricular vessels	Washio	Nose

Flap	Type of flap	Blood supply	Described by	Uses
Paramedian forehead	Axial fascio/ myocutaneous	Supratrochlear	Gillies, Millard, Converse, Menick	Nose, cheek
FAMM	Musculomucosal Ty 3 M&N	Facial artery	Pribaz	Defects of oral cavity
Buccinator	Musculomucosal Ty 3 M&N	Buccal Br of maxillary	Bozola	Palate defects

References

1. Ariyan S. The pectoralis major myocutaneous flap. A versatile flap for reconstruction in the head and neck. Plast Reconstr Surg. 1979;63:73–81.
2. Mathes SJ, Nahai F. Classification of the vascular anatomy of muscles: experimental and clinical correlation. Plast Reconstr Surg. 1981;67(2):177–87.
3. Bakamjian VY, Long M, Rigg B. Experience with the medially based deltopectoral flap in reconstructive surgery of the head and neck. Br J Plast Surg. 1971;24:174–83.
4. Morain WD, Hallock GG, Neligan PC. Internal mammary artery perforator flap. In: Blondeel PN, Morris SF, Hallock GG, Neligan PC, editors. Perforator flaps: anatomy, technique and clinical applications. St. Louis: Quality Medical; 2006. p. 429–39.
5. Baek SM, Biller HF, Krespi YP, Lawson W. The lower trapezius Island myocutaneous flap. Ann Plast Surg. 1980;5:108.
6. Pallua N, Wolter TP. Moving forwards: the anterior supraclavicular artery perforator (a-SAP) flap: a new pedicled or free perforator flap based on the anterior supraclavicular vessels. J Plast Reconstr Aesthet Surg. 2013;66:489–96.
7. Martin D, Pascal JF, Baudet J, et al. The submental Island flap: a new donor site. Anatomy and clinical applications as a free or pedicled flap. Plast Reconstr Surg. 1993;92:867.
8. Collar R, Zopf D, Brown D, Fung K, Kim J. The versatility of the temporoparietal fascia flap in head and neck reconstruction. JPRAS. 2012;65:141–8.
9. Lentz J. Resection du col du condyle avec interposition d'un lambeau temporal entre les surfaces de resection. Assoc Franc m de Chirur (Paris). 1895;9:113–7.
10. Washio H. Further experiences with the retroauricular flap. Plast Reconstr Surg. 1972;50:160–2.
11. Menick FJ. A ten-year experience in nasal reconstruction with the three-stage forehead flap. Plast Reconstr Surg. 2002;109:1839.
12. Pribaz J, Stephens W, Crespo L, Gifford G. A new intraoral flap: facial artery musculomucosal (FAMM) flap. Plast Reconstr Surg. 1992;90:421–9.
13. Bozola AR, Gasques JA, Carriquiry CE, Cardoso de Oliveira M. The buccinator musculomucosal flap: anatomic study and clinical application. Plast Reconstr Surg. 1989;84:250–7.

Free Tissue Transfer for Head and Neck Reconstruction

19

Takako Eva Yabe and Rahul Jayaram

19.1 Introduction

The range of defects in the head and neck region are widely variable. Defect types are broadly categorised into anatomical subunits such as craniofacial, skull base, orbital, maxillomandibular, oral and oropharyngeal defects and cutaneous soft tissue defects in the head and neck. They can also be broadly classed based on tissue types or combination thereof- such as skin, muscle, bone and nerve. Tumour resection without appropriate reconstruction may give patients disease control and survival, but they will be left with functional and aesthetic deficits. Lack of reconstructive options can also limit the extent of anatomical and functional resection.

Microvascular free tissue reconstruction is employed to optimally maintain function and aesthetics. Such reconstruction is complex and resource-intensive. Therefore, it is imperative that appropriate pre-operative planning has taken place before embarking on the journey.

Although widely used and clinically robust, occasional problems encountered with free tissue transfer surgery can include thrombosis of the arterial or venous anastomosis, infection, fistula, wound dehiscence, haematoma, and haemorrhage. Such complications prolong hospital stay, increase morbidity and mortality and decrease quality of life. The patient-centred approach to their pre-operative, peri-operative and post-operative phase is essential to maximise the surgical outcomes and minimise the complications.

19.2 Brief History of Free Flaps Relevant to Head and Neck

The free flap is a reconstruction method that refers to a vascularised tissue removed from a donor site and transplanted to a distant location. It has been utilised for the last four decades as an essential reconstructive method in head and neck surgery [1]. Before the 1950s, the ablative defect was typically restored using large regional flaps (e.g., pectoralis major) or not formally reconstructed.

The term "microvascular surgery" was first used in 1960 by Jules Jacobson, who described microvascular anastomoses on the vessels down to 1.4 mm in diameter. Jejunal, omental and groin flaps were developed from the 1950s to 1970s, but they grew out of favour through the 1980s as pedicle flaps were more reliable, more accessible and quicker to harvest. The trend reversed again in the 1990s when free flap techniques became the dominant reconstructive method after cancer

T. E. Yabe (✉)
Wollongong Hospital, Wollongong, NSW, Australia
e-mail: Takako.Yabe@health.nsw.gov.au

R. Jayaram
St George's University Hospital, London, UK
e-mail: rahul.jayaram@nhs.net

B. Ashford (ed.), *Head and Neck Surgery for General Surgeons*,
https://doi.org/10.1007/978-981-19-7900-2_19

resection [1]. In the head and neck region, microvascular reconstruction is now considered the gold standard for any complex reconstruction.

19.3 Work-Up of Patients/Investigations

Head and neck resection with free flap reconstruction typically take around 8 h. Free flap failure rates are less than 5%. Patients are reminded that approximately 1 in 4 will experience minor complications and 1 in 20 may have a major complication due to surgery. It is crucial to conduct appropriate pre-operative assessments to maximise success and minimise morbidity.

19.3.1 Physical Examination

A complete history and examination are essential to ascertain comorbidities and nutrition status. A detailed review of previous interventions, such as surgery, complications and radiation, is crucial. One of the key determinants for successful free tissue transfer is the quality of the vascular pedicle and the recipient vessels. The neck vessel health and tissue healing capacity can be predicted based on the evidence of neck and donor site operations that might influence vessel or flap selection. Scar from common traumatic injuries and elective surgeries in the hip, wrist, and inguinal region should alarm the surgeon regarding the potentially non-usable donor sites.

19.3.2 Imaging

Imaging in the form of computed tomography (CT) or magnetic resonance imaging (MRI) with contrast can be helpful to confirm vessel patency, calibre and length. A dual-phase CT angiogram is ideal for highlighting arterial and venous vasculature. Ultrasound examination can demonstrate vessel size and flow dynamics but is more user dependent than other modalities.

The advances in virtual surgical planning and pre-operative imaging optimise accuracy, shorten the operative time and increase the predictability of results for the reconstructive surgeon.

19.3.3 Nutrition

It is estimated that 35% of head and neck cancer patients are malnourished at the time of presentation [2]. This could be due to dysphagia, odynophagia or catabolic effect of malignancy. This can be compounded by alcohol related malnutrition in individuals with a history of alcohol abuse and excess. Pre-operative nutritional assessment by experienced speech pathologists and dietitians is strongly recommended by the Enhanced Recovery After Surgery (ERAS) Society [3]. The degree of dysphagia and risk of the refeeding syndrome should be addressed at the time of review.

Depending on the location and nature of pathology, oral feeding cannot be recommenced immediately post-operatively. Such an issue should be anticipated before surgery; therefore, a nasogastric tube or gastrostomy tube can be inserted at the time of surgery. Enteral feeding should be initiated within 24 h after surgery [3]. Gastrostomy tubes are typically used when prolonged nutritional support is anticipated or expected adjuvant therapies may worsen dysphagia [3].

19.3.4 Haematology

A routine pre-operative review should include a blood panel that may reveal underlying anaemia. Pre-operative haemoglobin values below 10 g/dL have been demonstrated to be a significant predictor of flap failure and thrombosis [4]. In our institution, the authors transfuse if haemoglobin is less than 80 g/L.

19.3.5 Flap Selection

Pre-operative flap planning is essential to avoid unanticipated intraoperative surprises and to optimise post-operative function. The surgeons should consider the tissue components, amount of tissue bulk and length of the vascular pedicle unique to different flap types. The characteristics of different flaps will be described later in this chapter.

Some flaps allow for simultaneous flap harvest and tumour resection, thus shortening the overall operative times. Prolonged operative times, specifically longer than 18 h, have been significantly associated with increased rates of free flap failure [5]. Therefore, the logistical organisation between the ablative and reconstructive team is critical when deciding the free flap of choice.

Knowledge of the vascular supply to the neck is fundamental to avoiding flap ischemia or loss. Knowing the dose and fields of any prior radiation therapy will facilitate a prudent choice of skin incision and recipient vessel selection.

19.3.6 Tracheostomy

The indication for tracheotomy is dependent on the presence of cardio-respiratory comorbidities, tumour stage, location and planned resection, the planned extent of neck dissection and previous head and neck radiation. Elective tracheostomy is a relatively safe procedure for adults; however, can be associated with risks, more extended hospital stays and increased costs of care [3]. Many institutions have a policy and procedure regarding the management of tracheostomy patients. Ward staff and junior team members should be equipped and trained to manage such patients in an emergency. Many studies report that patients can often be successfully decannulated within 2 weeks after surgery, but reports vary on the appropriate pathway to decannulation. Nearly all studies agree that a patient should pass a capping trial before decannulation [3].

19.4 Subsite Use of Free Flaps

Each ablative subsite poses unique anatomical and functional challenges in free flap reconstruction. The table below shows the suggested flap choice for different subsites. This is not prescriptive by any means and each defect should be examined to identify the ideal flap that can address its deficits (Table 19.1). Common soft tissue and composite flaps are described later in this chapter.

Table 19.1 Suggested free flaps for each ablative subsite

		Ablative subsites				
		Oral cavity/ oropharynx	Pharyngolarynx	Maxillomandibular	Craniofacial	Cutaneous soft tissue
Free flap	RF	✓	✓	✓	✓	✓
	ALT	✓	✓		✓	✓
	LD				✓	✓
	MSAP	✓				✓
	RA	✓			✓	
	Fibula			✓		
	DCIA			✓		
	Scapula			✓		

Abbreviations: *RF* radial forearm, *ALT* anterolateral thigh, *LD* latissimus dorsi, *MSAP* medial sural artery perforator, *RA* rectus abdominus, *DCIA* deep circumflex iliac artery

19.5 Common Soft Tissue Free Flaps

19.5.1 Radial Forearm

The radial forearm fasciocutaneous flap (RFFF) was originally developed in 1978 and reported in 1981. The flap with a rich axial pedicle consisting of the radial artery, venae comitantes and cephalic vein made reconstructive surgery breakthroughs. It can be harvested as a composite flap incorporating muscle, tendon, nerve or bone. Once the radial artery is harvested, the perfusion to the hand depends on the continuity of the palmar arch. It is therefore important to perform an Allen's test to assess an adequate inflow from the ulnar artery. It is a workhorse flap for head and neck reconstruction and is commonly used for the reconstruction of oral tongue, cheek, floor of mouth, laryngopharyngeal, oesophageal and surface defects (Fig. 19.1).

19.5.2 Anterolateral Thigh

The anterolateral thigh (ALT) flap was described by Song et al. The application to the maxillofacial region was described in the 1990s. It is generally raised as a fasciocutaneous flap based on the septocutaneous perforators of the descending branch of the lateral circumflex femoral artery and venae comitantes. The other variations of this flap include adipofascial, myocutaneous, muscle only (Vastus lateralis Flap), or a combination as chimeric option with the anteromedial thigh flap. The body habitus of the patient should be considered when choosing this flap. An increased adiposity will make the flap unexpectedly bulky which can impair function and cosmesis. This is another workhorse flap for the head and neck reconstruction and has particular advantages of large surface area, a discrete scar and minimal donor site morbidity. The neurotised version can be used for dynamic reanimation of the face [6] (Fig. 19.2).

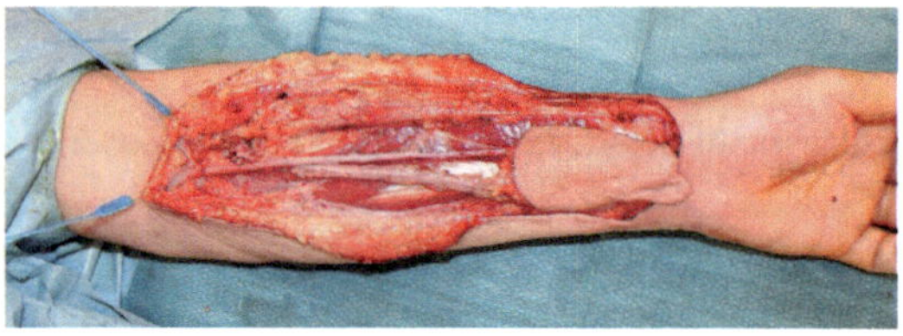

Fig. 19.1 Radial forearm free flap with associated vascular pedicles

19.5.3 Latissimus Dorsi

Latissimus dorsi (LD) was first reported as a free flap in 1979 for breast reconstruction. Reports of its use in the head and neck soon followed, with Fujino et al. reporting a case of successful reconstruction of a total cheek defect in 1981. It is particularly useful for defects of the entire scalp where a defect requires broad soft-tissue coverage. The pedicle comprises the thoracodorsal artery, a terminal branch of the subscapular artery, and its accompanying venae comitantes. The muscle flap is typically covered with a split-thickness skin graft which will give an excellent cosmetic result. Most commonly used for large surface defects coverage as a free flap, it can also be used as a pedicle flap in a recipient vessel depleted neck or salvage scenarios. Despite the size, donor functional deficit is minimal. The rotation axis and the pedicle length limit the reach of the pedicled flap but allow for reconstruction of defects on the neck or parotid region (Figs. 19.3, 19.4, 19.5, and 19.6).

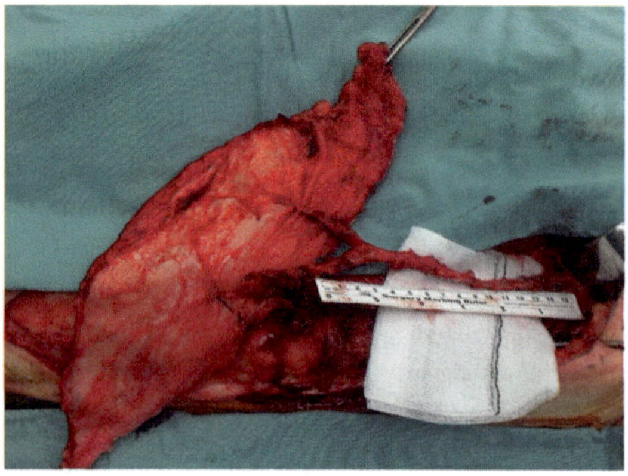

Fig. 19.2 ALT free flap demonstrating fasciocutaneous flap with two perforators

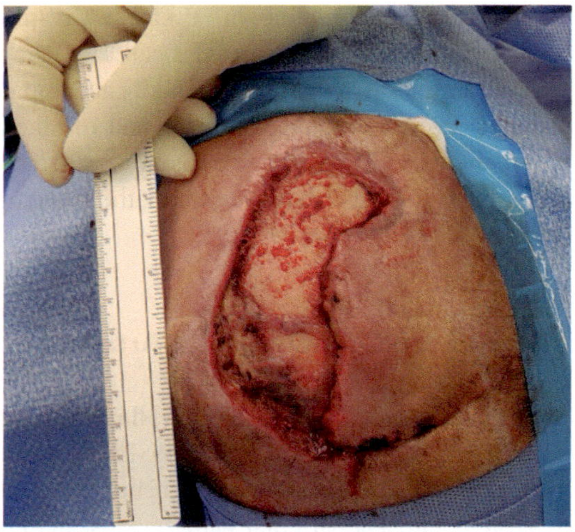

Fig. 19.3 Scalp defect

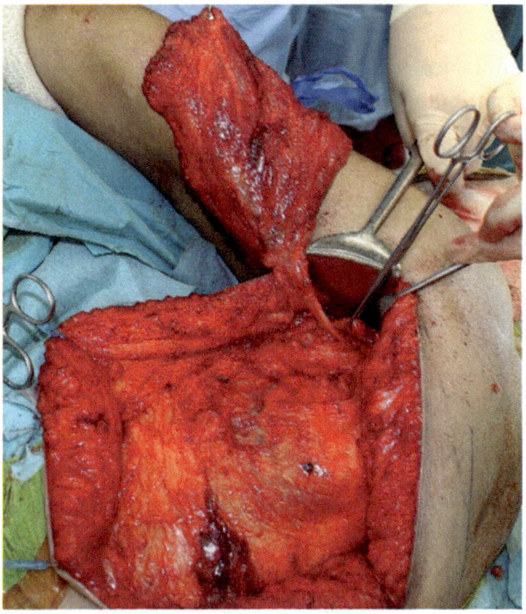

Fig. 19.4 Latissimus dorsi free flap with associated pedicle

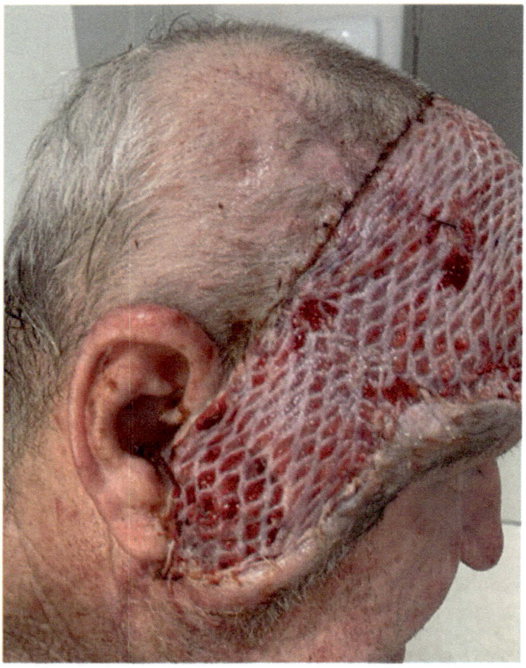

Fig. 19.5 Two weeks post latissimus dorsi free flap and split skin graft

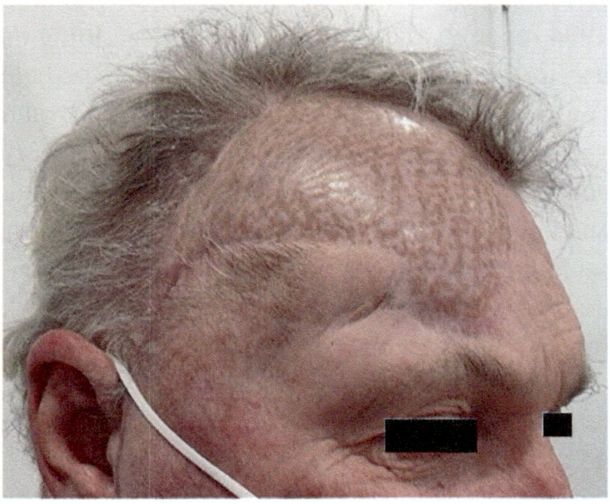

Fig. 19.6 One year following latissimus dorsi free flap and split skin graft in the same patient

19.5.4 Medial Sural Artery Perforator Flap

Medial sural artery perforator flap (MSAP) was first described by Cavadas et al. in 2001. It was first used for lower limb reconstruction, and then the clinical application was increased to include head and neck. MSAP flap has low donor site morbidity, adequate vascular pedicle length and a thin fasciocutaneous component even in obese patients. The pedicle consists of a medial sural artery and two venae comitantes. The greater saphenous vein can also be used as drainage. The versatility of MSAP comes from its ability to be elevated as a thin fasiocutaneous flap or elevated with the underling gastrocnemius muscle to fill

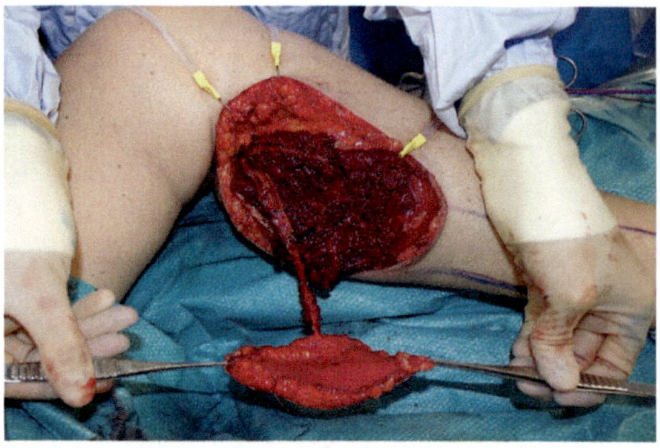

Fig. 19.7 Medial sural artery perforator flap with associated vascular pedicles

the deep defect, or it can also be elevated as a chimeric flap. The sural nerve, the lesser saphenous vein or the plantaris tendon can also be harvested within the flap (Fig. 19.7).

19.5.5 Rectus Abdominus

The first free rectus abdominis flap was performed by Holmstrom in 1979. Hasegawa et al.in 1994 reported a first clinical report describing its use in the head and neck. The vascular pedicle consists of the deep inferior epigastric artery and venae originating from the external iliac artery and vein. The main advantage of this flap is bulk and hence is used for reconstruction of total glossectomy and skull base defects. This flap has generally been superseded in head and neck reconstruction by the ALT.

19.6 Common Composite Flaps

The composite free flap contains more than one tissue unit such as skin, muscle and bone.

19.6.1 Fibula

The fibula free flap was first described independently in Japan and Australia in 1973. The work of Wei et al. in 1986 employing this flap as a chimeric flap expanded its utility in complex composite head and neck reconstruction. The mandibular reconstruction with this flap was first reported in 1989 by Hidalgo. The vascular pedicle consists of a peroneal artery and its accompanying two venae comitantes. Care must be taken to protect peroneal nerve and ankle joint stability by leaving at least 5 cm of proximal and distal fibula bone intact (Fig. 19.8).

19.6.2 Deep Circumflex Iliac Artery

Deep circumflex iliac artery (DCIA) flap was first reported, as a bony flap, in 1979 by Taylor et al. then as an oromandibular reconstruction in 1989 by Urken et al. The vascular pedicle consists of a deep circumflex iliac artery from the external iliac system, accompanying venae comitantes. It provides an alternative to the fibula and scapula free flaps with thicker bone more suited to implant placement. At least six vascular systems contribute to the iliac crest, and free flaps have been reported based on all 6 (Fig. 19.9).

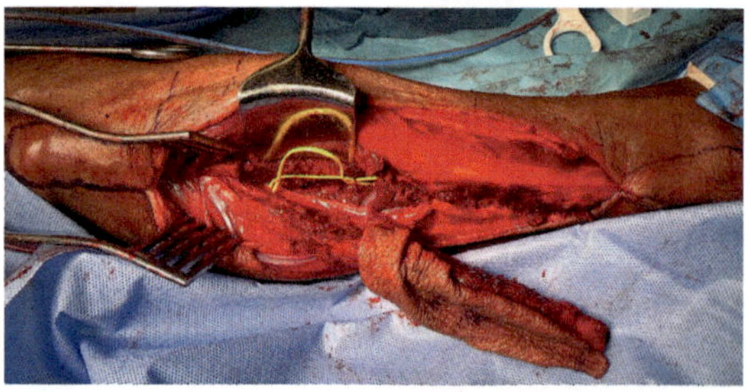

Fig. 19.8 Fibular free flap with associated vascular pedicles

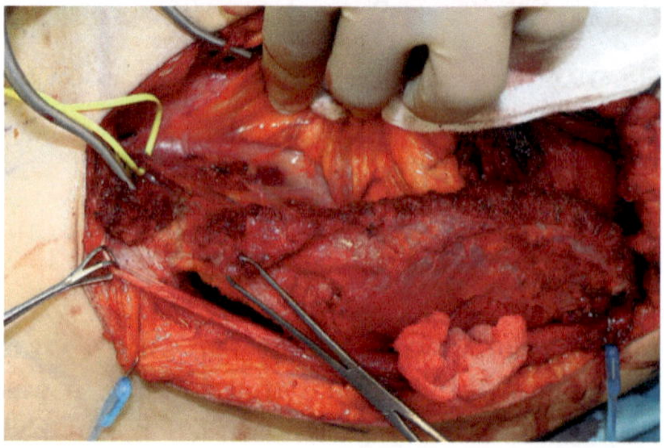

Fig. 19.9 Deep circumflex iliac artery free flap with associated vascular pedicles

19.6.3 Scapula

The scapular fasciocutaneous free flap, based on the circumflex scapular artery, is a part of the subscapular system. It was initially described in an anatomic study by Saijo in 1978. Batchelor and Sully used a scapular and latissimus dorsi free flap to reconstruct a scalp defect in 1984 (Figs. 19.10, 19.11, and 19.12).

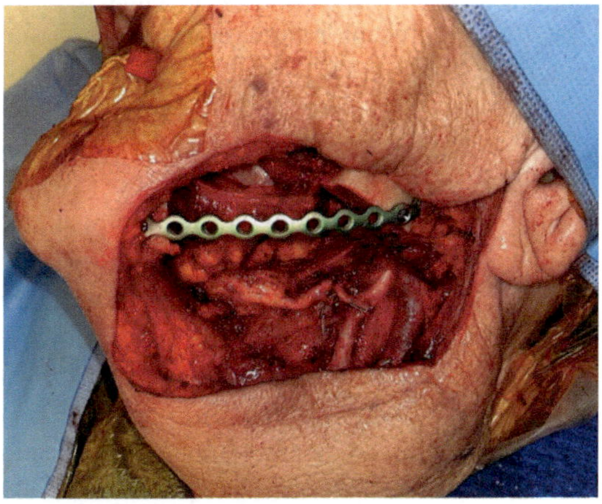

Fig. 19.10 Segmental mandibulectomy defect with reconstruction plate in situ

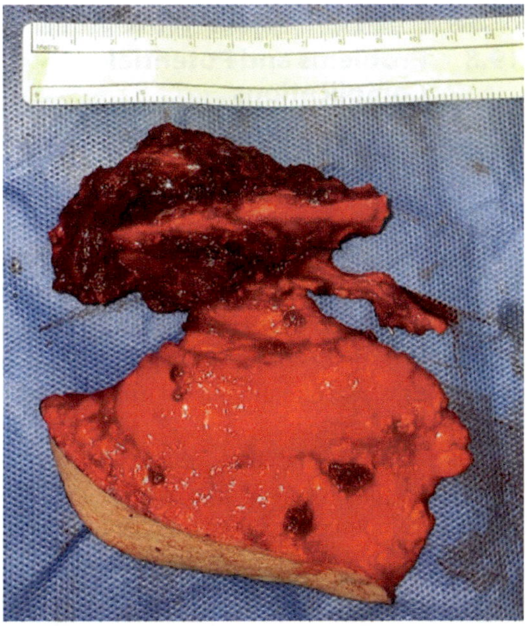

Fig. 19.11 Chimeric scapula free flap

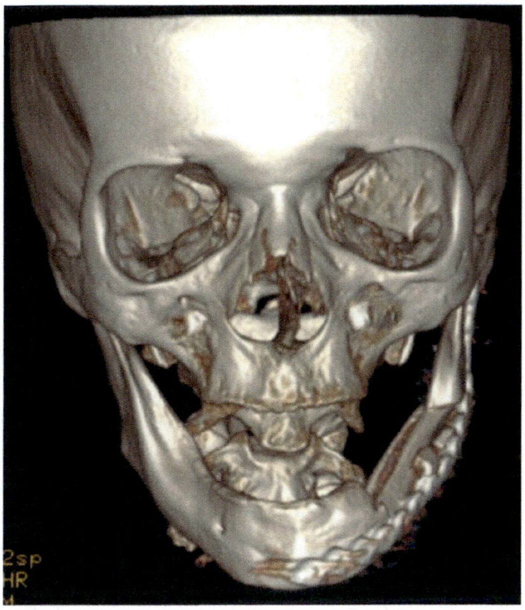

Fig. 19.12 Reconstructed post-operative CT image

19.7 Post-operative Management

19.7.1 Intensive Care

Most head and neck free flap patients are admitted to the intensive care unit (ICU) post-operatively, to monitor the patient's early recovery, undertake high frequency flap observations, and to manage the airway as required.

Vasopressor use is often frowned upon due to concern that vasoconstriction caused by such agents could compromise the flap blood supply. There is conflicting evidence regarding the use of vasoactive agents in free flap surgery. Vasoactive agents can cause vasoconstriction and decrease flap perfusion, while others suggest no adverse outcomes. The judicious use of such vasopressors should be employed with input from intensivists, as fluid overload can compromise the flap's viability. Fluid overload is thought to cause pedicle thrombosis from endothelial damage, extravasation, oedema and venous stasis. Furthermore, free flaps are more sensitive to oedema from loss of lymphatic drainage and autonomic innervation. It is imperative there is clear communication between the surgical, anaesthetic and ICU team so that everyone is aware of when the medication is started and when it is stopped. Notwithstanding technical surgical issues, if the patient is well, the flap will not be harmed.

19.7.2 Flap Monitoring

The purpose of flap monitoring is the early detection of vascular compromise (venous or arterial) and to prevent flap loss. The highest risk for vascular compromise is during the first 24 h, when the intimal injury is the highest, and the risk significantly drops after the first 3 days following surgery [7]. The free flap monitoring should be performed hourly for the first 24 h with tapering of intensity after the initial 24 h [3]. The assessment should include a physical exam of flap warmth, turgor, capillary refill, colour, and Doppler assessment of the vascular pedicle. Handheld or implantable doppler devices are routinely used.

19.7.3 Anticoagulation

Immediate to early thrombosis is mainly attributed to technical failure. There are no pharmacologic measures that have been proven to reduce free flap anastomotic thrombosis or flap necrosis [3].

After surgery, maintaining a neutral head position can prevent kinking or pressure on the pedicle with the subsequent flow compromise. Ties around the neck (i.e., tracheostomy ties, oxygen mask) can have a tourniquet effect and should be avoided. Advanced atherosclerotic disease, diabetes mellitus, prior radiotherapy, and prior neck dissection can also contribute to poor vessel quality [8], compromising the integrity of the anastomosis. In our practice, head and neck free flap patients receive either subcutaneous injection of unfractionated heparin or low-molecular weight heparin depending on their body weight and renal function.

19.7.4 Antibiotics

Oropharyngeal surgery is classified as a Class II Clean/Contaminated procedure. Infection risks inherent in head and neck free flap surgeries are long duration, malnutrition, use of a bone flap, prior radiotherapy and tracheostomy. Pre-operative antibiotics at induction and 24 h of post-operative antibiotics (usually cephazolin 1 g three times a day with or without metronidazole 500 mg twice a day) have consistently demonstrated a significant reduction in surgical site infections [9].

19.7.5 Nutrition

Following an initial nasogastric or gastrostomy feeding, there should be a multidisciplinary approach to the commencement of oral feeding. There is a theoretical risk of wound breakdown and fistula formation when the reconstruction involves the oral cavity and pharynx. A return to oral feeding as early as the sixth post operatively day is observed to be safe without increasing the risk of orocutaneous fistula or flap related complications [10, 11].

19.8 Problems and Potential Complications

19.8.1 Wound Infection and Dehiscence

Head and neck operations often breach the upper aerodigestive tract, and hence are considered clean-contaminated procedures. This means a 20–30% risk of developing a wound infection justifying the use of antibiotics during the early post-operative period.

When wound dehiscence occurs, the principles of care involve managing drainable collections by aspiration or exploration, regular sterile dressings, wound culture, appropriate antibiotic therapy and attention to nutritional support.

Extensive tissue loss may require a skin graft, myocutaneous or a further free flap for cover (Figs. 19.13 and 19.14).

19.8.2 Flap Ischaemia

Regular and frequent monitoring of flap health is to recognise the vascular insufficiency early and to prevent a flap loss. Prompt re-exploration and revision are crucial as most flaps fail to recover after 10–12 h of ischaemia. Venous insufficiency is more common than arterial and tends to develop later. Venous congestion gives the flap a bluish appearance with swelling, oedema, and on the needle prick test, a brisk dark venous ooze. In contrast, the flap with arterial ischaemia is pale, cool to touch and does not blanch. The thrombosed vessel should be resected to a healthy vessel wall before re-anastomosis. If that is not possible, an alternative recipient vessel should be sought. Authors often use external carotid artery (for more proximal and better calibre) or transverse cervical artery (for non-radiated field) in the vessel depleted neck when more distal branches of vessels are of inadequate calibre. Other causes of early flap failure are haematoma and recipient vessel problems. Late flap compromise (>48 h) is usually due to infection or mechanical stresses on the pedicle leading to compromise. Prior radiotherapy to the recipient neck, significant medical co-morbidities such as diabetes, hypercoagulable states and alcohol withdrawal may also contribute to flap failure [12] (Fig. 19.15).

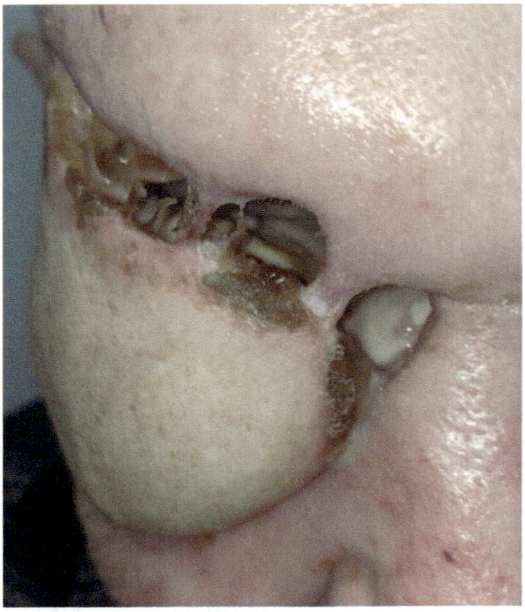

Fig. 19.13 Wound dehiscence during adjuvant radiotherapy following extended orbital exenteration and ALT free flap

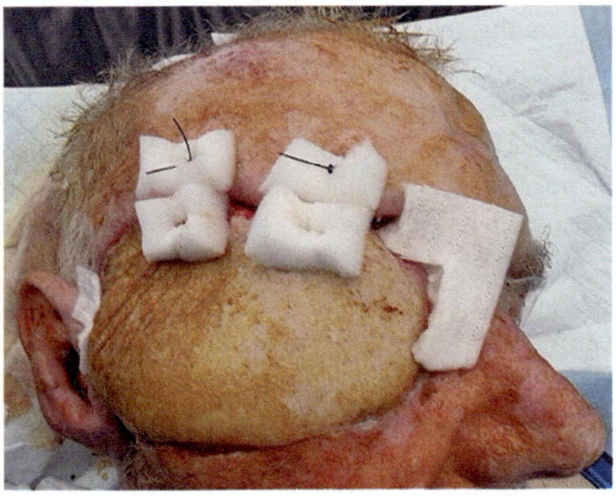

Fig. 19.14 Bolstered flap as a temporary measure to complete adjuvant radiotherapy

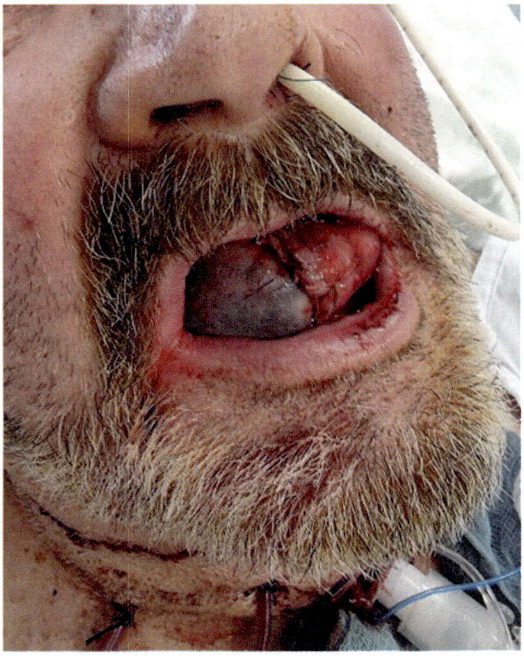

Fig. 19.15 Venous ischaemia of RFFF for right hemiglossectomy on day 1 post-op

19.8.3 Fistula

Orocutaneous fistula is a complications of major head and neck surgery that may delay much needed adjuvant treatment and place a patient's life at risk with neck sepsis. The reported incidence is up to 20%, and a large percentage of fistulas received a major second operation to achieve wound healing. The vacuum-assisted closure (VAC) device is useful when the flap is viable, not infected or is a low-output fistula. The authors advise against using VAC when the major vessels are exposed or within the wound bed.

When the defect is too large to be closed by secondary intension, a second free flap or regional flap depending on prognosis, tissue quality, and fistula size should be planned within a week after the first debridement.

When patients present with the fistulae while on radiotherapy, radiotherapy should not be interrupted, and the fistula managed conservatively by less aggressive but effective wound care until radiotherapy is completed and a definite reconstruction planned. However, this is only true if there is no risk of carotid blowout. Many of these patients present not only with fistula but also with other coexisting unfavourable conditions such as tissue atrophy, plate exposure, trismus, or even occult recurrence, which ideally can be addressed at the same time.

Hypothyroidism can complicate head and neck cancer treatment and is an under-recognised cause of failure to heal following surgery. Thyroid function should be tested for and corrected in all head and neck cancer patients, especially those with free flap reconstruction.

19.8.4 Carotid Blowout

Carotid blowout is a rare but significant complication following major neck surgery. In a series of 280 patients who underwent major head and neck surgery, 3% suffered carotid artery rupture. Of the 3%, most died, and 11% survived but with adverse neurological outcomes [13]. Neck sepsis and previous radiation are the most significant risk factors. The management depends on its acuity of presentation.

In the event of life-threatening massive bleeding on the ward, the focus should be on arresting life-threatening haemorrhage with direct pressure and securing the airway. Definitive exploration and repair will follow in the operating theatre. Angiography with embolization can offer a safe and rapid alternative method of achieving vascular control in patients with spontaneous rupture of the common carotid, carotid bulb or external carotid system once the patient has been stabilised.

19.9 Tips and Tricks

19.9.1 Vessel Selection and Orientation

The availability of recipient vessels can be predicted pre-operatively based on presenting pathology and the planned extent of neck dissection. There are common vessels that are used based on location in the head and neck region. The superficial temporal artery and vein are used in the upper third of the head, the facial and superior thyroid artery and vein for the lower third of the face, and the external carotid artery branches and jugular veins in the neck. In the vessel depleted neck, finding a vessel in the contralateral neck, outside the previous radiation or surgery fields (e.g., transverse cervical) or more proximally (e.g., external carotid) can help prevent arterial problems (Table 19.2).

The free flap pedicle often has more than one vein as a draining vessel. If the separate veins can be traced to a confluence, a single venous anastomoses can be achieved. If no confluence and both veins have good flow and calibre, both these vessels should be anastomosed to suitable recipient veins. If the pedicle geometry permits, they should be anastomosed to separate systems (i.e., internal and external jugular). In this arrangement, one will act as a backup drainage system if the other one fails.

Table 19.2 Extent of neck dissection, associated common pathology and typical recipient vessels

Neck dissection levels	Primary pathology	Typical recipient vessels
1–3/1–4	Tongue, floor of mouth	Artery: Facial, superior thyroid, lingual Veins: Common facial vein/internal jugular vein
1–4/1–5	Metastatic SCC of neck	Artery: Facial, superior thyroid, occipital artery, transverse cervical artery Vein: Internal jugular, external jugular
1–4/2–4	Parotid	Artery: Superficial temporal, facial, superior thyroid, transverse cervical artery Vein: Superficial temporal, internal/external jugular vein

19.9.2 Perforator Based Chimeric Flaps

The chimeric concept for free tissue transfers in the head and neck setting was initially proposed by Koshima et al. Chimeric flaps consist of multiple spatially independent units with their own vascular supply, joined to a common vessel. Such vascular arrangement is particularly useful for complex defects needing tissue of varying structural and or functional components simultaneously. These are also useful when surgeons are presented with vascularly depleted necks due to previous surgery or radiotherapy. Compared to employing multiple free flaps, chimeric flaps offer good versatility while maintaining a similar complication rate (Fig. 19.16).

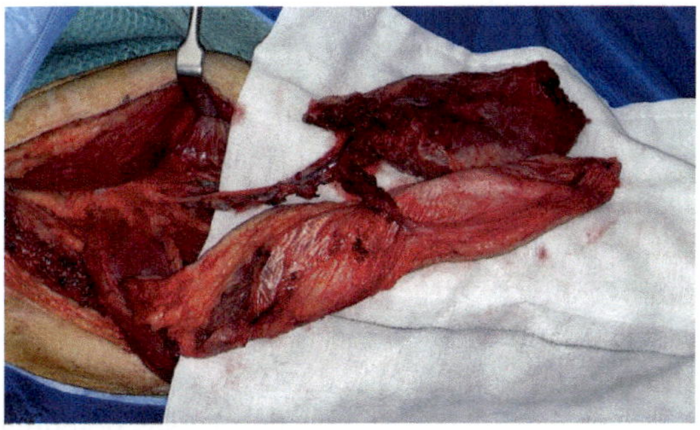

Fig. 19.16 Chimeric ALT free flap with vastus lateralis muscle and fasciocutaneous paddle

19.9.3 Reanimation

Functional and psychological morbidity caused by facial paralysis should not be underestimated. Facial reanimation can be categorised into primary versus secondary procedure and dynamic versus static reconstruction. The aetiology and duration of facial paralysis are the most important considerations when determining what kind of reanimation surgery would most benefit the patient. In general, younger patients with viable facial musculature and an intact neuromuscular junction who had an intentional sacrifice of facial nerve would benefit more from nerve transfer to achieve dynamic reanimation. In the setting of radical parotid surgery with a need for free tissue transfer, donor nerves are often available in reconstructive flaps. For older patients with multiple comorbidities, static facial suspension with tensor fascia lata (TFL) graft, tarsal strip and eyelid gold weight are often used to achieve oral competence and corneal protection.

Key Take Aways

1. Free tissue transfer is a key component of head and neck reconstruction.
2. This is a common procedure with very low failure rates in high volume centres.
3. A very thorough history and examination of both the neck and proposed donor site enhances free flap success.
4. No flap survives without adequate arterial inflow.
5. Venous anastomotic thrombus is more common than arterial.
6. Early free flap compromise or failure is usually technical, and regular post operative observation of a free flap provides early opportunity to address insufficiency of perfusion.

19.10 Conclusion

In this chapter, we have outlined the variety of free flaps commonly used in head and neck reconstruction and salient points in managing patients who need free tissue transfer to achieve biologically robust, functional and cosmetic reconstruction. Familiarity with these reconstructive options will give ablative surgeons the skills to balance the extent of resection versus potential outcome. The mutual understanding and collaboration between ablative and reconstructive surgeons will produce the best possible outcomes in head and neck surgery.

References

1. Steel BJ, Cope MR. A brief history of vascularized free flaps in the oral and maxillofacial region. J Oral Maxillofac Surg. 2015;73(4):786.e1–11.
2. Leung JS, Seto A, Li GK. Association between preoperative nutritional status and postoperative outcome in head and neck cancer patients. Nutr Cancer. 2017;69(3):464–9.
3. Dort JC, Farwell DG, Findlay M, Huber GF, Kerr P, Shea-Budgell MA, et al. Optimal perioperative care in major head and neck cancer surgery with free flap reconstruction: a consensus review and recommendations from the enhanced recovery after surgery society. JAMA Otolaryngol Head Neck Surg. 2017;143(3):292–303.
4. Motakef S, Mountziaris PM, Ismail IK, Agag RL, Patel A. Perioperative management for microsurgical free tissue transfer: survey of current practices with a comparison to the literature. J Reconstr Microsurg. 2015;31(05):355–63.
5. Ishimaru M, Ono S, Suzuki S, Matsui H, Fushimi K, Yasunaga H. Risk factors for free flap failure in 2,846 patients with head and neck cancer: a national database study in Japan. J Oral Maxillofac Surg. 2016;74(6):1265–70.
6. Hasmat S, Low TH, Krishnan A, Coulson S, Ch'ng S, Ashford BG, et al. Chimeric vastus Lateralis and anterolateral thigh flap for restoring facial defects and dynamic function following radical parotidectomy. Plast Reconstr Surg. 2019;144(5):853e–63e.
7. Kroll SS, Schusterman MA, Reece GP, Miller MJ, Evans GR, Robb GL, et al. Timing of pedicle thrombosis and flap loss after free-tissue transfer. Plast Reconstr Surg. 1996;98(7):1230–3.
8. Vincent A, Sawhney R, Ducic Y. Perioperative care of free flap patients. Semin Plast Surg. 2019;33(1):5–12.
9. Rodrigo JP, Alvarez JC, Gómez JR, Suárez C, Fernández JA, Martínez JA. Comparison of three prophylactic antibiotic regimens in clean-contaminated head and neck surgery. Head Neck. 1997;19(3):188–93.
10. Aires FT, Dedivitis RA, Petrarolha SM, Bernardo WM, Cernea CR, Brandão LG. Early oral feeding after total laryngectomy: a systematic review. Head Neck. 2015;37(10):1532–5.
11. Kinzinger MR, Bewley AF. Perioperative care of head and neck free flap patients. Curr Opin Otolaryngol Head Neck Surg. 2017;25(5):405–10.
12. Novakovic D, Patel RS, Goldstein DP, Gullane PJ. Salvage of failed free flaps used in head and neck reconstruction. Head Neck Oncol. 2009;1(1):33.
13. Stell PM. Catastrophic haemorrhage after major neck surgery. Br J Surg. 1969;56(7):525–7.

GPSR Compliance

The European Union's (EU) General Product Safety Regulation (GPSR) is a set of rules that requires consumer products to be safe and our obligations to ensure this.

If you have any concerns about our products, you can contact us on ProductSafety@springernature.com

In case Publisher is established outside the EU, the EU authorized representative is:

Springer Nature Customer Service Center GmbH
Europaplatz 3
69115 Heidelberg, Germany

Batch number: 10732801

Printed by Printforce, the Netherlands